STRESS IN POST-WAR BRITAIN, 1945–85

Studies for the Society for the Social History of Medicine

Series Editors: David Cantor
Keir Waddington

Titles in this Series

1 Meat, Medicine and Human Health in the Twentieth Century
David Cantor, Christian Bonah and Matthias Dörries (eds)

2 Locating Health: Historical and Anthropological Investigations of Place and Health
Erika Dyck and Christopher Fletcher (eds)

3 Medicine in the Remote and Rural North, 1800–2000
J. T. H. Connor and Stephan Curtis (eds)

4 A Modern History of the Stomach: Gastric Illness, Medicine and British Society, 1800–1950
Ian Miller

5 War and the Militarization of British Army Medicine, 1793–1830
Catherine Kelly

6 Nervous Disease in Late Eighteenth-Century Britain: The Reality of a Fashionable Disorder
Heather R. Beatty

7 Desperate Housewives, Neuroses and the Domestic Environment, 1945–1970
Ali Haggett

8 Disabled Children: Contested Caring, 1850–1979
Anne Borsay and Pamela Dale (eds)

9 Toxicants, Health and Regulation since 1945
Soraya Boudia and Nathalie Jas (eds)

10 A Medical History of Skin: Scratching the Surface
Jonathan Reinarz and Kevin Patrick Siena (eds)

11 The Care of Older People: England and Japan, A Comparative Study
Mayumi Hayashi

12 Child Guidance in Britain, 1918–1955: The Dangerous Age of Childhood
John Stewart

13 Modern German Midwifery, 1885–1960
Lynne Fallwell

14 Western Maternity and Medicine, 1880–1990
Janet Greenlees and Linda Bryder (eds)

15 Human Heredity in the Twentieth Century
Bernd Gausemeier, Staffan Müller-Wille and Edmund Ramsden (eds)

16 Biologics, A History of Agents Made From Living Organisms in the Twentieth Century
Alexander von Schwerin, Heiko Stoff and Bettina Wahrig (eds)

17 Bacteria in Britain, 1880–1939
Rosemary Wall

18 Health and Citizenship: Political Cultures of Health in Modern Europe
Frank Huisman and Harry Oosterhuis (eds)

19 The Politics of Hospital Provision in Early Twentieth-Century Britain
Barry M. Doyle

20 Institutionalizing the Insane in Nineteenth-Century England
Anna Shepherd

21 Psychiatry and Chinese History
Howard Chiang (ed.)

22 The Development of Scientific Marketing in the Twentieth Century: Research for Sales in the Pharmaceutical Industry
Jean-Paul Gaudillère and Ulrike Thoms (eds)

Forthcoming Titles

The Rockefeller Foundation, Public Health and International Diplomacy, 1920–1945
Josep L. Barona

The Politics of Vaccination: A Global History
Christine Holmberg, Stuart Blume and Paul R. Greenough (eds)

STRESS IN POST-WAR BRITAIN, 1945–85

EDITED BY

Mark Jackson

Routledge
Taylor & Francis Group
LONDON AND NEW YORK

First published 2015 by Pickering & Chatto (Publishers) Limited

2 Park Square, Milton Park, Abingdon, Oxon OX14 4RN
711 Third Avenue, New York, NY 10017, USA

Routledge is an imprint of the Taylor & Francis Group, an informa business

First issued in paperback 2017

BRITISH LIBRARY CATALOGUING IN PUBLICATION DATA

Stress in post-war Britain. – (Studies for the Society for the Social History of Medicine)
1. Stress (Psychology) – Great Britain – History – 20th century. 2. Mental health policy – Great Britain – History – 20th century. 3. Public health – Great Britain – History – 20th century.
I. Series II. Jackson, Mark, 1959, editor.

362.2'0941'09045-dc23

ISBN-13: 978-1-8489-3473-3 (hbk)
ISBN-13: 978-1-138-63013-0 (pbk)

Typeset by Pickering & Chatto (Publishers) Limited

CONTENTS

LIST OF CONTRIBUTORS

Nicole Baur is an Associate Research Fellow in the Centre for Medical History at the University of Exeter. She holds a PhD in Health Geography from Heidelberg University, Germany (2005). She has worked extensively within interdisciplinary teams to pursue a long-standing interest in the interactions between society, the natural environment and human health. Specific work has included spatial analyses of weather patterns and mental illness, people's perceptions of place and local conditions in their experience of illness and people's social interpretations of illness-related memories. Her latest research focuses on knowledge generation and translation into medical practice. Her publications include: *Die Diphtherie in medizinisch-geographischer Perspektive* (2006); 'Public Policy and Patient Privacy: Archiving Patients' Mental Health Records from the Age of the Great Hospital, *c.*1948–1970', *Archives*, 36 (2012), pp. 36–49 (with J. Draisey and J. Melling); and 'Family Influence and Psychiatric Care: Physical Treatment in Devon Mental Hospitals *c.*1900–1970', *Endeavour*, 37 (2013), pp. 172–83.

Ali Haggett is a Wellcome Trust Postdoctoral Fellow and Lecturer in the Centre for Medical History, University of Exeter, where she received her PhD. She is currently researching the history of male psychological and psychosomatic illness, in Britain, since the Second World War and the place of notions of balance in shaping experiences and understandings of mental health. Her broad interests are in the cultural and social histories of mental illness, gender, psychiatry and psychopharmacology, and her work on housewives and neurosis in Britain was published with Pickering & Chatto in 2012 as *'Desperate Housewives': Neuroses and the Domestic Environment 1945–1970*. Her new book, *A History of Male Psychological Disorders in Britain 1945–1980*, will be published by Palgrave Macmillan in 2015.

Sarah Hayes is an Associate Research Fellow in the Centre for Medical History at the University of Exeter. Her PhD thesis, 'The Medicalization of Maladjustment: The Conceptualization and Management of Child Behavioural Disorders in Britain, 1890–1955', focused on the history of child psychiatry and psychology, exploring historical perspectives on the mental and emotional well-being of children in the nineteenth and twentieth centuries. She has recently completed a Wellcome Trust-funded project on occupational health, examining the impact of workplace design on the physical, mental and emotional health of factory workers in Britain in the second half of the twentieth century.

Mark Jackson is Professor of the History of Medicine at the University of Exeter. He is a Senior Academic Adviser (Medical Humanities) at the Wellcome Trust, was a member of the History Sub-Panel for REF 2014, and has recently been appointed to the WHO European Advisory Committee on Health Research. He has taught modules in the history of medicine and the history and philosophy of science for over twenty years at undergraduate and postgraduate levels, and has also been involved in teaching medical history to GCSE and A level students. His books include *Newborn Child Murder* (1996), *The Borderland of Imbecility* (2000), *Infanticide: Historical Perspectives on Child Murder and Concealment 1550–2000* (ed., 2002), *Allergy: The History of a Modern Malady* (2006), *Health and the Modern Home* (ed., 2007), *Asthma: The Biography* (2009), *The Oxford Handbook of the History of Medicine* (ed., 2011), *The Age of Stress: Science and the Search for Stability* (2013) and *The History of Medicine: A Beginner's Guide* (Oneworld, 2014). He is currently editing *The Routledge History of Disease* and developing a project on the history of the midlife crisis.

Edgar Jones is Professor of the History of Medicine and Psychiatry at the Institute of Psychiatry and King's Centre for Military Health Research, where he is programme leader for the MSc in War and Psychiatry. He originally trained as an historian at Nuffield College Oxford, before completing a doctorate at Guy's Hospital in clinical psychopathology and training as an analytical psychotherapist. His research has explored how individuals, both soldiers and civilians, cope with the intense stress of war and how they seek to adjust to peacetime existence. In particular, he has studied the conceptualization and treatment of shell shock in the First World War and battle exhaustion during the Second World War. His research into psychosomatic disorders in the context of war led to papers on peptic ulcer and Gulf War syndrome. He has also written on the use of medical film to educate doctors in the treatment of psychiatric casualties. Edgar Jones is co-author of *Shell Shock to PTSD, Military Psychiatry from 1900 to the Gulf* (Hove: Psychology Press, Maudsley Monograph, 2005).

Jill Kirby is a researcher in the History Department at the University of Sussex specializing in twentieth-century British social history. Her research examines the experiences of stress in Britain in the twentieth century and draws on self-help literature, the Mass Observation Archive and oral histories. Previous research looked at household medicine in the first half of the twentieth century. She has a MA in Contemporary History from Sussex and MSc in Organizational Behaviour from London University. Most recently she managed a JISC-funded digitization project, *Observing the 1980s*, working with colleagues at Sussex and the British Library to create an open educational resource based on Mass Observation Project writings, contemporary ephemera and British Library oral history collections.

Joseph Melling has completed research in the history of the workplace and is interested in the health and welfare of workers across the world. He has undertaken studies of managers as well as workers. His recent publications include work on the history of silicosis and pneumoconiosis as well as the history of mental illness in the past two centuries. He is currently working on trans-national organizations and health, including the dissemination of ideas of occupational stress in the modern world.

Chris Millard is a Wellcome Trust Postdoctoral Research Fellow at the Centre for the History of the Emotions, Queen Mary, University of London. For his MA at the University of York, he researched the history of deliberate self-harm in Britain and America, tracing current archetypes of forearm cutting by females back to the 1960s and 1970s. His PhD at the Centre for the History of the Emotions at Queen Mary analysed an epidemic of attempted suicide, read as a 'cry for help', in post-1945 British psychiatry. This was found to be rooted in the flourishing of social psychiatry and attempts to integrate psychiatric practice into general hospital settings. His current project traces the development of Munchausen syndromes in the late twentieth century – Munchausen syndrome, Munchausen syndrome by proxy and Munchausen by internet. These shifting and contested categories are used to interrogate and contextualize one part of a pervasive organizing category of contemporary thought – 'the social' – which underwrites social medicine, social psychiatry, social history and sociology.

Debbie Palmer is currently a nurse at Tavistock Hospital, Devon. After qualifying in nursing at the London Hospital, Whitechapel, in 1985, she took an extended career break in 1989 to raise four children. Returning to academic study in 2001 as a mature student, she developed an interest in the history of nurses' occupational health. Her monograph *Who Cared for the Carers: The History of Nurses' Occupational Health, 1890–1948* was published by Manchester University Press in 2014. More recently, she has worked on the history of occupational stress among airline pilots and civil servants and has recently returned to nursing, specializing in the care of terminally-ill and elderly patients.

Pamela Richardson is an honorary Fellow at the University of Exeter where she was awarded a PhD on the history of West Country Quaker families in 2007. She is currently researching the care of long-term child patients with bone disease and the specialization of orthopaedic nursing in the early twentieth century.

Matthew Smith is a Senior Lecturer and Director of Research for History at the University of Strathclyde and a member of the Centre for the Social History of Health and Healthcare. In addition to an imminent monograph on the history of food allergy (Columbia University Press), the research for which was funded by the Wellcome Trust, he has written two books on the history of hyperactivity (*An Alternative History of Hyperactivity: Food Additives and the Feingold Diet* and *Hyperactive: The Controversial History of ADHD*), also funded by the Trust. He is a past winner of the Roy Porter Prize and the Jack D. Pressman-Burroughs Wellcome Career Development Award and was named an AHRC/BBC New Generation Thinker in 2012. He has presented his research on Radio 3's Night Waves, spoken at the Free Thinking Festival and blogged for PsychologyToday.com. He serves on the executive committee of the Society for the Social History of Medicine as Publicity Officer, and is a book review editor and editorial board member for the *History of Psychiatry*. His next project will be on the history of social psychiatry.

ACKNOWLEDGEMENTS

The contributions to this volume were first presented as papers at a conference entitled 'The Stress of Life: Gender, Emotions and Health after the Second World War', organized by the Centre for Medical History at the University of Exeter in April 2012 and supported by a grant from the Wellcome Trust, No. 082834/Z07/Z. I am grateful to members of the Trust for both financial and intellectual support. The conference was made possible by the organizational skills of Claire Keyte and the continued sponsorship provided by the Department of History and the College of Humanities at Exeter. I would also like to thank the speakers and participants at the conference, all of whom contributed substantially to the quality and congeniality of the discussions. Material from the Mass Observation Archive quoted in Chapter 4 is reproduced with permission of Curtis Brown Group Ltd, on behalf of The Trustees of the Mass Observation Archive, © The Trustees of the Mass Observation Archive. David Cantor, the series editor, has been a wonderfully constructive companion in the process of developing and producing the volume, as have members of the editorial and production team at Pickering & Chatto, in particular Mark Pollard, Eleanor Hooker and Sarah Thomas. I am deeply grateful to my son, Riordan, for compiling the index entries at a moment when I was under particular pressure to fulfil other commitments.

The strain of editing this volume has been mitigated by the presence in my life of Siobhán, Ciara, Riordan and Conall, who unfailingly manage to cope with the stresses generated by my unhealthy preoccupation with work.

STRESS IN POST-WAR BRITAIN: AN INTRODUCTION

Mark Jackson

There was no single post-war Britain, no intrinsic British culture or identity to be rebuilt, no simple pattern of social reconstruction, no straightforward pathway to either personal or collective recovery after nearly six years of global conflict. When the Second World War ended in 1945, British people, like those of many other nations, were struggling to reconcile themselves to the appalling consequences of war: over 450,000 British soldiers and civilians had been killed and many more severely wounded; families and communities had been destroyed; cities and homes had been reduced to rubble; and welfare services were struggling to cope with the burden of physical and psychological illness, not only amongst members of the armed forces but also amongst civilian populations. Peace brought little immediate relief from stress or any swift return to normality. Rather there followed a gradual process of individual and communal readjustment to social and political conditions only partly recognizable to previous generations. Obstacles to recovery were not limited to the domestic stage. The perpetuation of global instability during the Cold War, evident in Western responses to the consolidation of Soviet power, the Korean War and the arms race, as well as the humiliation of the Suez crisis in 1956 and the migration of workers and refugees, amplified the anxieties and fears of men and women already rendered vulnerable by the cumulative stresses of separation, injury and loss.

Commenting on the difficulties faced by post-war families in 1946, the Hungarian psychoanalyst Therese Benedek (1892–1977) warned that war veterans and their families would struggle to cope with peace because 'readjustment to civilian life may put the already exhausted adaptability of the individual under a new stress'.[1] Benedek's caution resonated with widespread convictions that careful reconstruction at many levels of British life was necessary in order to re-establish a sense of safety and security and to boost the health and productivity of a stressed nation. In 1945, contributors to a volume entitled *Rebuilding Fam-*

ily Life in the Post-War World, edited by the philanthropist Sir James Marchant (1867–1956), had set out the particular challenges facing the British population, including the need to reverse the declining birth-rate, restore economic stability, improve nutrition and education, and promote psychological and spiritual well-being.[2] In a concluding chapter that focused explicitly on the adverse effects of the war on family life, Sir Arthur MacNalty (1880–1969), who had been Chief Medical Officer between 1935 and 1941, cited the British historian Lord Elton (1892–1973) in order to emphasize the centrality of the family in any post-war plans for social reconstruction: 'The end in view is to restore a land in which families can live together in happiness and contentment in a sense of security'.[3]

Concerns about boosting family stability and economic confidence shaped post-war social and welfare policies aimed at enhancing physical health, psychological well-being and social equality on both sides of the Atlantic.[4] During the 1940s and 1950s, successive British governments, both Labour and Conservative, introduced a series of initiatives and legislative reforms designed to rebuild towns and landscapes ravaged by bombs, to restore psychological and physical well-being, and promote family life. The Olympic Games held in London in 1948, widely known as the 'Austerity Games', and the Festival of Britain in 1951 constituted deliberate attempts on the part of the government to improve morale and promote confidence in British science, technology and the arts. Health-care services were reorganized under the terms of the National Health Service Act of 1946, legislation that made medical treatment free to all at the point of delivery. Although economic constraints soon began to limit the provision of free prescriptions and free dental care, the National Health Service transformed the organization and availability of medical services across the country and was regarded proudly by patients and contemporary commentators as emblematic of progressive post-war commitments to reform.

Other substantial social changes were more piecemeal and gradual, triggered not only by the war but also by the continuation and modification of inter-war social and cultural shifts. Although many servicemen returned to jobs that they had vacated during the war, women became increasingly important and more visible members of the workforce. Young women also began to benefit from the expansion of higher education, with increasing numbers of school-leavers enrolling in universities and teacher-training colleges. Combined with the commitment of second-wave feminists to challenge cultural and political inequalities, such changes served to redefine gender relations and family dynamics, triggering fierce debates amongst politicians and doctors about the impact of working mothers on personal and family health. It was in the wake of emergent shifts in working practice and family expectations that work-life balance was adopted as a key concept in endeavours to instil greater resilience to stress amongst post-war populations, and to reconstitute the determinants of domestic stability and occupational productivity.[5]

The political challenge of coping with change and reconfiguring social relations was also evident in patterns of, and responses to, immigration. In 1948, approximately 30,000 people in Britain were from British colonies, often living in close communities in major cities. By 1962, that number had risen to 500,000 as many of those who had served in the British forces during the war arrived from India, Pakistan and the Caribbean in order to find employment, reconnect with families or avoid persecution. Immigration was partly encouraged by government policies aimed at addressing labour shortages, supporting members of the colonies by granting British citizenship and improving the economy: during the post-war decades, immigrants to Britain contributed substantially to the capacity of the National Health Service and the transport system in particular.[6] While such processes benefited many migrants and their families, as well as bolstering post-war efforts to rebuild Britain, they also triggered substantial tensions as both immigrants and local communities attempted to adapt to new occupational and living conditions that could adversely affect physical and mental health.[7] These changes were not confined, of course, to immigration to Britain after the Second World War, but constituted a health and welfare challenge to populations around the world.[8]

Post-war developments in health and welfare services undoubtedly improved conditions and prospects for many people. Yet members of, what has been termed, the 'transitional generation', that is the men and women whose 'formative years straddled the late 1950s and early 1960s', were clearly confronted with a particular constellation of new stresses and strains.[9] According to Lynn Abrams, women were torn between the traditional conservative discourse of 'social duty', linked to their roles as mothers and wives, and the opportunities for freedom, choice and self-fulfilment generated by more liberal approaches to women's education and careers.[10] As well as coping with memories of conflict, young men too struggled to adapt to shifting patterns of work and home life, to adjust to the changing conditions of industrial labour and to re-establish relationships with their families that had been disrupted by the war. First and second generation immigrants faced prejudice, hostility, violence and the difficulties of cultural assimilation. Between the 1950s and 1980s, rapid advances in science and technology and new avenues for recreation and relaxation wrought further pressures on people of all ages: while developments such as space travel, nuclear power, television, the contraceptive pill, organ transplantation, pop music and the increased availability of domestic appliances may have enhanced the living standards and aspirations of many, they also posed new ethical dilemmas and threatened to overwhelm the capacity of post-war populations to cope with the accelerating pace and complexity of life.[11]

Broad and indiscriminate national accounts of the transition from war to peace or of the processes and patterns of post-war reconstruction should be tempered by an awareness of the extent to which people experienced and articulated change in different ways. Whether regarded primarily in positive or negative terms, welfare reforms, cultural shifts and technological advances were not distributed evenly across time and space. Nor did they affect all classes, sexes, ethnic groups or ages equally. The manner in which the recovery of individuals, families and communities varied has rarely been revealed by sweeping social histories that have foregrounded national trends, political achievements, welfare reforms or scientific progress. Just as nostalgic images of the 'swinging sixties' as a decade of unparalleled sexual freedom and youthful rebellion have tended to obscure the reality of many people's lives, so too any over-simplified or celebratory account of the nation's recovery from war neglects the real stresses and strains that continued to inflect the lives of many people in post-war Britain.[12]

Attempts to reveal personal stories of endurance and resilience, in the face of social upheaval and cultural change, have largely mobilized oral history or sources from the Mass Observation Archives, a project that was established in the 1930s as a means of capturing the attitudes and experiences of individuals, families and communities. For Abrams, although all personal testimony should be regarded as contingent, one of the values of oral history lies in its capacity to generate a more finely grained understanding of how individual life stories cohere with or contradict 'more generalized and longer-term accounts of social change'.[13] As several chapters in this volume illustrate, individual narratives of adjusting to change and coping with stress offer what Abrams refers to as 'the opportunity to make connections between biography and history, the personal and the social'.[14] At the same time, both oral history and Mass Observation sources remind us that the effects of change were neither inevitable nor uniform; rather, different people adopted different, and variably successful, strategies for survival in the face of apparently similar stresses.

In a revealing account of her own childhood during the late 1940s and 1950s, Carolyn Steedman has further highlighted the value of merging biography with historical analysis. What emerges from her juxtaposition of experience and context is a firmer understanding that there are many lives for which 'the central interpretative devices of the culture don't quite work', lives such as Steedman's that were lived 'out in the borderlands'. As Steedman shows throughout her account, personal interpretations of the past 'are often in deep and ambiguous conflict' with the more formal explanatory tools of a culture: there are many people to whom the dominant models and values do not apply, for whom there is no place in the official narratives of social recovery and cultural change in the post-war period. According to Steedman, we must refuse to let individual lives be 'absorbed by the central story'.[15] Yet, the clarity of Steedman's critique should not lead us to exaggerate differences between individuals or to overstate apparent disjunctions between experiences of hardship and distress, on the one hand, and prominent scientific and political models of stress, resilience and reform, on the other. As the chapters in subsequent sections of this volume demonstrate, personal and collective experiences of coping were often linked to scientific models of stress through a social and cultural matrix that defined both.

Chronologies of Stress

Recent histories of stress share much in common. Historians, sociologists and anthropologists have all been largely preoccupied with accounting for the development of physiological and psychological models of stress in the modern period, focusing in particular on the theories of stress and adaptation developed by scientists and psychologists, such as Walter B. Cannon (1871–1945), Hans Selye (1907–82), Harold G. Wolff (1898–1962) and Richard Lazarus (1922–2002). These studies have emphasized the ways in which, during the twentieth century, the concept of stress became an increasingly popular means of explaining the onset of illnesses such as arthritis, peptic ulceration, diabetes and heart disease, the capacity of men and women to cope with combat and bombardment, the fragility or resilience of workers under demanding and dangerous occupational conditions and the ability of modern populations to adapt to dramatic social and cultural disruption. At the same time, historians have agreed that the term stress was often applied in ill-defined ways, used indiscriminately by scientists, clinicians and patients to capture a range of symptoms and signs, such as fatigue, anxiety, indigestion, sleeplessness and worry, or to describe both the causes and consequences of psychological and physiological maladjustment.[16]

Historians of stress have disagreed, however, about precisely when stress emerged as a conceptual tool for explaining distress and disease. Some scholars have highlighted the long history of stress as a concept, tracing its use from sixteenth-century accounts of hardship and distress, through seventeenth- and eighteenth-century studies of structural deformity in mechanics and nineteenth-century attempts to link the pressure and pace of modern life to the appearance of heart disease and insanity, to its role in twentieth-century studies of the impact of modern patterns of work and warfare on minds and bodies. There is much evidence to support this interpretation. The term stress was certainly widely employed from the early modern period to refer to adversity or affliction, a vernacular usage that was consolidated in the late nineteenth century by British and American clinicians, such as George M. Beard (1839–83), Thomas Clifford Allbutt (1836–1925) and Charles Arthur Mercier (1852–1919), who used stress to describe the environmental circumstances responsible for triggering neurasthenia, diabetes, hypertension and insanity. In 1922, an emphasis on stressful situations was reinforced by the British *Report of the War Office Committee of Enquiry into 'Shell-Shock'*, in which 'the stress of battle' served as a short-hand for the fatigue, sleeplessness, fear and sense of responsibility induced by prolonged periods of combat.[17]

In these historical narratives of continuity, popular and scientific accounts of stress are thought to have emerged from the traditional matrix of modernity: the language of stress and stability reflected an urge to impose order and control on what were regarded as unstable natural, social and cultural systems; experiences of stress were dictated by modern rhythms of work and leisure; and scientific formulations of stress were rooted in laboratory studies of physiological and emotional balance, as well as in capitalist endeavours to enhance productivity and enforce military efficiency in the face of anxiety and fatigue. Stress and its attendant disorders thus emerged as one of the principal costs of Western civilization: the modern pursuit of scientific knowledge, technological advances and political freedom generated new kinds of trauma, tension and tiredness. Although historians who emphasize continuity recognize the remarkable proliferation of stress discourse across the late twentieth century, they regard this primarily as a manifestation of 'high modernity', that is as a product of the consolidation of the military strategies, occupational routines, technological transformations, bureaucratic processes and social relations characteristic of modern nation states.[18]

Conversely, some historians and social scientists have tended to locate the origins of stress, as well as the emergence of scientific studies of stress, more clearly in the years immediately following the Second World War.[19] It was during the post-war years, they argue, that the collapse of social order served to generate new experiences of illness and to precipitate new ways of exploring and explaining disease. From this perspective, stress in all its guises emerged, not as a product of the patterns and processes of modernity, but as a potent manifestation of an unsettled and fragmented post-modern world. There is also some evidence to substantiate this interpretation of the recent history of stress. During and after the Second World War, military and medical authorities were increasingly concerned about identifying and managing 'flying stress' amongst pilots.[20] From the 1950s, the language and concept of stress were mobilized in the popular press to explain the proliferation of chronic physical and mental illnesses and rising levels of sickness absence in a world where traditional values appeared to have collapsed. Prompted by the publication of books and journals dedicated to exploring the physiological and psychological parameters of stress, clinicians in Europe and America began to refer to 'stress diseases', to implicate stress in the aetiology of anxiety and heart disease, in particular, and to refer more widely to families, communities and nations under stress.[21] By the 1980s, scientists and journalists alike were proclaiming that people were living in an 'age of stress': post-war populations, they argued, were being engulfed by a 'stress epidemic' triggered by the challenge of adapting to the uncertainty, instability and 'unwanted tempo' of life.[22]

These seemingly contrasting accounts of the history of stress, one emphasizing the gradual transmission and evolution of ideas through the nineteenth and twentieth centuries, the other highlighting a marked moment of transition after the Second World War, are not necessarily mutually exclusive. Rather, they can be reconciled in a narrative that acknowledges both continuity and change. Tracing the transmission of ideas about stress or the shared experiences of stress across generations should not preclude recognition that the Second World War constituted some form of watershed, or turning point, in the history of stress. Research into combat stress during the war, particularly into the links between stressful circumstances, individual constitution and psychological breakdown, encouraged novel conceptualizations of the relationship between the environment and mental health, and raised the visibility of stress as a causative factor in disease. Concerns about the effects of rapid social and cultural change, about the impact of global political instability on health and welfare and about the consequences of new patterns of work and family relations served to push stress, as an explanation for anxiety and illness, to the forefront of clinical, political and popular consciousness. Not for the first time, but perhaps more forcefully than previously, identifying, preventing and alleviating stress became key objectives for governments, employers and health-care authorities striving to improve military efficiency, encourage community cohesion, enhance productivity and reduce the burden of chronic, supposedly stress-related, diseases. In the post-war years, stress became an increasingly prominent indicator of social distress and the effective reduction of stress became a measure of the success of social, economic and welfare reforms.

Current historical scholarship has so far done little justice to the complexity of changing patterns and shifting models of stress, especially the manner in which relatively well-established formulations of stress were manipulated in particular moments for particular purposes, making possible new meanings and interventions. Historians have also failed to capture or explore, in any detail, personal experiences and memories of coping with stress or how these persisted or varied across time and space or between different occupational and demographic groups. We know little about what stressed individuals and families or about how people perceived and managed stress in the past. We have few studies of how people assessed the relative impact of war and peace or work and family on patterns of stress or how employers and employees differed in their attitudes to workplace stress. There are few attempts to determine whether stress has (or has not) been distributed unevenly or experienced and manifested differently according to age, class, gender and ethnicity. And we have little historical understanding of the relationship (if any) between scientific models of stress, on the one hand, and personal perceptions of stress and its consequences, on the other.

Based in part on the findings from a large-scale research project on the modern history of stress, carried out at the University of Exeter, this edited collection examines such issues in more depth.[23] Research carried out so far at Exeter has focused primarily on the elaboration of scientific formulations of stress and on the intersections between professional, private and state accounts of stress at work. This volume aims to expand the parameters of historical investigation by exploring both personal formulations and organizational models of stress in post-war Britain. The chapters are not intended to be comprehensive: they do not, for example, address stress and ill-health associated with immigration, which constitutes a fruitful direction for further research.[24] The contributions presented here focus particularly on the period between the Second World War, when stress was coming to the fore as a means of articulating the impact of circumstances on health, and the 1980s, by which time stress had become part of a common language of illness and distress.

Chapters in Part One explore the effects of the transition from war to peace, the relative impact of work and family life on health and the different experiences of, and approaches to, stress in men and women. These studies rely not only, or indeed primarily in some cases, on clinical, industrial or government sources relating to stress and health, but also on a range of interviews, letters and family archives analysed to identify attitudes and responses to stress. Together, they testify to the manner in which warfare, social change and new patterns of work and leisure created pressures that often adversely affected the health and well-being of post-war populations. Part Two examines some of the contemporary physiological, psychological and sociological models that were used to explain the experiences and consequences of stress. In particular, they explore the ways in which neuropsychiatric, psychosomatic and industrial formulations of stress were strongly shaped by a variety of presumptions and assumptions about gender and class. The extent to which these models were informed by, or in turn influenced, individual and family perceptions of stress remains open to question, but chapters in the second section of the book highlight the manner in which post-war theories, just like experiences, of stress were closely fashioned by social context.

Stress at Home and Work

The outbreak of the Second World War in 1939 and its conclusion in 1945 inflicted both anticipated and unforeseen traumas on individuals, families and communities in Britain. As Pam Richardson demonstrates in her chapter on the lives of two families, people responded to war and its aftermath in different ways. Just as there was a variety of stressors, including separation, loneliness, tiredness, illness, bereavement and repatriation, so too there was a range of adaptive strategies that individuals and families employed to cope with stress. Collated, in this instance, from letters and interviews, personal narratives suggest that some of the most important buffers against stress in the post-war period were family support, faith and occupation. Although faith figured rarely in scientific and clinical accounts of stress, the importance of work and family in mitigating the effects of stress were well-recognized by contemporary commentators. In a series of publications that were widely distributed around the world, the Hungarian-born scientist Hans Selye emphasized the manner in which occupation and distraction might alleviate stress and promote health. Similarly, the left-wing American writer Alvin Toffler (b.1928) highlighted the need for post-war generations to develop 'new buffers and balance wheels', such as families, work and communities, in order to reduce stress and achieve happiness.[25] In this regard, personal experiences and scientific theories were mutually constitutive of the post-war emphasis on stress as a threat to the balance and stability of family life.

As Nicole Baur's chapter makes clear, however, families did not always serve to diminish stress and preserve health, but instead constituted on occasion the cause of stress and disease. The language of stress first appeared in asylum procedures and patient records in Devon in 1907, and the term was subsequently regularly used, along with worry, strain and shock, to explain the onset of mental illness. Personal and family narratives demonstrate how any hopes that peace would reduce stress after the Second World War were not always reflected in experiences. As families struggled to rebuild domestic life after the war, psychological distress was often blamed on a variety of stressful circumstances: financial difficulties; the loss of employment; marital problems and divorce; pressures at work; the challenges of parenting; illness and bereavement; and domestic violence.[26] Conversely, illness in one member could place a whole family under stress, as partners, parents and children struggled to cope not only with the behaviour and needs of their relatives, but also with the stigma associated with a diagnosis of mental illness. Although hospitalization might remove some of the stress of caring for a relative, it could deepen the sense of shame. Many families did welcome patients home from hospital, but in some cases the trauma and distress occasioned by a period of mental illness proved to be an insuperable obstacle to marital reconciliation.

Coping strategies varied. According to many post-war stress theorists, smoking and alcohol offered some relief from stress and had often been used fairly effectively by soldiers and civilians to cope with the stress of war.[27] As Ali Haggett reveals, however, awareness and understanding of the relationship between work and home stress, on the one hand, and alcohol abuse, on the other, developed slowly in the post-war years. When doctors and health-care authorities did begin to address the perceived problems of alcohol abuse, their aetiological models and therapeutic approaches differed according to whether they emphasized the role of personality or the significance of wider social, domestic and occupational problems, and whether they were concerned primarily with the impact of drinking on the health of patients or on industrial productivity. Explanations for, and the manifestations of, alcoholism were gendered. In part this may have reflected lived experiences: women appeared to drink because of stressful domestic circumstances, while men's drinking seemed to lead to marital breakdown; women presented largely with psychiatric problems such as anxiety and depression, while men failed to seek help or complained only of somatic symptoms such as indigestion.[28] Yet, patterns of behaviour and explanation were themselves shaped, and reinforced, by gendered stereotypes, behavioural norms and occupational expectations.

Work figured strongly in personal accounts of the stress, strain, tension and anxiety felt by post-war generations. Jill Kirby's analysis of oral history interviews and Mass Observation sources suggests that work played a crucial role in providing people with a sense of status and identity. As a result, both a lack of work and stress at work threatened health and economic security. Many employees demonstrated stoicism and resilience, but others succumbed to workplace stress, developing both physical and psychological symptoms attributable to poor working conditions or to what were seen as unrealistic pressures to perform. Evaluations of stressed workers varied. As in previous and parallel discussions of shell shock and combat stress, some employers and their welfare officers regarded difficulties coping with work and high levels of absenteeism as products of individual weakness rather than the structure or processes of the workplace. In some cases, this led organizations and the government to establish treatment and rehabilitation centres for distressed workers in the hope that this would restore them to health and productive employment. Constrained by masculine stereotypes and internalized norms of masculinity, stressed male workers preferred to blame their ill-health on a personal inability to cope with a competitive world rather than on working conditions or managerial failings.

Industrial and economic competition, as well as technological developments, led to fundamental transformations in working practices during the post-war years. Foremost amongst these changes was the widespread adoption of automation in the British manufacturing industry and the rising popularity of Time and Motion studies to monitor workers' outputs. Using examples from the automobile, tobacco and boot and shoe industries, Sarah Hayes reveals two dominant features of post-war debates about stress: firstly, a persistent preoccupation with the impact of modernization and mechanization on mental health and emotional well-being and on the capacity of individuals to adapt to shifting industrial practices and processes; and secondly, the increasingly significant relationship between occupational health and managerial control. Within these ideological and practical arenas, personal experiences of stress and illness at work, triggered by boredom, noise, monotony and the need for increased machine speed, accentuated disputes between trade unions and employers and contributed to the breakdown of industrial relations in the 1970s. At the same time, they encouraged closer attention (on the part of both employers and employees) to domestic circumstances as an alternative cause of stress that could be blamed on the worker, thereby deflecting attention away from the perils of hazardous workplace conditions.[29]

Distinctions between domestic and occupational causes of stress and illness were drawn elsewhere in the post-war years. As Debbie Palmer argues in the final chapter in this section, stress-related illnesses were of particular interest to the Civil Service, where the managerial and economic impacts of sickness absence were emerging as key concerns. Studies of absenteeism carried out in the 1960s by Sir Daniel Thomson (1912–76), the Service's Chief Medical Advisor, implied that stress levels were linked to the workers' inability to adapt to cultural, social and managerial change and that stress-related sickness absence was far more common amongst lower grade workers and women. Married women appeared to be particularly prone to taking time off sick, a pattern linked by Thomson, and many other contemporary commentators, to their 'divided loyalties' between family and work.[30] Thomson's harsh evaluation of workers' personal responsibilities for health, which identified the home rather than work as the principal determinant of stress, reflected a reality for many women who were struggling to balance work and family pressures, or to adapt to substantial changes in the social and domestic relations between men and women. In the context of heavily politicized debates about the impact of work on women's health, it is no coincidence that it was precisely at this moment that the notion of work-life or work-family balance was gaining traction in sociological studies of health and happiness.[31] At the same time, however, preoccupations with the domestic setting betrayed a persistent prejudice against women entering the workforce and a managerial fixation with exonerating work and social conditions as causative factors in stress-related disease. Subsequent surveys challenged Thomson's conclusions, gradually shifting emphasis from inherent gender differences to inequalities in class but, as chapters in the second section demonstrate, many of these normative assumptions about the behaviour of men and women under stress continued to shape physiological, psychological and social models, as well as experiences of stress in the post-war years.

Models of Stress

If the Second World War and its aftermath substantially reconfigured the stresses and strains of domestic and working life, it also encouraged scientists and social scientists to reframe their models and theories of stress and its impact on health. One of the principal arenas for clinical accounts of stress was the armed forces, particularly the Royal Air Force, where 'flying stress' had been a focus of research since the early 1920s. Both during and after the Second World War, military psychiatrists on both sides of the Atlantic attempted to identify more precisely the particular combination of personal temperament and situational stressors that was liable to lead to psychological breakdown and, as a result, threaten morale and efficiency. As in many other domains, individual responsibility figured strongly in British military understandings of stress, leading to the identification of pilots as 'lacking moral fibre'. Accounts of flying stress (and indeed most post-war studies of behaviour under stress) focused almost exclusively on men as the primary, or exemplary, experimental subjects. Although women served in the armed forces and were exposed to much the same stressors, there was little recognition of the stress experienced by women. When women were considered in the context of flying stress, it was usually simply in terms of their capacity to mitigate or exacerbate the stress experienced by husbands and sons. As my discussion of flying stress in Chapter 7 suggests, experiments on men and the rare accounts of women under stress mobilized and consolidated normative notions of masculine strength and female frailty in the face of danger. One of the consequences of this process, often perpetuated by historians, has been to highlight differences, rather than similarities, between the experiences of men and women under stress during and after the war.

Recognition of the shared nature of stress across gender, age and class boundaries should not prevent us from recognizing that the effects of stress could present in different ways. In his analysis of clinical formulations of psychosomatic disorders amongst veterans, Edgar Jones (like Ali Haggett in her analysis of gender and alcohol consumption) points out that men in particular tended to somaticize their distress, presenting to their doctors with symptoms of indigestion or peptic ulceration, which had become key causes of morbidity and invalidity amongst both soldiers and civilians during the war. Military clinicians had tended to dismiss diet or smoking as aetiological factors, but in the post-war years, when indigestion and peptic ulceration appeared to be more common than during the war, opinions differed about the causes of the rising incidence of stomach disorders: ulceration was variably blamed on unemployment, social deprivation, work pressures, and alcohol and cigarette consumption. As in previous and parallel debates of occupational stress and gastritis, notions of 'constitutional weakness' as a product of both physiology and personality shaped models of gastric disorders: the traumas of war and the emotional challenges of post-war reintegration were seen as potential threats to the physical and mental health of especially vulnerable individuals.[32] In the 1950s, models of stress-related indigestion and ulceration were of particular economic significance in the context of growing financial constraints on the National Health Service. As Jones suggests, trends in stomach disorders may well have been fashioned partly by new patterns of recording clinical data, novel diagnostic procedures and the increased availability of services, as well as by exposure to stressors. Whatever the cause, the prevalence of gastrointestinal symptoms created logistical problems for general practitioners and hospital doctors coping with finite resources and with the difficulties of determining whether patients with indigestion and abdominal pain should be treated primarily by gastroenterologists or psychiatrists.

The relationship between mind and body, and between environmental and constitutional factors, also figured in clinical disputes about how to explain the role of food allergies and stress in shaping physical and mental health. Some allergists emphasized the role of certain foods or environmental toxins in causing allergic conditions such as asthma and eczema as well as various psychiatric symptoms. Others adopted a psychosomatic framework within which allergic manifestations and psychological distress were regarded more often as the product of what increasingly became known, during the 1960s and 1970s, as 'stressful life events'.[33] As Matthew Smith argues, disagreements between proponents of these conflicting models of allergic disease and mental illness were not simply the consequence of contrasting interpretations of the empirical evidence or different diagnostic procedures. They were also the result of professional differences, moulded by ideological and political factors, that shaped doctor-patient relationships, attitudes to social and environmental reform, and beliefs in the predictive power of stress. These differences were not entirely resolved by the discovery of IgE as the mediator of many allergic reactions in the late 1960s. Certainly clinical and scientific attention began to shift towards elucidating the immunological mechanisms behind life-threatening allergic reactions, such as anaphylaxis triggered by exposure to nuts. Diverse practitioners also began to develop a shared language of allergy that recognized both emotional and physical origins of allergic reactions. The place of psychological stress in these discussions, however, remained open to question.

If stress operated as a concept that mediated between alternative models of stomach disorders and allergies, it also functioned as a mechanism for framing disputes about well-being at work. At the heart of investigations into sickness at work were disagreements about the relative contributions and responsibilities of the organization and its employees. In Chapter 10, Joseph Melling demonstrates how social conditions, workplace cultures and personal temperament were variably indicted as factors leading to workers' failure to adjust to, and cope with, work pressures. These disputes were not new: during the inter-war years, industrial psychologists and social reformers had been interested in identifying the combination of situational and constitutional factors that appeared to drive patterns of chronic disease, sickness absence, lowered productivity and social unrest; an approach encapsulated in the notion of 'psychosocial medicine'.[34] After the Second World War, these issues were reframed in the increasingly popular language of stress. Although the term was rejected by some investigators, largely because of its vagueness and elasticity, stress increasingly provided a conceptual model for understanding and representing a range of physiological and emotional symptoms and signs triggered by the working environment. Moving away from previous historical preoccupations with stress in the laboratory and clinic, Melling argues that the visibility of stress in the post-war years was not dependent primarily on the promotion of the concept by scientists, but on a constellation and conjunction of circumstances linked to Western perceptions of psychological distress and the transformation of the global economy.

The prominence of occupational, environmental and domestic factors in both personal narratives of stress and scientific, clinical, military and occupational models of stress should remind us of the importance of recognizing the centrality of the social context in shaping the prevalence and force of stress as an organizing concept. In his account of post-war explorations and explanations of attempted suicide, Chris Millard pushes contingent notions of the 'social' to the foreground of historical analysis. After 1945, the tools and techniques of psychiatric epidemiology were applied by clinicians and social scientists to clarify the links between individual instances and population patterns of mental illness. The elaboration of a psychosocial space, within which environment and illness were regarded as mutually constitutive in this way, was facilitated by widespread adoption of the concept of stress. In a move away from psychoanalytical models of distress that continued to prioritize the pathological nature of inner fantasies and conflicts, many psychiatrists conceptualized mental illness as a product of social stress. The key personnel responsible for identifying social stress, whether it appeared to reside within the family or at work, were psychiatric social workers, who visited patients and their families at home in order to provide psychiatrists with empirical evidence on which to base diagnosis and intervention. As in other iterations of stress and health, clinical formulations of attempted suicide were shaped by gendered experiences and expectations: according to the British psychiatrist Neil Kessel (1925–2003), whose interests encompassed research on alcoholism and suicide, attempted suicide was a communicative 'cry for help' articulated by young women who were struggling to cope with the stress of emotional isolation and domesticity. In this version of psychological maladaptation, the external social, domestic and occupational determinants of distress were combined with internalized normative images of the self to provide the concept of stress with compelling, if unstable, explanatory powers.

Conclusion

In 1980, Hans Selye claimed that widespread beliefs that people were then living in an 'age of stress' were misplaced. Post-war populations, he argued, had too readily forgotten that 'the caveman's fear of being attacked by wild animals while he slept, or of dying from hunger, cold or exhaustion' must have been at least as stressful as the fear of war, economic uncertainty and overpopulation that plagued the inhabitants of late-twentieth-century societies.[35] At one level, Selye was quite right: people in all periods and places have been distressed by personal circumstances; disrupted family and social relationships; the limited availability of resources; the inevitability of death; the instability of political and military regimes; and the difficulties of adapting to radical social and cultural change. Such distress has not always been expressed in the language of stress, but there is evidence of some experiential continuity across generations and cultures in terms of the demands to adapt that have been placed on people around the world.

At another level, however, Selye underestimated the extent to which 'something happened', as the American novelist Joseph Heller put it, in the mid-twentieth century to raise the visibility of stress as a language and conceptual apparatus capable of articulating and explaining the distress and illness experienced by individuals, families, communities and nations.[36] Many of the reasons for the remarkable surge of popular and scientific interest in stress can be traced to the trauma of the Second World War, which continued to cast its shadow over subsequent decades. As British populations, like their counterparts throughout the world, struggled to cope with physical danger, bereavement, injury, repatriation, economic insecurity and political instability, the language of stress served effectively to capture a collective sense of anxiety and unease. Although (or perhaps because) the term stress was imprecise, it became a convenient means by which to express bodily and psychological discomfort, to identify the external circumstances or internal constitutional characteristics responsible for causing ill-health, and to provide a link between life events, personal experience and scientific theories of disease. By the 1980s, stress had become a familiar and pervasive component of the modern vocabulary of hardship, suffering and pain. From this perspective, understanding experiences and formulations of stress is fundamental not only to historical accounts of physical and mental health after the war, but also to our attempts to comprehend the full range of social, economic, political and cultural challenges faced by post-war populations as they adjusted to the transition from war to peace.

Adopting a wide range of sources, methods and perspectives, contributors to this volume collectively challenge simplistic narratives of stress and distress in post-war Britain. Tracing the language, concepts and experiences of stress through the post-war decades, the chapters explore the manner in which work and home, as well as war and peace, dictated patterns of mental and physical health. They reveal how employers and doctors, as well as employees and patients, measured and disputed the relative impact of external circumstances and individual temperament on the capacity to adapt to social and cultural change, how normative accounts of masculine strength and feminine frailty determined how men and women were seen to cope with stress and how scientific investigations of mind and body were integrated into a complex model of disease that has continued to prescribe approaches to health and happiness well into the twenty-first century.

1 FROM WAR TO PEACE: FAMILIES ADAPTING TO CHANGE

Pamela Richardson

In the decades following the Second World War, researchers from different disciplines began to explore and analyse the causes and effects of stress in more detail. Scientific studies of stress were dominated by Hans Selye (1907–82), who introduced the concept of the 'general adaptation syndrome' or 'stress syndrome', which established links between the biochemical and physiological consequences of stress, on the one hand, and disease, on the other.[1] Psychological accounts of stress were also developed in the post-war years, particularly through the work of the American psychologist Richard Lazarus (1922–2002) on the perception and appraisal of stress and coping.[2] Lazarus later emphasized the importance of narratives or proto-typical stories as a means of exploring emotional responses to stress, urging scholars to use 'emotional narratives to understand what is stressful for people, why and how they cope ... the gold is in people's stories'.[3] His theory was that emotions reflected the fate of personal goals and that appraisal of emotions and managing the attendant stress were crucial for physical, social and psychological well-being. For Lazarus, stress and coping were reciprocal processes: when coping was effective, stress was controllable.

Subsequent research by Lazarus and others suggested that the hassles of personal every-day life were arguably more stressful than major life events, a perspective that 'presented an important counterpoint to the then prevalent view about the significance of major life stressors',[4] such as war and deprivation. In 1945, Roy Grinker and John Spiegel had argued that the 'stress of war tries men as no other test they have encountered in civilized life ... valuable lessons can be learned ... regarding the methods by which men adapt themselves to all forms of stress, either in war or in peace'.[5] Although some authors, such as Reuben Hill, recognized the manner in which the functional ability of families was compromised by a failure to cope with life stress,[6] British researchers in the post-war period rarely explored family histories of stress in any form. Yet, when peace returned in 1945, it was soon evident that emotions engendered by experiences throughout five years of war had changed individuals and rendered traumatic the rebuilding of family units. Further stressful events made it difficult, if not impossible, for families to re-establish relationships as they had been before the war.

In order to expose and understand the variety of difficulties that faced parents and their children during and after the war, this chapter will contrast the experiences of two families in the period 1939 to 1950. The first family comprised William, who was 41 years old in 1939 and had been in the army since he was fourteen, his wife May, aged 43, and their three daughters, Lizzie, Nancy and Rose, aged 11, 9 and 7 respectively. Alternative perspectives on the stress of war and its aftermath are provided by the second family, which demonstrates the transition into manhood and family life of 20-year-old Robbie, who had to overcome emotional, physiological and psychological stress in his naval career and in his personal life with Maria, whom he married during the war. The analysis draws on written and oral histories.[7] Although the word 'stress' did not always figure in personal recollections, terms such as 'strain', 'worry', 'concern', 'depression' and 'anxiety' recurred, indicating common experience of conditions and emotions that we now refer to in terms of stress.[8] Both oral interviews and written recollections demonstrate some of the stresses associated with war and peace and the role of age, gender, personality and culture in shaping reactions to events, often beyond people's control. They also illustrate a key feature of post-war discourses on stress, namely the adaptive ability of people faced with changing circumstances.

'This Country is at War with Germany'

The declaration of war in September 1939 had little immediate effect for most of the population, but for those in the armed forces changes began at once.[9] William and May were living in the garrison town of Aldershot, and civilians were evacuated within the first forty-eight hours. The Cambridge Evacuation Survey, edited by child educationalist Susan Isaacs (1885–1944), illustrated the immediate, and potentially long-term, effects of mass evacuation and how the war shaped thinking on the damaging results of separation.[10] It particularly emphasized the importance of mothering in a child's development. Isaacs, child psychiatrist John Bowlby (1907–90), paediatrician and psychoanalyst Donald Winnicott (1896–1971) and psychoanalyst Anna Freud (1895–1982) all argued that evacuation was a story of stress and tragedies, with children becoming emotionally distant, especially from the mother, and that physical separation was a pathogenic factor in future relationships.[11]

May's children were not evacuees, since she took her eldest and youngest daughter to stay with her sister in Dorset, while Nancy, the middle child, remained in hospital at Alton in Hampshire, where she had been a patient since

1937.[12] Nevertheless, it is apparent that separation and relocation were distressing for May. She left her home, parted from her husband not knowing when she would see him again and was moving further away from her sick child, who was already suffering from her own estrangement and lack of mothering. A disciplined home and nursing life had made May a practical and positive person. In her married life, she had adapted to the rootlessness of the army's three-year postings, but this time was different; family life was fractured and the future uncertain. She could manage her own stress, which was exacerbated by the added financial strain of Nancy's treatment and the anxiety which became evident in Lizzie and Rose, but coping with being unable to help her middle daughter proved more difficult.[13] As Rose later recalled, removal to Dorset was an anxious time:

> I was only seven but I had to look after the cat. It was difficult with my gasmask as well and the cat was heavy. She escaped from her basket while we were waiting for the train and ran away. I can remember my screaming, and Mum had to stop me from running after her. I always wondered what happened to that cat.[14]

After a nightmare journey, the house was in darkness when they arrived so they slept on the doorstep, where they were discovered next morning. May had, what was then termed, 'a nervous breakdown' and needed rest and care for several weeks. In the contemporary stress terminology popularized by Selye, May's 'adaptive energy' was spent.[15] Her determination and faith helped her: she took no drugs but, like many others found during the war, smoking offered relief.[16] The family's nomadic lifestyle meant that the girls had also learned to cope with changes of friends and schools, but now they struggled to adapt to farm life and the severe discipline of a childless aunt. As the oldest child, Lizzie did her best to help, always trusting that God would look after them. By contrast, Rose developed psychological symptoms: she was rebellious and difficult, having temper tantrums and stomach aches, especially on the days when her mother was away visiting Nancy. Nancy rarely saw her father, had only monthly contact with her mother and none with her sisters during her time in hospital, a situation that created long-term problems for the whole family.[17]

William was under different pressures. Serving in the Royal Army Service Corps, he was sent where his logistical expertise was most needed. He could do little to alleviate family worries, except write reassuring letters and telegrams. Although he was able to visit once during the four months that May and the girls were in Dorset, he was not welcome because of a past disagreement with his brother-in-law, bringing an extra strain for May.

Early in 1940, May, Lizzie and Rose settled in a house near Nancy's hospital. Talking about this period, Lizzie welcomed the resultant continuity of schooling. She had attended eight different schools before she was ten and felt educationally disadvantaged. Nancy returned home later that year, in callipers and on crutches, but in remission. It was difficult for her to adapt to the rhythm of family life and its close relationships after the impersonal discipline and ordered routine of a large and busy hospital, which fostered emotional independence.[18] After more than three years of institutional life, Nancy could not identify with her sisters. Her behaviour embarrassed them and she rejected their offers of help. By her own admission she was a maladjusted, ill-educated child, violent and had fits of uncontrollable rage, which needed physical restraint:

> I was a horrible child, angry, confused and uncertain about everything and I now can recognise that my behaviour at that time was a release of frustration and pent up emotion caused by the loss of so much of my childhood.[19]

She had not felt resentful during her time in hospital, eighteen months of it strapped to her bed on traction; resentment came later, when she was back in the family and realized what she had missed. In her study of maladjusted children, Sarah Hayes has described similar reactions in returning evacuees: 'Long periods of separation brought a wealth of emotional difficulties ... Most had to adjust to changes in family structures, different family routines and new domestic, social and educational environments'.[20] Disruptions to family life were manifest in other ways. Rose embarked on a bout of petty pilfering. Although she offered no reason for this behaviour, evidence suggests that she was jealous of the attention paid to her sister.[21] She later admitted that and said: 'It was worse when she arrived home, because Mum really fussed over her. I think I felt my place as the baby of the family was threatened and my reaction was to be naughty'.[22] Rebalancing the family dynamics took time and it was the strength and patience of their mother, in the absence of professional support, that restored a sense of order. May's coping strategy centred on her own supportive siblings and on William's younger brother, who was a strong influence on the girls. Continuity of contact between family members, as well as good friends and neighbours, provided stability for them all, an experience shared by others in this period.[23] May made light of her worries to William, knowing of his army responsibilities and perhaps feeling he might think she was not coping well, although this may have partially excluded him from his children's lives.[24] He was in London during the Blitz, and then posted first to France and later to Gibraltar. He suffered a breakdown and was invalided home to a sanatorium in Scotland. It could have been a result of heavy drinking, but May never discussed this 'illness' with their girls.

In 1972, Maurice North emphasized the importance of religious belief, highlighting the 'manner in which ... the decline of religious belief seemed to have produced ... the loss of security and certainty'.[25] In common with many people in that period, this family were members of a strong church community, which provided comfort, security and group activities for adults and children to enjoy.[26] William was a passing visitor to the tight-knit female group and the emotional distance between them grew. The girls recorded May's sense of humour, her enthusiasm and encouragement of their plans for the future and her unfailing support to family members. Her resourcefulness and practicality helped to maintain her mental well-being, but she suffered from bouts of illness. The constant worry of her children being hungry caused her to give them much of her own ration, a situation that may well have exacerbated the effects of prolonged stress and led to recurrent infections.[27]

William and May's experiences during the war can be compared and contrasted with those of Robbie and Maria. Robbie joined the Royal Naval Reserve in November 1940 when he was almost twenty-one. He was a qualified marine engineer, but enlisted as an ordinary seaman rather than serve as an officer in a ship's engine room. He wrote to his parents: 'went through yet another medical examination and was told that in three weeks I would be called up to do six months in Bell-bottoms ... and if I was of any use would have a chance at a commission ... and then would be fit for work'.[28] Like most young men, he felt ready for adventure. His father had been a Naval Officer during the First World War and had instilled discipline and stoicism in his son.[29] Life had run smoothly for Robbie until his younger sister had died while he was away at boarding school. He could not share his grief even with his elder brother; when he returned home for the holidays no trace of her remained and no one spoke of her or acknowledged his distress. His feelings remained unresolved for many years.

Away from home, life on a battleship was disciplined and busy, but nothing had prepared him for being detailed to help clear the human debris in an anchored ship that had been bombed, an experience that he also repressed.[30] After officer training, he joined a corvette on convoy escort duty in the Atlantic, the Mediterranean and the Arctic, adapting to physical discomfort in extremes of weather. As the sea war intensified, he learned the value of friends, helping each other to cope and, as all his friends did, began to smoke to relieve the tension that was part of their lives. It became increasingly difficult to write cheerful letters home, so he wrote about pre-war activities, trying to hold on to the normality that he had known.[31] The seasickness that plagued him may well have been a physical manifestation of the strain of constant readiness for action from an enemy largely unseen beneath them. As Hans Selye pointed out in 1957, and as a number of historians have subsequently suggested, 'the gastro-intestinal tract is particularly sensitive to general stress ... and this may be accompanied by vomiting', caused by high levels of hormones released in response to stress.[32]

In foreign ports, time off from shipboard life was a precious respite. Rare home leaves were opportunities to escape pressure and enjoy normality and the company of family and his girlfriend, Maria, whom he had known for several years through her friendship with his sister. Her difficult early life meant she had no close family of her own and so she was independent and practical, good at sport and a fine musician, which provided solace.[33] She and Robbie corresponded regularly and met during his periods of leave. Their friendship grew into a deeper relationship. They married when she became pregnant, but Robbie had to return to sea, feeling guilty and anxious about leaving Maria to cope alone.[34] His mother's distress was evident only in that in all his letters written to her throughout the war and preserved, none relating to the pregnancy remain. She knew and liked Maria and she and his father were generous and practical in their help and support, but it was a difficult situation for them all.[35] Robbie's discomfort is evident in later letters. It was several months before he referred to Maria as his wife. Although she was well-looked after by his family, she was facing something unknown and frightening and was also living with the anxiety of knowing that Robbie was in constant danger.

The experiences of Robbie and Maria were common during the war and provide evidence of the emotional reaction to the uncertainties of the time. Perhaps until the 1960s, the social and moral code of the inter-war years remained strong, particularly in the middle classes, and children conceived out of wedlock were perceived as evidence of sexual laxity. The resultant strain, which reverberated through many families, broke relationships and some girls were shamed and disowned.[36] There were frequent wartime marriages, often to legitimize the babies. This may have contributed to the rise in the divorce rate in 1947, which is discussed in the second part of this chapter.

At twenty-three, Robbie's relatively carefree bachelor life was over and, when off duty, he had time to reflect on his future and worry about the responsibilities of being a husband and a father. His life seemed to be in two separate compartments, each equally demanding, but it did not seem so bad when he heard that his brother was also going to be a father.[37] He and Maria had to find their own answers to the pressures. This was perhaps easier for Robbie, for whom unrelenting hard work in tough conditions was an antidote, but Maria had to overcome loneliness and poor health and remain strong and optimistic in preparation for her baby.[38] According to Selye and others writing about stress at this time, 'deviation' from one form of stress to another constituted an important strategy alleviating pressure and 'for combating purely mental stress. Everyone knows how much harm can be caused by worry'.[39] Robbie heard of the birth of his son when the baby was six weeks old but, except for photographs, did not see him for a further eighteen months. For Robbie, the last half of the war was a period of rapid transition from carefree boyhood to responsible manhood.

The experiences of these two families demonstrate a variety of wartime stressors and adaptive strategies. For the men, conflict carried its own stress. In addition, William struggled with a sick child, family worries and alcohol dependency. Inexperienced at relationships, Robbie was apprehensive about his future responsibilities and work prospects. May and Maria both had to cope with the anxiety of separation from their husbands and the challenges of their day-to-day lives, May trying to balance the varying needs of her children while Maria was learning the meaning of motherhood. For the children, war meant that a young infant did not know his father and three young girls struggled to understand and cope with the changes taking place in their lives.

'The ... War is ... at an End'

In May 1945 the conflict in Europe was over. Four months later there was world peace.[40] Writing at the time, Grinker and Spiegel questioned whether peace would automatically lessen individual stress.[41] In a similar vein, other commentators acknowledged that, in the 1950s, people were only beginning to comprehend 'the adaptation of the human organism to stress'.[42] The trauma of the transition from war to peace was evident in all lives and particularly distressing when expectations were so high. In 1939 no one had known how long the war might last, but people recognized that life would be difficult. They adapted to growing privations and coped as well as they could. There was a general feeling of fighting the common cause. But when the war was won, everyone expected that peace would bring better things. However, with the fabric of society ruptured, peace triggered a series of different stressors which, in many cases, precipitated personal life-changes. As Reuben Hill pointed out in 1949, the ripple effects of stress and trauma affected wider kinship groups and damaged 'the functional stability of families'.[43]

Replicated throughout the country was the hope and expectation of the mothers and children in these case studies. In preparation for William's return, May had her hair done, spring-cleaned the house and prepared what food she could, given the rationing. The girls recalled their preparations many years later.[44] When William did return, he was thin and frail and needed compassionate leave for some weeks. This was not the homecoming that May and the girls had anticipated. By contrast, Robbie's repatriation was more joyful. When he arrived home in July 1945, he was eager to meet his son and reunite with his wife and family. Maria had made him a familiar part of the baby's life through photographs and talking about 'daddy', so his son greeted him with affection.

Most men returning home had high expectations. After the exigencies of war, they looked forward to comfort, good food and a loving welcome. Starved of familial affection for long periods, they wanted to make up for that loss. They expected families to welcome them as heroes, but in reality they were strangers to their children, who had grown up in their absence. For some men, they returned to no home at all, just a bombed-out shell. Family members had been killed or injured and love had often died. In 1988 Julie Summers based her book *Stranger in the House* on interviews with men and women who lived through that post-war period. Each chapter presents a different viewpoint of events and emotions. The women had become more independent, used to doing things their way, and families were functioning well without a man. There were national shortages, of work, housing, food and fuel. The challenge was how to rebuild relationships and restore family strength.[45]

There have been different historical interpretations of homecoming. American historian Geoffrey Field emphasized the preoccupations of the British government with family and children, expressed in various forms of official advertising, once the war was over:

> smiling responsible parents and healthy, carefree children … symbolic of the nation's 'social capital' and a better future … domestic and mothering images of women … the family … the chief incubator of citizenship and community values.[46]

While these attitudes reflected growing political intervention in, and influence on, family life, Julie Summers has portrayed a different picture by focusing on more personal and social themes:

> Men were uneasy with the freedom from order and discipline; thrown into a state of uncertainty about how they would fit back into civilian society. They were confused by women who had grown older, who had become independent. Then there were the children who didn't recognise their fathers … jealous of attention now lavished on mothers.[47]

Both scenarios were potential sources of stress for the two families in this study. William remained in the army, where order and discipline continued to structure his life. His peacetime role was less stressful, but his relationship with his wife was brittle and that with his daughters was difficult. Robbie was free from naval control but apprehensive about his role as husband and provider.[48] For different reasons both men were anxious about the future.

Despite previous experiences during and after the First World War, military authorities took scant account of the traumatic psychological effect of the war on men, women and children, and the medical profession and public continued to underestimate the results of delayed shock and the weariness of the population. In January 1945, the magazine *Women's Own* published an article 'Back to Real Life' by Nora James, in which she pointed to the importance of re-instatement of the home as a family unit and placed the onus of tackling the post-war years on women.[49] That was not an easy task for those who, like May, were tired and unwell as a result of their wartime experiences. In 1946, the Hungarian psychoanalyst Therese Benedek (1892–1977) described the struggles that families were continuing to have in readjusting to civilian life because their capacity to cope was exhausted; a point also made by Summers in her historical accounts.[50]

The government was aware of the social problems that would come with the war's end. In 1942, Winston Churchill had appointed Ernest Bevin as Minister of Reconstruction and planners had begun to consider the post-war future.

Army psychiatrists, among them Thomas Forrest Main (1911–90), were particularly anxious about the mental and emotional problems that would arise.[51] Immediately after the war, Resettlement and Advice units were set up throughout the country with specially trained officers. Barbara Cartland (a Welfare Officer throughout the war) was outspokenly critical about the inadequacy of the training, arguing that official advice, albeit well-intentioned, did not address 'intimate personal problems and men were often referred to voluntary bodies such as the British Legion, the Salvation Army and the Church who, it was felt had more experience'.[52] In 1948 the Marriage Guidance Council (set up in 1938) stressed the urgent need for doctors to be more aware of the degree of marital discord at that time, and it offered the assistance of its counsellors to help and advise general practitioners.[53] There were other avenues of relief. At Regimental Associations men found reassurance in the company of other ex-servicemen. Robbie and William both enjoyed meeting up with friends to relax and discuss problems. For women, the Women's Institute and the Townswomen's Guild offered interest outside the home. May continued to work for the British Legion after the war. Maria had a daughter in 1946 and another in 1949, so her hands were too full to seek outside diversions, except for her music and tennis.

Although families could facilitate adjustment and adaptation, if family relationships were discordant or the home was broken by the loss of one parent, it became the greatest cauldron of stress, particularly for children. The psychologist Cyril Burt (1883–1971) emphasized the significant role of 'the social and domestic environment in the aetiology of maladjustment [of children]'.[54] This certainly appeared to be true in the case of William and May, for their children, especially Rose, were under great strain. One of the consultants treating Rose's back condition, before a firm diagnosis was reached, suggested that there could be a psychological element to her pain.[55]

The two mothers in these case studies had contrasting psychological experiences after the war. Previously balanced and optimistic, May was forty-eight years old and experiencing what her doctor called 'the change of life'. The motivation that had driven her throughout the war had diminished. She looked forward to 'the comfort of stability',[56] but the accumulation of the hormonal changes associated with menopause, continuing concern for Nancy and the effects of William's drinking on his health, compounded by anxiety and physical debilitation caused by wartime and post-war shortages, made it difficult for her to look forward to a happy future. By 1948, Lizzie was working in a local bank, Nancy had begun her training to be a nurse and Rose was in the fifth form of the local Grammar School. Although May became more depressed when the two older girls left home, she and William were not among the 60,254 divorces in 1947. The number did not reach that figure again until 1971 when a redrafted law made divorce easier. The large increase in the late 1940s (following the end of the Second World War) is considered to be attributable to women's increased participation in the labour force which meant couples were no longer as financially dependent on each other.[57]

William, posted nearby and living at home, did not know how best to help May. She behaved normally with the children, who sensed the tension in the home but did not know how to help. She found it difficult to talk to William about her feelings, he spent more and more time at the local pub with his male friends and the gap between them grew. Both parents were heavy smokers but May increasingly resented Will's drinking and the effects on the family. She threatened to leave him but divorce was difficult: the process was expensive and carried much opprobrium. In that post-war period, some men and women walked away from their marriage responsibilities, which created financial and social problems for the children deprived of a parent.

Later in 1948 May joined William in Germany, where he was serving with the British Army of Occupation of the Rhine, to give her a much needed break and for them to try to re-build their relationship. It was not a success and May was distressed by the bombed state of Hamburg and the appalling conditions in which people were struggling to live. It revealed the ruthlessness of Allied action and confirmed her opinion, expressed to the girls, that in war it was civilians, mostly women, who suffered and struggled to adapt. The experience added to her already disturbed mental state. When the family was re-united, they had another problem. Then seventeen, Rose was suffering with a damaged and painful back, which needed surgery. The orthopaedic surgeon wrote to William in July 1949:

> I do not think that the decision to carry out this operation should be arrived at too quickly as this is an unusual state of affairs in a girl of this age and I am sure that we ought to give every chance for the pain to be relieved in other ways.[58]

Conservative treatment was unsuccessful and in January 1950 William applied to his commanding officer for a posting back to the United Kingdom on compassionate grounds. An extract from his letter stated:

> I have been completely separated from my family since September 1939, except for periods of privilege leave and my continual separation is having a marked effect on my wife's health.
>
> My second daughter was a patient in an Orthopaedic Hospital for a period of 4½ years, being finally discharged in August 1944 following a major operation [she had a left hip arthrodesis]. During this period my wife had a very worrying time. Of this period I was serving in Gibraltar for 2½ years.
>
> My youngest daughter has been in the care of an Orthopaedic Specialist since January 1949 and is now awaiting early admission to hospital to undergo a major Spinal operation.[59]

May's family doctor sent a letter of support, setting out May's physical and mental state. He added: 'it is desirable that Mrs X does not have this added worry to cope with on her own'.[60] The request was granted. William arrived home on the day of Rose's operation to find that Lizzie was in the same hospital having an emergency operation to remove her appendix. Rose wrote:

> I woke up in the middle of the night ... my mother was there ... I immediately assumed she was there because I was going to die and it was very odd that it didn't worry me at all. She told me that Lizzie was a patient downstairs and she had had an operation ... In retrospect I cannot understand how my mother didn't break down after all the health problems we had. I suppose it must have helped that she had been a nurse. Perhaps all that strain caused her cancer.[61]

The inauguration of the National Health Service was an event which touched everyone in the United Kingdom and this family epitomizes the relief from anxiety and distress that it brought. After years of financial strictures imposed by the cost of Nancy's long treatment, there was nothing to pay for Rose. A significant cause of worry was removed.

According to Janet Finch and Penny Summerfield, central 'to the aims of the post-war social reconstruction was the desire to consolidate family life again after the disruptive effects of war and to build a future in which marriage and the home would be the foundation of a better life'.[62] But for some, family life had frequently been a battleground of emotional, mental and financial stress and this was even more so in the post-war period. Difficult relationships needed a catalyst and the good times, fondly remembered by 'Lizzie', 'Nancy' and 'Rose' tended to include the wider family.[63] The wartime absence of husbands left married women celibate at a time when they most needed the reassuring comfort of physical intimacy to combat their anxiety. That need was subsumed in hard work and keeping busy, and some found it difficult, or did not want, to resume such intimacy when their men came home. Men too were changed by war-time experiences and often suffered similar problems that were difficult to talk about. In the years between 1945 and 1960, the growing discipline of sociology concentrated increasingly on marriage and family life and some studies focused on the emergence of 'companionate marriage'. Couples like May and William stayed together but in a companionate marriage based on sharing and partnership; marriage as an *institution* rather than a *relationship* which involved physical intimacy. This preserved the status quo for the children.

Robbie was anxious to recreate the security he had known in a happy home and Maria was in the prime of life and longing to create the settled family life denied her. They faced challenges in the post-war period. Although they had been friends since their schooldays, they had not had an intimate relationship so there was much to learn. She was a proud and loving mother,[64] but Robbie quickly realized that she was psychologically insecure and suffered frequent episodes of ill-health. She needed his support, so he abandoned plans to continue his engineering studies and became involved in agriculture instead. They moved around the country as he changed jobs, but he refused a promotion because it meant greater devotion to company politics and more travelling. It would have eased their finances but, knowing Maria's frailty, he chose always to spend as much time as possible at home and it was a loving, supportive relationship for both of them. They had two more children and her whole life centred on the family.

These two men, one middle-aged, one young, found it impossible to share their experiences of war with their wives. The medical legacy of war for William was high blood pressure and alcohol dependency; for Robbie it was a legacy of stomach trouble as a result of chronic seasickness, varicose veins from long hours of standing, tinnitus caused by gunfire and recurring nightmares about the horrors that he had witnessed. Their wives also had anxieties they found difficult to share. In company with other women, they had carried the total responsibility of home and children. They had managed well and grown in confidence but then had to step back and allow their men to assume control. Although personal and marital discord were common after the war and although the consumption of psychotropic drugs was increasing,[65] May and Maria preferred to rely on their own resources.[66] Both women died of cancer, May in 1958 and Maria in 1969. May's smoking was a prime cause, perhaps aggravated by the accumulation of stress. Maria neither smoked nor drank, and she was rigorous about healthy food and enjoyed a happy marriage, but her childhood insecurities may well have left a legacy of anxiety and poor health.[67]

Conclusion

In 1946, Therese Benedek suggested that the stress of war would continue to impact on readjustment to peace.[68] In the lives of the two families in this study some of Benedek's fears, and those of other scientists and social scientists in the field, were realized. In the post-war period, effective coping relied heavily on the support and encouragement of family, neighbours and friends. May had her own extended family; without close family of her own, Maria was fortunate to have Robbie's kinship group to help her. The inner resources of these two women were developed through their life experiences,[69] and in May's case were strengthened by her deep faith and the help of her Christian community. The same faith prompted Robbie's parents to support Maria when she needed help. Talking about his war, Robbie remembered how most dying men, pulled from the sea, cried to God for help; he wondered whether humans were born with innate faith, which, though often buried, surfaced in time of desperate need.[70] Both women were practical in the home and garden. Outside interests, such as music, sport and the power of group commitment, also helped to alleviate stress and maintain self-confidence.[71]

Evidence from the Second World War and from the subsequent transition to peace facilitated a shift from the physiology to the psychology of stress. In the 1960s and 1970s, Lazarus and his colleagues explored strategies for finding emotional, mental and physical balance and enabling individual coping mechanisms in order to minimize the wear and tear of life.[72] In 1981, he joined A. K. Kanner, J. C. Coyne and C. Schafer in research that compared stress in relation to major life events and stress caused by smaller day-to-day problems, identifying the need for further, more refined, studies of the impact of different life stressors on health.[73]

The case studies described in this chapter suggest that change, whether good or bad, could be traumatic. It was the major, more visible events of this period, such as the outbreak of war, Dunkirk, D Day, the Peace declaration and the Cold War, that appeared to affect men more; they were the ones who fought and had to find work when peace came. For women and children, the hassles of day-to-day living resulting from those global events had greater significance in their lives at home and at school and work. These stresses are difficult to quantify historically, for the cumulative effect of one could cause the other or follow from it; they were bound together, as were stress and coping, with individual reactions based on a variety of circumstances.

Much has been learned about combatting stress from the trauma of the two major life transitions between war and peace. Nowadays returning service personnel, fewer in number and spread out over time, receive counselling and help to alleviate post-traumatic stress. The organization Combat Stress, which was established in the wake of the Second World War, offers 'a broad ranging therapeutic programme specifically designed to address Service related mental ill health that is often complex, chronic and enduring in nature'.[74] This programme encompasses treatment across a wide spectrum of symptoms triggered by the anxiety of anticipating negative outcomes of events, as well as the stress and distress caused by work or life changes. The emphasis in modern therapy is on restoring a sense of meaning and balance by addressing the fears of memory and rebuilding connections in marriage and in the wider circles of relatives and friends. This approach has served to save relationships with children and partners, but the current emphasis is not wholly on rebuilding families. It is now recognized, as it was not in the immediate post-war period, that family relationships are not always beneficial. Nevertheless, our early-twenty-first century commitment to mitigating the stress of war and to reducing the challenges caused by the transition from war to peace are very much a legacy of the experiences of soldiers and their families after the Second World War.

2 FAMILIES, STRESS AND MENTAL ILLNESS IN DEVON, 1940s TO 1970s

Nicole Baur

In October 1970, O. was admitted to hospital following an episode of mania believed to be caused by being 'under *stress* from unduly overlong visit by her mother-in-law owing to bus strike'.[1] However, surviving correspondence between O.'s husband and the psychiatrist sheds light on O.'s life before admission, painting a profoundly more complex picture. Following an unhappy childhood, her marriage was tainted by a miscarriage and by her mother-in-law's constant interference. Relocating to Scotland was hoped to be a move 'away from family constrictions'. Though a welcome relief, the move meant that 'from summertime in Devon, O. [woke] up to November in Glasgow – cold and foggy. Depression set in and [was] fought off and return[ed] only to be fought off again for six years'. Subsequent moves back to Devon and later Gloucestershire failed to bring relief, as the home became a holiday stop for the family on both sides. Determined to make these visits a success, O. kept up a brave front, but when a bus strike extended the mother-in-law's stay, she finally broke down.

Many elements of family stress theory are evident in O.'s story, which has to be understood in the context of her relationships with her extended family. She was affected by various major life events, leaving her emotionally deprived from childhood and in a job with little satisfaction. Her marriage was characterized by several losses, including an unborn child, and disruptions to her social networks. Additionally, she continued to be exposed to strained familial relations. Although her illness was attributed directly to her the mother-in-law's extended stay, it is more likely that the cumulative effect of all the above experiences triggered it. Her case notes further suggest that such experiences were exacerbated by O.'s worrying and emotionally unstable personality, making her vulnerable to developing a mental disorder. While O.'s family situation clearly impacted on her illness, the surviving documents tell us little about the stress her illness placed on her family. This chapter explores the more complex linkages between families, stress and mental health after the Second World War.

'Stress' Enters the Devon Case Files

'Stress' as a term began to feature in Devon case notes from 1907, following the adoption of the Medico-Psychological Association's 'Schedule of Causes and Associated Factors of Insanity' by the Commissioners in Lunacy. Amongst the bias towards physiological aetiologies, 'stress' – subdivided according to its duration into sudden and prolonged stress – was the only category that could cover any non-physiological cause. It is, therefore, not surprising that within a few months of its adoption 'stress' turned into an umbrella term for socio-environmental factors in the causation of mental disorders across England and Wales. As early as 1908 'mental stress' accounted for an averaged 20 per cent of admissions, often in combination with physical factors, setting the trend up to the middle of the twentieth century. During the decade between 1940 and 1949, Devon doctors nominated 'mental stress' as a cause of illness in just under one quarter of cases, ranking it third after hereditary influences and a patient's disposition and life cycle. In more than 87 per cent of cases stress had existed over an extended period of time prior to admission. Case notes also illustrate that stress continued to be considered a contributory rather than the sole aetiological component, as in over 40 per cent of cases stress was combined with other factors.

The new classification scheme introduced an interesting linguistic shift. Prior to 1907, when doctors used their own words to capture what they perceived to be the cause of the mental illness, expressions such as 'stress' or 'strain' hardly featured. Neither were they part of lay vocabulary. The introduction of the classification scheme appears to be responsible for the considerable increase in the term 'stress' amongst doctors from 1907, but interestingly lay people also began to describe causes more often in terms of 'shock, strain, worry'. As Mark Jackson has pointed out, the term 'shock' had been used in the late nineteenth century, particularly in novels, to refer to 'the colossal sense of shock generated by new industrial technologies, emerging modes of education, and novel forms of high-speed travel and communication'.[2] In the Devon data, whereas 'worry' could refer to any type of concern or upset, 'shock' was primarily used to describe news of either death or severe illness received by the patient and referring to either a close relative or the patient themselves. Later in this paper it will be shown that while the term 'stress' was common in doctors' vocabulary, in the post-war period, relatives tended to continue using words such as 'strain, shock, worry' or 'grief' to express their emotions about a patient's illness and sometimes to refer to the burden experienced in caring for the patient.

Unfortunately, case note entries tell us very little about what doctors meant by 'stress' or how they arrived at this conclusion. The most potent clue that the term was used as a collective for a large variety of socio-economical factors is the occasional supplementary comments by doctors, for example, 'stress – death of husband'. The reason for these additions is unclear, but we might presume that at least some doctors regarded the classification scheme with its distinct bias towards physiological explanations as deficient. Another indicator that doctors thought of 'stress' in socio-environmental terms can be obtained from listening to the views of lay people, whose testimonies are at the centre of this chapter.

Stress Research and the Family

Starting with the Great Depression and the effects of WWII in the 1930s and 1940s, family stress research examined how hardship and life events affected families.[3] Almost simultaneously, the role of families in mental disorders and their coping mechanisms began to be explored.[4] While early studies of family stress emphasized the family's pathological effects, research from the 1970s onwards focused on family strengths and support mechanisms.[5] While this work has provided historians with insights into contemporary approaches to the family as a system, we know very little about how families experienced stress. Family stress research was geared primarily towards understanding how families coped with stressful events, with little attention paid to the interpersonal processes in families under stress. Specifically, early post-war stress research did not pay serious attention to family testimony in its attempts to assess major life events and chronic stressors. Instead, it followed Reuben Hill's ABCX model. Hill, investigating the effects of war-induced separation and reunion, attempted to explain 'the crisis-proneness and freedom from crisis among families'.[6] Focusing largely on pre-crisis factors, the model proposes that if a stressor *A* (e.g. the death of a loved one) interacts with *B* (the family's crisis-meeting resources, such as, for example, family adaptation and integration) and *C* (the family's subjective definition of the stressful event), *X* (a crisis) may arise.[7] Hill's model emphasized two areas hitherto neglected, namely the importance of the family's subjective perception of the event as well as their resources to cope with it, thereby challenging previous strictly linear, deterministic notions that stressful life events inevitably resulted in crises. Converted into a theoretical framework for family stress research in 1973 and subsequently modified into the Double-ABCX model, Hill's model was foundational to all subsequent family stress research.[8]

Besides their over-reliance on quantifiable data, these models assumed that every person responded to a stressor in the same way, ignoring emotions and cognitions of patients and their families.[9] As Lazarus and others argued, however, more attention needed to be paid to individual perception and evaluation of a stressor, the appraisal of which was subjective, dependent on social conditions, structures and policies and did not always correspond with the objective situation.[10] Therefore, besides characteristics of the stressor, such as its duration, severity, controllability, predictability and novelty, an individual's social network and other social factors had to be taken into account.[11] An alternative approach, focusing on minor stressors affecting ordinary families on a day-to-day basis, was proposed by Kanner et al. in 1981, and greater focus on interactions between individuals and their environments led to the development of the diathesis-stress model, combining inherited predisposition with environmental vulnerability.[12] Despite such developments, family stress research has failed to explain fully the nature of the relationship between stress and mental disorders. Model-based studies have established stress as a process in a fully interactive system, whose social context is vital to understand its relationship to mental disorders.[13] Focusing exclusively on patients' views, however, ignores the perspectives of people affected by the patient's mental disorder, including close relatives and family members. This chapter argues that historians need to probe beyond medical models of stress to understand interpersonal relationships so crucial for the patient's hospitalization and return home. Such understandings can often only be gained from personal narratives, including those of the patient and those of their relatives and friends.

The importance of family testimony was recognized early in Devon and its significance increased after the foundation of the National Health Service. Social histories, introduced in Devon in the 1930s, provided doctors with more insight into patients' social backgrounds, and while families were sometimes reluctant to respond to the questions, letters addressed to hospital doctors revealed complex stories. In writing, many relatives felt free to address their view of the patient's mental disorder, not only providing clues to faulty domestic situations, but also detailing their experiences with the patient before admission and concerns about the patient's return into the family community. This paper is based on narratives of patients' biographies provided by patients or their relatives, shedding light on the nature of subjective experiences.[14] They have been gathered from a diverse range of archival sources, including admission papers, in particular Statements of Particulars (SoPs), and surviving correspondence of relatives with the hospital as well as social services. Contrary to much existing research, it uses the same set of data to investigate the stresses that patients experienced within their families and the strains that the mentally ill placed on their close relatives. The majority of existing research lacks this comparative angle by focusing on only one of these dimensions. It is also noteworthy that, contrary to many studies, the narratives used in this paper were gathered at the very beginning of the patient's hospitalization. This is a crucial stage when researching mental illness based on lay experiences because exposure to psychiatric knowledge can influence causal beliefs amongst relatives as well as amongst patients.

The Family as Causal Agent in Mental Illness

Surviving documents demonstrate that much of the stress experienced by Devon patients was domestic in nature. Such stress could result from life events, most notably bereavement, as well as on-going stressors. Similar to findings of contemporary studies, the Devon materials illustrate that life events were more prominent as causative agents in patients diagnosed with depressive disorders than disorders such as schizophrenia.[15] Most stressful life events contained an element of actual or perceived loss. Bereavement affected over one third of Devon patients with a perceived aetiology of domestic stress.[16] Over 80 per cent of patients suffering from the effects of bereavement were women, the majority having lost their husbands, while considerably fewer were mourning the loss of their mother or a child. The death of a child in particular triggered feelings of guilt or inadequacy, of being unable to properly care for or even bear a child. The age range from 24 to 79 years suggests that a number had lost their husbands at a relatively young age, possibly due to the Second World War, compared to male admissions which ranged from 50 to 78 years. Consequently, while depressive conditions headed the list of diagnoses on the female side, many male patients were diagnosed with various forms of senile changes. Existing research has shown that men are often at higher risk of mental illness after an experience of loss due to smaller social networks, but the Devon data from the post-war period does not necessarily corroborate these results. Although most patients were admitted within one year of the death, the permanent loss of a close person could have long-lasting effects. Admission figures show that for some patients anniversaries of deaths, such as birthdays or upcoming holidays to be spent without their loved ones, could act as reminders and render people vulnerable to an attack or recurrence of a mental disturbance.

Similar to O.'s story, surviving documents illustrate that aetiological entries on case notes frequently referred only to the most immediate event before admission, although patients had been suffering for a longer period of time from various stressors. For example S., whose depressive illness was allegedly triggered by her husband's recent death, had been exposed to various stressors well before that, including the suicide of her eldest son, whom she found hanging, and a court case about the divorce of her youngest son.[17] In other cases, bereavement was coupled with deep feelings of anger, as in B.s' frustration at her husband's brother's failure to attend his funeral.[18] Similarly, 35-year-old C., mourning her father's passing, was described by her husband as being rather frustrated and disappointed at the father's will.[19] In other cases the death was preceded by a long period of nursing the partner or parent, which adversely affected the patient's physical health and social life. Correspondence with relatives and patient testimony clearly illustrate that the 'shock' of losing a loved person or the 'worry' following it was frequently not the only adversity patients had to cope with. In addition to the emotional burden, death often resulted in further losses. Financial hardship, even the loss of the home, was not uncommon after the death of a family member. In other instances, widows had to take on the responsibility for money matters and businesses after the death of their husbands – for which tasks they often felt ill-equipped.

The effects of the stress of the Second World War were still clearly felt in Devon during the following two decades. 41-year-old A.'s admission in 1949, for instance, was attributed to the death of her baby at birth.[20] Closer inspection of her social history, however, reveals that she had been suffering from war strain owing to being bombed out of her house and subsequent frequent house moves; her husband, being on war service, was unable to support her when the child was born. War stress impacted on families through more than the loss of goods and chattels, as both Reuben Hill and Therese Benedek argued at the time.[21] Food shortages prevented mothers from feeding their children adequately and millions were separated from their loved ones. It is therefore not surprising to read that 'it is entirely through the war, that her [A's] nerves have given way'.[22] Further corroborating Hill's and Benedek's findings, the Devon documents illustrate that seemingly joyful events, such as a husband's return from war, could lead to stress – both in the returning soldier who had to adjust to civilian life again as well as in the family to which he returned.

Life events made up only one category of environmental stressors. They were conceptualized as datable, single events requiring a change in the individual's daily routine. While such events increased the risk of developing a mental illness, they excluded 'ongoing noxious environmental factors which are a commonplace and repetitive feature of the subject's routine life world'.[23] Daily strains resulting from family interaction or perceived overwork could have similar effects, rendering the relationship between the family and mental illness notoriously complex.[24] In Devon, many such strains concerned the marital relationship. About half of the patients whose mental disorder was traced back to domestic stressors felt trapped in an unsatisfactory marriage. Reasons for this feeling remain mostly obscure with couples simply considered to be 'incompatible'. Often, women put domestic stress down to the husband's ill-treatment of the family, his drinking habits and financial irresponsibility.[25] Statements taken from men were more likely to blame sexual problems caused by the 'patient['s] unhealthy attitude to life and people' or 'being frigid and afraid of getting pregnant'. Women seemed to have regarded such situations from a different perspective. Their descriptions often detailed the husband's insatiable sexual appetite. One female patient described graphically the many instances of sexual abuse she had endured from her husband, all the while functioning as his wife before she refused him sexual contact two years before her admission. She confided in her husband's family, but was refused help and felt trapped in her marriage, knowing that 'when I [left] him on my own accord, I [could] not claim any maintenance from him'.[26] The letter also implies that many women would not talk openly about such problems with medical staff, but felt able to write to the doctor instead. Neglect or ignorance could also be at the bottom of family conflicts; as in R's case, who confided that she was 'as pleased as punch with [the first birthday card she had ever received from her husband] as it is the little things that count'. She received it – while hospitalized – because 'I kept reminding him not to forget me'.[27]

The role of women as housewives was not perceived detrimental to mental health. This corroborates Ali Haggett's findings that depressive disorders in married women were caused primarily by unsatisfactory marriages rather than by suburban isolation and women's roles as homemakers.[28] Housework was, however, mentioned by husbands who felt that their wife's illness prevented them from fulfilling these duties. As we will see later in this chapter, such attitudes seemed to have impacted negatively on women who felt poorly supported by their husbands, particularly during periods of physical weakness, and felt regarded as a housekeeper rather than a wife.[29] Similarly, the ability to carry out housework to the expected standards was regarded as a potent sign of recovery by social workers during their after-care visits.

Domestic stress was triggered to a lesser extent by parental concerns, particularly in the case of women, by disagreements with their children, children's unhappy marriages, custody battles or children taken into care. In some instances patients and relatives listed conflicts with the extended family as the cause of the illness, particularly when living under the same roof provided little private space. Girlfriends or boyfriends were also frequently considered the cause of the illness: 'we now feel sure that it was worry that at first upset [our son]. About three-and half years ago he worried a good deal over a girl and at times fainted'.[30] It was not unusual for relatives to blame illness on the state of wider society. One husband, for example, opined that: 'We live on the corner opposite to the casual ward entrance of the local Poor Law Institute. We get quite a few casuals lining up every evening and perhaps that, coupled with my being so much away evenings, has had a distressing effect, although she has never said anything about it'.[31] In many such cases relatives went to great lengths to protect the patient from the detrimental influence: 'I think [her husband] is the cause of all her trouble and if you could make it convenient for the nurse to ask her if she would wish to see him before he came, it would not be such a shock for her'.[32]

Families Under Stress

Many patients were looked after by their families for a considerable time before being admitted. The stress of caring for a relative and its impact on the patient's future as a member within the family community often only became evident (or acknowledged) after the patient's hospitalization. Families were often unprepared for caring for a mentally ill relative and the task influenced family life profoundly, since it frequently necessitated shifts in family roles. Eruptions of deviant behaviour required frequent adjustments from all family members with respect to help-seeking strategies and responsibility for the patient's continuing care. The strain of such adjustments often only emerged after the patient's admission to hospital, demonstrating that the family's evaluation of their loved one's mental illness was a complex process. Correspondence from Devon illustrates that attending to the patient's needs proved not only physically and emotionally draining, but that patients' unpredictable or bizarre behaviour – often resulting from delusions – gave rise to fears amongst family members, particularly children.[33] With hindsight, some families referred to the decision about home care as 'perhaps unwise'. Continuous disruptive behaviour, resulting in interruptions to sleep and social life, as well as difficulties with neighbours, resulting from the patient's behaviour, could lead to anger and family resentment owing to the increased strain.

Families had to cope with feelings of embarrassment and stigmatization resulting from mental illness. In the early 1960s, Erving Goffman suggested that being associated with a stigmatized person 'taints' people, a notion that has continued to shape research into the social determinants and consequences of mental illness.[34] In the post-war decades, stigmatization was such that families would tell their neighbours that the patient had gone 'away on business [or holiday] for some time' rather than admitting to their hospitalization.[35] Others would admit to a patient being hospitalized, but would lie about the nature of the hospital. Letters composed by patients during hospitalization illustrate that sometimes even the family was prejudiced against mental illness. R., mentioned before, for example, pleaded with the doctor: 'My elder daughter still gets on her capers and when she gets worked up she still calls me "mental deficient". Also my husband lets her say what she likes, so I am asking a favour of you, will you try to convince them as to the real nature of my staying with you'.[36]

Other letters reveal that sometimes mental illness was concealed even from the closest family members: 'I understand from his sister that he was certified some years before I married him. Of course I did not know this until after I was married'.[37] The degree of stigmatization might explain why, despite the obvious burden experienced by families, the Devon case files give evidence that many families were slow to view their family member as ill and even slower to accept that the illness was psychological. Often, the behaviour was put down to the patient's temperament, for example, as being 'sensitive' or 'taking everything to heart'. Direct references to violent tempers were few, as relatives preferred to describe the patient as 'a little excitable' instead. In other instances the violence was not only downplayed, but the victims blamed themselves for it, as this wife who stated that 'although [her husband] threatened to harm me, it was always in the manner of a man who was intoxicated and never viciously. Also some of the trouble was my own timidity because I was alone with him'.[38] Other relatives were adamant that the patient was not suffering from a mental illness, but simultaneously blamed themselves for waiting so long before getting help: 'It is not a case of insanity with [our daughter], but nervousness and sensitiveness, which developed into her thinking there was some scandal concerning her. If we had only realised the consequences, we would have had treatment for her years ago. My wife is grieving terribly on her account, altogether it is a great worry to me'.[39]

A patient's expulsion from the family and into the hospital was only occasionally preceded by violent behaviour. More often, family members felt 'overworked', 'physically drained' and no longer able to cope with the patient at home. From the numerous letters written to hospital doctors we can deduce that many families regarded hospitalization as necessary and often overdue, or carried some hope that the discipline in hospital would benefit the patient.[40] Yet, the family was no longer regarded as an initiator of treatment, but was seen merely as delivering the patient to the hospital and handing over all responsibility.[41] One woman, whose son was admitted, wrote that since his discharge with 'war hysteria' he 'has been nothing but a source of worry'.[42] Another emphasized that she had been doing her best to give her husband a comfortable home, but admitted that her 'whole life for 12 years was entirely given up to looking after him, as he would not allow me to have any friends to see me'. The contents of her letter reveal how trapped she felt in this marriage. Nevertheless, when she asked whether it might be possible to obtain a divorce, she claimed that she would be doing so for the benefit of her husband:

> I have been looking after him myself until about 1.5 years ago when he got so restless and made life so difficult for me [that] I agreed to give him his freedom and let him live his own life and making my own living so that he could have his income to spend on himself. I thought if he had this sense of freedom it might improve his health. I had really tried everything else. I could not possibly go through this again and I wonder if it would be possible for me to get a separation or divorce. I think he might be much better if entirely free from all domestic responsibilities'[43]

While it was unusual for a woman to seek divorce, the topic was by no means rare. Although housework did not feature prominently in women's accounts of mental illness, a wife's failure to cope with domestic duties was amongst the most frequent reasons nominated by husbands seeking a divorce. Usually men claimed that the patient's failure to carry out responsibilities at home duties would have a negative impact on children: 'I want to give [my three children] a proper chance when the war is over and I am out of the army. [My wife – whom he addressed as 'Mrs XX' rather than by her name] is not capable of looking after the children or myself. So I hope you will understand the importance of this vital matter [his divorce on grounds of her insanity]'.[44] In general, husbands seemed to be able to cope with one or two admissions, but if further occurred, they tended to withdraw from their wives. Contrary to women whose husbands were hospitalized, husbands seemed unwilling to take over the wife's role in the household and filing for divorce while their wives were hospitalized caused great distress.

Relatives' attitudes towards the patient could change with their hospitalization and recognition of the burden the patient had presented prior to admission. Evidence of a family's attachment to the patient can be gathered from correspondence and visits. Contemporary research in this area focused on the frequency of visits a patient received.[45] Such studies revealed some interesting points, including the fact that contacts decreased with prolonged hospitalization, that total abandonment was usually related to chronic illness and that patients who were visited were more likely to be discharged.[46] Total abandonment was rare in Devon but, when it occurred, families ceased to regard the patient as one of them and felt no obligation for their future care. In some cases the hospital had great difficulties in discharging such rejected patients, even to the extended family. Surviving documents illustrate that patients were all too aware of being unwanted. G., for example, asked the doctor how she might obtain some weekly pocket money from her husband: 'For nearly two years I have been a patient in this hospital and have not received one cent from him. He has not been in to see me once. He is looking after my little girl, she is nearly 9 years old and I have never seen her once [since being hospitalized]. I have not bothered except for writing to him a few times, but he never answered'. She put her slow progress in hospital down to her constant worries about these family matters: 'If I was more settled in my mind, I am almost certain I would improve much more quickly'.[47] More common were mutual feelings of abandonment – not always congruent with the objective situation. Often, for example, family members wrote to the hospital because they had not heard from the patient for considerable time, despite sending several letters with stamped envelopes.[48] They expressed distress about the patient having developed a dislike to them and excluding them from their life. Letters from patients were often taken as a sign of recovery, as the patient 'sounded so much better', and were therefore eagerly awaited.

Drawing conclusions about the integration of patients into their families merely on visiting data has its flaws in a rural county like Devon. Visiting a hospitalized relative was not always possible owing to long distances and the lack of, or expense, of transport. Many relatives had to save money before they could make the journey. Others had to arrange for time off work to come to the hospital.[49] Therefore, the hospital received numerous requests for out-of-hours visits, as relatives tried to combine them with other commitments in and around Exeter, or whenever a lift was available. Limited visits were made up for by correspondence – often with apologetic messages regarding the failure to visit to be passed on to the patient. These letters suggest that the majority were concerned about the well-being of their relatives in hospital. As a consequence, many patients received cards for special occasions, 'tuck boxes' for birthdays and a supply of goods they used to like at home, including cigarettes and tobacco.[50] During the war, many families rationed their own allowances to be able to send food to a hospitalized patient. Other ways of showing patients that they had not been forgotten was to take them out for a day, such as a short break over Christmas or Easter, or take them to the theatre.[51]

Many patients were keen to leave hospital and return home, sometimes to 'please [their] families'.[52] Some patients wrote to the doctor claiming that their 'people would like them to go as soon as possible' or that they have found employment, promising they could now relieve the financial burden on the family.[53] Other patients begged their relatives to remove them from hospital, sometimes falsely claiming that the doctor had granted discharge from the following week. Such requests could leave families in deep distress, as one mother stated that 'it is worrying to get all these pleading letters and not know what to do'.[54] Sometimes patients continued to feel responsible for their families when hospitalized, such as the man who repeatedly requested discharge to attend to his sick wife at home.[55] Some felt indebted to their families because of the support they had received during their illness and felt they ought to return home to help out in emergencies.[56] Others felt financially responsible for the family while in hospital. One male patient sent home his 'few shillings every week', fully aware that his wife's earnings would not pay for the upkeep of the house. He feared that 'the strain of my wife endeavouring to maintain the home and the extra expense is proving too much for her and I should not like to have my wife breakdown [sic], as this would cause a complete disaster to my home for which we have both worked very hard to provide'.[57] Sadly, this relationship did not survive as his wife fell in love with another man and left him while he was still in hospital. This decision impacted significantly on the patient's relationship with his daughter. While his wife claimed that she had never stopped the girl from receiving his letters, she 'strongly object[s] to letters [of her father] being sent to the school for the embarrassment they might cause'. The patient, in turn, claimed that the only way to reach his daughter was through the school, as letters sent to the home address were not forwarded to her. There are also instances when relatives requested a patient's discharge to help with family matters, as in the case of young girl whose father died while she was hospitalized, leading to her mother's breakdown. She was needed to support her mother and look after the rest of the family.[58]

In Devon, most families welcomed the patient home after discharge, as contemporary commentators also reported.[59] Many readily agreed that a change of environment could only be conducive to the patient's further recovery. Some regarded the hospital as initiating emergency treatment: 'I have observed [my wife's] satisfactory progress and it would seem that at this stage a change from her present environment is now necessary to effect her complete recovery'.[60] Others were somewhat unhappy with the living conditions in hospital: 'I am extremely anxious as to whether it is still necessary to keep [my daughter] confined to one room, as on my last visit she seemed normal enough to be up and about'. The father's views were expressed more strongly in a follow-up letter a month later: 'I feel certain that it would be in [my daughter's] own interest that a complete change of surroundings would be most helpful to restore her back to health and strength. I certainly think the change would be most beneficial to her. For her, when she seems so well it is a great worry to her to have to remain in hospital'.[61] Efforts to transfer the patient to an institution closer to home also indicate that families wanted their relatives closer to them.[62] Many families, such as O.'s, were prepared to make great sacrifices to have the patient back home, including moving house, arranging for a live-in nurse or giving up work. It is not evident from the documents whether such radical changes impacted further on the patients or their families in the longer term.

Some patients, however, were not welcome at home anymore. Apart from the stigma that patients could bring to the family, there were other reasons for not letting them back into the family. Amongst the most important were financial aspects.[63] A number of relatives claimed that they would be willing to provide a home for the patient, but were unable to for financial reasons. In some cases families had to give up their homes when husbands were admitted and were living in overcrowded conditions with relatives which made it impossible for the patient to return home.[64] A minority expressed fears that the patient would continue to be a financial burden on the family, as 'once certified [they] would not be able to take up any work outside the house'.[65] Social pressures on the family, optimism about recovery, a patient's role in the family and their stage in the life cycle also profoundly influenced whether a patient would be welcomed home again. The refusal to have the patient home after hospitalization does not necessarily mean that families were uncaring, but by placing the patient in the hospital they had absolved themselves from responsibility and regarded the doctor as the main figure in the patient's care. In an attempt to protect themselves from further stress, some relatives feared a recurrence of mental illness and refused to have the patient back home. It is noteworthy that few families were willing to be the bearers of such bad news; most used the doctor as the mediator to deliver the message that they were not welcome anymore.

According to contemporary studies, whether the return of the patient into the original domestic settings was the best strategy depended on family attitudes towards them and whether they were regarded as dangerous.[66] It was also shown that the return to a family where there were strongly expressed emotions could be detrimental to the patient.[67] From a historical perspective, we know little about the fate of patients in their own home after discharge except in situations when they were re-hospitalized and families described the burden involved. Such letters reveal that patients sometimes returned to families, whose members were themselves suffering from despair, resentment and isolation as a result of the patient's illness.

Conclusion

The aim of this chapter has been to investigate the incorporation of family interaction into stress research. Post-war studies on the aetiology and effects of stress were strangely devoid of discussion about family interaction or testimony. The Devon case notes, however, illustrate families' crucial roles in the onset of illness and the care and recovery of patients. Contrary to much published research on the history of stress, this chapter is based on qualitative data obtained from narratives by patients and their relatives. Examining these documents has revealed several key points that can enhance our understanding of the connections between families, stress and mental health. In the first place, the archival sources echo Reuben Hill's call to consider the importance of mediating factors, such as family resources and a family's subjective perception of events in the emergence of crises, thereby challenging the often proposed linear process between stressful events and a period of mental illness. Besides attesting to families' vital roles in a patient's development and their progression through a mental health crisis, the letters and testimonies also illustrate that, in turn, the patient's illness could profoundly impact on family life, functioning and coherence. Many patients, for example, experienced a prolonged period of stress prior to admission, either in the form of a sequence of stressful life events or persistent daily stressors, or a combination of both. Nursing patients at home for long periods required families to make substantial allowances in order to accommodate the patient's needs. As a consequence, hospitalization became a key stage regarding decisions about the place of the patient within their family.

The style of letter writing suggests that the absence of family testimony in case notes is not only to be blamed on the physicians, but that relatives tended to express their views and anxieties more freely in letters than in personal encounters. Many letters, particularly those written by women, contained explicit requests to keep the contents strictly confidential. Others started with apologies for not having addressed the letter's content during the interview with the doctor, then admitting to feelings of guilt resulting from the inability to cope with the stress the patient had been causing at home. Many authors went on to say that they had nobody to talk to and that this lack of intra-familial communication seemed to have caused additional stress and drained coping resources. Such confessions transform correspondence from mere adjuncts, to case notes, to invaluable documents when investigating the causes and progression of a mental health crisis.

In the current climate of concerns about mental health, close inspection of these letters to and from patients in institutions in Devon, during the post-war years, draws attention to the various contexts in which mental health crises can arise and the manner in which they can be managed. Contrary to the priorities of much post-war stress research, which was beginning to focus on major stressful life events, mental health crises were usually caused not by one individual stressful event. Much more frequently, as in O.'s story, multiple stressors worked together to cause a crisis. Although institutionalization was not always successful, such historical evidence suggests that it was multi-level approaches to mental illness, involving close collaboration between patients, their families, doctors and welfare and social services, that were more effective in easing levels of stress amongst patients and their families and in adequately addressing mental health problems.

Acknowledgements

Research for this article was carried out under three consecutive Wellcome Trust grants (081752/Z/06/Z, 085857/Z/08/A, 090836/Z/09/Z) with PI Professor Joseph Melling and in collaboration with John Draisey from the Devon Record Office.

3 GENDER, STRESS AND ALCOHOL ABUSE IN POST-WAR BRITAIN

Ali Haggett

Much has been written about the history of alcohol and its abuse. However, although historians have analyzed the ways in which governments have responded to alcohol abuse, in policy terms and on medical and psychiatric of theories of alcoholism,[1] far less is known historically about drinking behaviour – that is, about which individuals drank in the first place, and why. In recent research men have been identified as more likely to drink to damaging levels than women, but to be diagnosed less frequently as suffering from psychiatric disorders such as depression and anxiety.[2] A MIND survey in 2009 reported that men were 'twice as likely as women to report using alcohol as a coping strategy when they were feeling low or worried', suggesting that for men drinking is a possible manifestation of emotional distress.[3] However, with the notable exception of Mark Micale's *Hysterical Men* (2008), historical analyses of gender and mental illness continue to be dominated by accounts that emphasize the common association between women and psychological illness.

This chapter will examine alcohol abuse as a 'coping mechanism' in post-war Britain. I shall argue that a wide range of psychological symptoms were experienced by men, but that men exhibited different symptoms than women, if medical advice was sought at all. Whereas women tended to present with symptoms of low-mood, anxiety, lack of motivation and sadness, which were easy to recognize, men were more likely to self-medicate with alcohol or present with psychosomatic symptoms, including a spectrum of ill-defined disorders affecting the stomach, digestion, sleep and general well-being. Drawing on published reports, archival sources and interviews, the chapter explores a range of clinical, social and cultural forces that influenced debates about gender, alcohol abuse and psychological symptoms in three broad areas: medical surveys of alcohol use and abuse; general practice; and the workplace. I shall argue that the failure to examine drinking as a coping mechanism in men has had important implications for the broader interpretation of patterns of psychological illness since the 1950s.

Clinical and Social Surveys of Stress and Alcohol use in Men and Women

The decades following the Second World War marked a period in which a popular language of stress emerged, resonating with contemporary concerns about political instability and social change.[4] Building on the earlier work of Walter Cannon (1871–1945), Adolf Meyer (1866–1950), Harold Wolff (1898–1962) and Hans Selye (1907–82), post-war stress researchers developed and explored the parameters of stress within general medicine, psychiatric epidemiology, psychology, psychosomatic medicine and occupational health.[5] Mark Jackson has argued that, although the terms worry and anxiety did not disappear completely from medical and popular discourse, the term 'stress' increasingly began to dominate debates about the negative health consequences of the pressures of modern living. Such concerns about rising levels of stress were mobilized by those with interests in preserving health and restoring productivity after the Second World War.[6] Given the significant interest among stress researchers, psychiatrists and clinicians in the social and economic determinants of health, and into the constitutional and personality factors which might dictate responses to stress, it is perhaps surprising that the role of alcohol as an 'escape' mechanism was largely absent from debates until the late 1970s. It was not until 1978 that the British psychologist Tom Cox, for example, noted explicitly that an individual's capacity to cope could be altered or manipulated by the consumption of alcohol, drugs and nicotine – and that these coping strategies were not unproblematic.[7] Discussions about coping were similarly absent from professional debates about the use and abuse of alcohol.

Medical and philosophical theories about alcoholism and problem drinking have a long history which has been examined in detail elsewhere.[8] Thom has shown how a major shift took place in the mid-twentieth century from a 'moral' model of alcoholism, which tended to see the problem as one of individual deficiency or 'moral worth', towards a disease model requiring medical treatment.[9] The American biostatistician and physician Elvin Morton Jellinek (1890–1963) published his seminal piece 'Phases of Alcohol Addiction' in 1952 in which he highlighted the notion of 'loss of control' which progressed through a set of stages towards 'rock bottom'.[10] These principles were further developed by the German-born neurologist, Max Glatt (1912–2002), into a 'U shaped' chart depicting a 'slippery slope' with an upward path to recovery.[11] In the 1970s, the British psychiatrist Griffith Edwards (1928–2012), who became an internationally renowned expert on addiction, coined the term 'alcohol dependence syndrome' which was incorporated in the World Health Organization's *International Classification of Diseases* in 1979. Edwards outlined the dependence syndrome in an article published in the *British Medical Journal* in 1976, co-written with the American psychiatrist Milton M. Gross.[12] Edwards's influence on addiction studies was manifest in a prolific range of publications directed at both academic and popular readerships.[13] The model of alcoholism eventually adopted by the British National Health Service (NHS) in the post-war years was based on the work of Max Glatt at his therapeutic treatment unit at Warlingham Park, Middlesex, during the 1950s.[14]

Although there was increasing acceptance that alcoholism was a 'disease', developments in policy and treatment in Britain were fragmented and piecemeal. While some commentators articulated concerns about alcohol abuse, there was still widespread denial of the problem. The first branch of Alcoholics Anonymous (AA) was founded in London in 1948, but aroused little interest among the medical profession.[15] Three years later, in 1951, a consultant psychiatrist applied for funds to attend a World Health Organization conference on alcoholism. However, his application was rejected, on the grounds that 'there was no alcoholism in England and Wales'.[16] Glatt himself recalled that when he first 'got into alcoholism' in the early 1950s, he knew 'not a thing about it' and that 'nothing much was written' about it in Britain.[17] Foreign visitors to his unit who came to learn about his treatment methods often remarked that when they had previously asked the Ministry of Health what methods were available for alcoholics in England they had all received the same response: 'We have not got any alcoholics'.[18] Despite the fact that men were significantly over-represented in statistics for alcohol abuse, prior to the 1970s there was no organized discussion about gender in British debates about alcoholism; it was simply noted to be less common in women. Efforts instead focused on establishing an accurate national estimate of alcoholics, on how best to treat the condition once diagnosed and on how to deal with the social problems caused by drunken offenders.

During the early 1960s, a number of social initiatives such as the Joseph Rowntree Steering Group on Alcoholism and the Camberwell Council on Alcoholism (CCA) were set up to examine the problem and, ostensibly, to promote preventative measures. As Thom has noted, the CCA eventually became nationally influential, partly because of the lack of other strong policy-relevant interest groups in the alcohol arena.[19] The stated aim of the CCA was 'to gauge the extent of the problem and to investigate personal, social and economic factors concerned in the *causes* of alcoholism'.[20] However, discussion tended instead to be dominated by its 'impact upon the life of the nation', in particular the deleterious social consequences of alcoholism: crime, social disturbance and family breakdown. Although the condition appeared to affect men in much larger numbers than women, discussions rarely mentioned why this might be. Occasional individual accounts from alcoholics themselves illustrate the widespread denial and failure to confront the problem. One former alcoholic whose contribution was published in the *Journal of Alcoholism* recalled that none of his friends, work colleagues or his employer ever took him aside and spoke seriously to him. Instead, he noted that they 'all connived in covering up ... what now appears to be serious drinking bouts and their attendant hangovers'.[21] This man concluded that ultimately, the situation in which he found himself was 'all part of the rich pageant of life as we know it', adding that, where alcohol was concerned, he was 'slightly more blind in a whole kingdom of the partially sighted'.[22]

Although researchers eventually acknowledged that much problem drinking remained unreported in the community, figures that existed in 1950 suggested that alcohol consumption was comparatively low.[23] This contributed to the official view from the Ministry of Health that alcohol abuse was 'not a problem'. However, as Thom has shown, a number of other factors framed the discourse on alcohol abuse. Firstly, the power of the temperance movement had waned considerably and thus, policy action, when it came, focused on the medical aspects of alcoholism and not on preventative measures. Secondly, the general disarray of mental health services following the introduction of the NHS resulted in a lack of resources for alcohol treatment. Thirdly, and perhaps most importantly, the disease model of alcoholism legitimized medicine's role in treating the condition, viewing it as a 'disease of the unfortunate minority'.[24] Debates failed to investigate many of the social factors and life stressors that might have contributed to individual drinking habits. Indeed, the Ministry of Health was explicitly concerned to limit enquiry strictly to treatment issues, since prevention would open 'very wide vistas' which were thought to be quite outside the scope of the Department'.[25]

Accounts from those working in medicine certainly reflected this approach. Casualty doctors noted that cases of alcoholism usually presented at the 'emergency end of the disease', and, because they were admitted to general hospitals, not psychiatric wards, as soon as they were 'physically well' they were discharged.[26] Emphasis on the physical nature of the condition was evident in accounts by hospital doctors, one of whom noted that alcoholics rarely presented in 'such a mental state' that would honestly warrant compulsory detention under Section 25 of the Mental Health Act.[27] During a series of seminars held by the CCA in 1970, the Registrar in charge of Casualty at King's College Hospital described his experience of treating intoxicated patients:

> Should someone present himself as very depressed, we try and find a physical reason to account for this ... such as an overdose of drugs ... or some overwhelming disease – I wouldn't spend too long on it. If it's an acute problem, we treat them, but if it's not, then they have to go. Overdose is seen as a psychiatric emergency – alcoholics are not.[28]

The remaining seminar discussion focused on the physical treatments that were available, such as stomach irrigation for alcohol poisoning and the use of vitamin injections. 'True' psychiatric cases, one doctor noted, were assured a consultation at the Maudsley Psychiatric Hospital; however, he added, 'you have got to find out what is the matter with him, to assess whether he should be chucked out or kept in'.[29] These attitudes were in contrast to the approach taken by alcohol experts such as Glatt who, although not underestimating the importance of personality, emphasized the 'great influence of social problems on the causation and development of alcoholism'. Indeed, one of his methods of treatment involved patients telling their 'life stories' – a technique he had developed previously when working with neurosis patients.Glatt worked closely with AA and claimed his methods complemented those employed by the organization.[30] Despite his notable influence, the eventual development of alcohol treatment units between the early 1960s and the 1980s was slow and patchy, and treatment methods were diverse.[31] Glatt noted himself that he faced considerable inertia and that 'many doctors and professionals [were] only too keen to avoid involvement with alcoholic patients'.[32] Indeed, by the late 1970s, research indicated that the majority of alcoholism referrals were not to specialist units.[33] However, it is notable that, although some provision was made for women, those who were referred to treatment units were predominantly male, likely to be in their forties and from the higher social classes. 'Skid row' drinkers were less likely to call upon services provided and consultants were less likely to admit them to inpatient wards, a pattern that, according to Thom, remained stable until the 1980s.[34]

During the early 1970s, a small group within the CCA put forward a proposal to investigate women alcoholics. Although numbers of women were thought to be very small at a ratio with men of one to four, a review of the literature suggested some specific concerns – among them evidence that, within the family unit, women were usually the primary carers of children and that regular 'drinking at home' made it harder to detect.[35] The nature of this investigation is particularly illuminating. Concerns clearly reflected long-established moralistic overtones about women and alcohol. As historians have shown, the focus has commonly been 'not so much on women as women, but on women as mothers, and on the notion of maternal neglect'.[36] The framework of the investigation into women drinkers was entirely different to that of the seminars, symposia and enquiries into drinking problems in men. To begin with, the group of professionals invited to contribute included not only medics, but sociologists and marriage guidance counsellors.[37] Specific areas for research included: the role of femininity; recent changes in the social role of women; the relationship between drinking and marriage; and how conditioning, upbringing and consequent life expectations might influence drinking. The onset of drinking was noted to be regularly triggered by marital breakdown, in contrast to the assumption that alcoholism in men was likely to lead to divorce. Research questionnaires distributed via staff to patients at treatment centres asked explicit questions such as: Why did your drinking become a problem? Do you think that being a woman makes a difference to your drinking problem? Was depression a factor in your drinking?[38] Staff at treatment centres were asked specifically about factors that might be unique to women in case histories, referrals and treatment. In one other rare article published on the subject, A. B. Sclare, a psychiatrist in Glasgow, had also noted that alcohol problems in women were often correlated specifically to environmental factors related to employment or domestic stress.[39]

Contributors to the CCA's project noted that women were more likely to be labelled as 'depressive', with the alcoholism treated as a secondary disease, if it was diagnosed at all.[40] Hospital doctors and general practitioners (GPs) were more likely to diagnose psychoneurosis to shield a woman from the stigma of alcoholism. Because of this propensity to be diagnosed as 'depressed' and not 'alcoholic', women were more likely to appear in statistics for psychiatric referral, treatment and psychotropic drug prescriptions. Specific focus was also directed towards the role of menstruation, menopause and hysterectomy in triggering the onset of drinking, as well as possible problems associated with homosexuality, sexual identity and loneliness. In addition, conclusions from this research suggested that women reported drinking when life 'got them down' or when they were 'restless and tense', because it helped them 'forget their worries'.[41]

These points of reference and formulations were in stark contrast to those examined and developed in debates about male alcoholics, which did not explore what was unique about being a 'man' in relation to drinking. Personal testimonies from men suggest that they were not comfortable with reflective analysis of their feelings and did not link drinking to emotional worry or anxiety in the same ways as women. This is illustrated perfectly by the testimony of one recovering male alcoholic who noted, 'The question I am often asked is "do you know what caused your drinking?"' to which he added, 'I am not able to isolate any particular cause or causes in myself … I am drawn to the conclusion that the most likely hypothesis is that I was conceived on the back of a brewer's dray'.[42] In psychiatric settings, 'marital discord and domestic stress' were specifically observed as 'precipitating factors for hospitalisation in women',[43] whereas, alcoholism was less likely to result in a man being referred for psychiatric assessment at all. In addition to analysis of the social consequences of alcoholism, the CCA's enquiry into women was thus structured around a set of research questions that were much more likely to identify social, cultural and economic factors – including life stressors – that prompted problem drinking.

Alcohol and Stress in General Practice

Some patients with alcohol problems presented in primary care. However, general practitioners (GPs) were largely concerned with how to diagnose the problem and deal with sickness certification than with why their patients might drink in the first place.[44] Many felt that there was so much stigma surrounding alcoholism that they were justified in falsifying certificates when a true diagnosis might lose the patient their job. Max Glatt conceded that hospital doctors were inclined to do the same thing.[45] Correspondence from the Rowntree Trust Steering Grou-pon Alcohol also suggests that GPs felt 'services on the NHS were so inadequate that many h[ad] decided not to waste their own time or that of their patients by attempting further use of them'.[46] GPs confirmed the general picture that alcoholic patients were usually male and that they would be most likely to present with some kind of somatic disorder that would indicate an alcohol habit – or their wives would make a visit to the family doctor to report the problem.[47] Griffith Edwards warned GPs that the alcoholic often came into the surgery asking for something for 'bad nerves' or something for 'his stomach', concluding that abnormal drinking may in fact cause, precipitate, imitate or be secondary to every known psychiatric syndrome.[48] The ability to recognize alcoholism, particularly in its earlier stages, was further complicated by the fact that physicians were socialized into a culture of heavy drinking at medical school. This resulted in a blurring of boundaries between abnormal and normal drinking. Indeed, by the 1980s, research had begun to uncover a significant problem with alcohol, drugs and mental illness in the medical profession. By 1982, the standardized mortality ratio for cirrhosis in doctors was three times that of the general population.[49]

There was little doubt among GPs, reflecting on their time in general practice, that the over-use of alcohol was commonly used by men as a coping mechanism.[50] There was also a consensus among them that men tended to present with psychosomatic symptoms that were more 'acceptable' and less stigmatizing. John Fry (1922–94), post-war pioneer of general practice-based research, kept meticulous personal notes about his patients which were also regularly interspersed with references to male patients with dyspepsia and 'epigastric pain', a term used to describe pain in the gastric region (often aggravated by alcohol), for which no organic cause could be found. Such patients were often additionally described as 'agitated', sometimes 'depressed', but seldom 'neurotic', a term that was largely reserved for anxious women.[51] Many men were diagnosed with duodenal ulcers. Fry was particularly interested in the clinical and social aspects of peptic ulcers and published widely from his observations in general practice.[52] Although not considered to be the only cause of ulcers, anxiety was seen as a precipitating factor for gastric disorders, and men were thought to be less likely to 'admit to pressures causing psychological stress'.[53] Indeed, wives commonly complained to their doctors that their husbands refused to visit the surgery at all and would bemoan 'Oh, he'll never come doctor. But if he does ... '.[54] Many GPs lived in their patients' communities and were often quietly aware of existing marital or familial problems. With tact, they were sometimes able to use this knowledge to elicit details about such matters from their patients.

Women, in contrast, emerged in consistently larger numbers in statistics for depression and anxiety. C. A. H. Watts, a GP who published widely from research undertaken at his own practice on the subject of neurosis and depression, found that between the ages of thirty-five and fifty-five, women were at least twice as likely to consult a doctor with depression or a neurotic reaction.[55] However, he also noted that men were far more prone to take their own lives and that addiction to alcohol was a 'very common factor among suicides'.[56] Although studies varied in the overall percentage of patients diagnosed with psychiatric disorders, the sex differential remained across surveys.[57] However, psychosomatic and alcoholic presentations of psychological illness were not always included in data, perhaps obscuring a more accurate picture of gender patterns and differences. Anthony Ryle, for example, explicitly omitted psychosomatic disorders from his study of neurosis in general practice, arguing that the inclusion of 'all stress disorders' in a survey of neurosis would say more about 'the doctor's enthusiasm for psychosomatic concepts' than about the real 'prevalence of disease'.[58] Unsurprisingly, his findings included significantly greater numbers of women with neurosis than other studies, perhaps also reflecting his interest in obstetrics and postnatal conditions. Other research also featured anomalies that could affect the accuracy of the gendered distribution of psychological illness. Logan and Brook's *Survey of Sickness*, published in 1957, for example, featured greater numbers of women with psychoneurosis, but the study included a large group of unspecified 'ill-defined illness' and evidence that male patients attended their GPs more regularly for 'indigestion' and 'gastrointestinal disturbances'.[59]

The difficulties involved with providing an accurate assessment of numbers with psychological disorders did not go unnoticed. Dr H. J. Walton, a psychiatrist from the University of Edinburgh observed in 1969 that the inclusion of 'psychosomatic' or 'stress' disorders in research would significantly alter the picture.[60] He argued that it was possible GPs were missing psychosomatic symptoms because of their training at medical school, which placed 'great emphasis on basic scientific investigation ... physical factors or theoretical matters'.[61] He added that, among medical students, 'suspicion and scepticism about psychiatry [began] early' and that many viewed psychiatrists as 'emotionally unstable, confused thinkers'.[62] Furthermore, he argued that the personality of individual doctors influenced their patterns of diagnosis, with some young graduates showing a lack of concern about the psychological components of illness.[63] Some 'physically orientated' graduates actively disliked patients who presented with psychogenic aspects to their illness. Among a survey of GPs attending a postgraduate course in psychiatric medicine, Walton also discovered that over half of the attendees found alcoholics a category of patient that was 'unacceptable'.[64]

This situation was widely reflected in the oral histories of GPs who noted in interviews that the ability to detect a psychosomatic complaint lay entirely in the self-taught skill of the family doctor. One doctor admitted that the only thing he could recall about training in psychological medicine was that a psychiatrist had once told him 'the golden rule is, if you don't know whether the patient's mad, or you are – *he* is'. He added, 'it gave me no insight into the cryptic or hidden psychological symptoms'.[65] He also admitted that 'the idea of hysteria as a woman's condition was still very much a popular concept in medicine, and menopausal and menstrual changes of mood ... so it was very easy to be patronising'. Additionally, he proposed that his 'ignorance' was undoubtedly 'moulded by the kind of habits of the practice and the habits of presentation of the practice, so [he] picked up what they were expecting and responded accordingly'.[66] This particular doctor also noted that alcoholism and gastric disorders were a significant problem among male patients:

> In those days, [for] what was called spastic colon [and] is now irritable bowel disease, we prescribed medicines like the 'double-strength nerve tonic' as a mild sedative as we thought people might be worrying. But, I don't think we really, well speaking for myself, I don't think I penetrated very far into their psychological disorders. Nor do I think they would be very willing to admit them themselves, because you know, men don't complain do they? Not much.[67]

In 1966, Michael Shepherd (1923–95), an influential consultant psychiatrist, noted that the average GP was 'unlikely to invoke a psychogenic factor in any case, unless he detects in the patient signs of current psychological or emotional disorder'.[68] Observing that psychosocial factors were identified more regularly in women, he suggested that this might be because doctors were simply 'more readily able to identify them as such'.[69] He argued ultimately that there was reasonable confidence among GPs about recognizing psychiatric disorder, but that there was much less confidence in their ability to relate it to causal or precipitating factors.[70]

Work, Stress and Alcohol

During the early 1960s, the CCA had highlighted alcohol abuse in the workplace as one major area of concern. Keen to draw attention to the hazards, experts on the effects of alcohol contributed increasingly to professional journals; however, the focus was primarily on the cost of drinking *to* industry and the government. Questions were rarely raised about why workers drank in the first place. A number of GPs attending an 'information week' coordinated by the CCA were critical of industry for failing to take the issue seriously. One doctor described industry's 'ostrich-like attitude' and suggested that companies were reluctant to confront alcohol abuse because of the stigma and bad press the reputation might bring.[71] Griffith Edwards explicitly advised that 'alcohol was an important industrial disease'.[72] At an industrial symposium held by the CCA during the early 1960s, one contributor recalled that a reformed alcoholic and colleague of his had personally written to twelve firms, whose employees cumulatively totalled 120,000, to ask, in confidence, what policies they had adopted towards alcoholic employees.[73] About one third 'didn't bother to reply'; one company 'took exception to the insulting suggestion that a firm of their acknowledged repute would ever employ an alcoholic'; others replied that 'drunkenness in their area was happily a thing of the past'.[74]

Professional journals that focused on alcoholism nonetheless identified a number of occupations in which individuals might be vulnerable to over-drinking. Concern was directed in particular on executive workers and those with jobs in the hospitality trade where alcohol was widely available. Other types of employment that allowed abuse to go undetected were also noted. Sickness absence among casual labourers, for example, might remain hidden since workers could simply resume work when they had recovered from a drinking bout. Employers were warned to be suspicious of repeated sickness certificates for gastritis, signs of irritability, decreased performance and poor time-keeping.[75] They were also advised to be alert to absences on Monday mornings, particularly 'if a wife phoned in', since this might indicate a weekend of heavy drinking.[76] Such concerns did not go entirely unnoticed by the media, as occasional articles were released in the press highlighting the issue of sickness absence due to alcohol. One headline in 1970 warned that 'Monday is hangover day for British Industry', claiming that 'a quarter of a million men in Britain will be off sick today, when all they have is a bad hangover'.[77] Another item described the problem as 'a secret illness' and as 'the complaint that nobody wants to talk about'.[78]

These problems were debated at a seminar attended by doctors, magistrates and members of industry, organized in as part of the information week, held in 1967, by the CCA. However, the debate remained focused on the consequences of drinking to industry and society, prompting one member of the audience to observe that, 'all the talks assume that the presenting problems – familial, social and so on – were as a result of the alcohol. Can't we assume it might be the other way around?'[79] The response from a magistrate was firmly that the problems that presented before him in the courts were largely the result of people ending up in trouble *because* of alcohol. One delegate suggested that changing social habits and increasing leisure time 'were particularly difficult', because men had 'not learned to use their leisure time to do anything but drink'.[80] Another made references to 'nagging wives ... worries, or whatever', from which drink was a refuge; however, discussion continued to emphasize the way in which problems arose from the alcoholism, not the other way around.

Debates on absenteeism and sickness absence within industrial medicine were well-established by the 1960s, but focused primarily on 'theories' of absenteeism and on improving techniques in data collection and analyses.[81] The motive behind such work was primarily the protection or enhancement of productivity. Most researchers employed a 'disease-centred' approach which underplayed social and emotional factors that might influence sickness patterns.[82] Although numerous studies illustrated that psychoneurotic and psychosomatic illness existed among workers, few British researchers were willing to discuss alcohol, despite the fact that international studies (often published in British journals) indicated that a clear correlation existed with neurosis.[83] International authors were more open about the problems of alcohol in industry and were explicit about its link with sickness absence and absenteeism. Studies from the USA, Sweden and Australia all emphasized the importance of identifying and addressing alcohol abuse in workers. W. Donald Ross's book *Practical Psychiatry for Industrial Physicians* (1956), for example, contained a whole chapter on 'Alcoholism', predicting that four million Americans were in 'some stage' of alcoholism. Ross noted that six out of seven of these were male and that much of the neurosis seen among women at work was a direct result of contending with an alcoholic family member at home.[84] A British review of this publication acknowledged that this was a much needed book since industrial medicine was unfortunately still 'antagonistic' towards psychiatry. However, the reviewer cited 'national differences' as a 'drawback' of the text, noting that 'alcoholism would hardly be considered a major problem amongst workers [in Britain]'.[85] A similarly titled British publication *Mental Health and Human Relations in Industry* (1954), compiled from research undertaken at the Roffey Park Institute, made no mention of alcohol abuse whatsoever. This was despite the fact that the book emphasized the emotional needs of workers and that the Roffey Park Institute itself focused holistically on the well-being of industrial workers.[86]

By 1974, 34 per cent of major American industrial employers had adopted some form of programme to provide assistance to alcoholics.[87] Some companies developed ambitious and innovative schemes offering confidential support to workers on any aspect troubling them, not just relating to alcohol abuse, but also to family or marital problems and indebtedness. The aim was thus to 'get to the root cause ... and save the employee's job'.[88] In contrast, by 1979 commentators in Britain were forced to acknowledge how 'slow' they had been to recognize the problem.[89] Herbert Berger, a physician from New York, speaking to an international audience of physicians and AA, was critical of the broad emphasis on treatment because it underplayed the causative aspects of alcoholism.[90] He argued that alcohol was only a secondary aetiology, and that the primary condition was the patient's inability 'to cope with the vicissitudes of his environment', warning that medics and AA were failing in the arena of prevention by waiting for the patient to 'hit rock bottom'.[91]

Women rarely featured in debates about industry and alcohol, although they were a source of concern in research on absenteeism and sickness absence. Most studies indicated that women were more frequently absent than men and that this was broadly the case across many different types of employment. For women, frequent absenteeism (a short period of undefined absence, which may or may not have been due to illness), was explained by their need to undertake family responsibilities in addition to their paid work.[92] Thus, it was assumed that one of the ways in which women coped with shouldering dual responsibilities was to take short periods of time off work to look after sick children or when other family members needed them. A well-cited study of industrial workers in France, published in 1962, argued that 'frequent absence means that there is a conflict between life at work and outside', and that 'female absenteeism cannot be explained by elementary biological or family factors alone'.[93] Although a number of factors emerged as important influences, including the nature of the work performed and the distance women lived from their place of work, a key conclusion was that many women felt that their 'proper place would be, and should always have been, at home'.[94] Home responsibilities nonetheless could only account for part of the explanation, since women also appeared in certified sickness statistics for psychological disorders more frequently than men. However, many of the reports in industry were affected by the methodological anomalies of general practice-based research. The classification of disorders differed greatly between studies, a problem exacerbated by the unreliability of doctors' certificates.

One key theme that emerged in research on sickness absence was that men appeared more frequently in data for gastric disorders and in groups of illnesses labelled as 'vague' or 'ill-defined'. Fraser's study of neurosis in factory workers in 1947 found that, although women outnumbered men significantly in numbers of 'definite neurosis', men predominated in the group of 'disabling psychosomatic illness' which included dyspepsia.[95] Ager and Raffle's study of London transport workers also identified a growing tendency for absences attributed to vague diagnoses (gastritis, fibrositis, sprains, and anxiety states), an observation supported in the report *Off Sick* (1971), published by the Office for Health Economics.[96] Ager and Raffle concluded that this general rising trend of 'sickness' was counter to 'generally improved health' and was therefore more likely to be a reflection of broader discontent with the social system than a true picture of morbidity.[97]

Literature on industrial health during the period suggests that where nervous strain and mental illness were explicitly correlated with stress, it was usually occupational stress that featured in analysis. In 1976, Cary Cooper and Judi Marshall argued that there were three separate dimensions to stress-related disease: the personal characteristics of the individual; stress related to the workplace; and pressures external to the work environment, such as family problems and financial difficulties. Their 'model of stresses at work' aimed to establish how these aspects combined to create symptoms of occupational ill-health, such as raised blood pressure, drinking and depression, sometimes leading to coronary heart disease and mental illness.[98] During the 1980s researchers increasingly began to acknowledge that studies had placed too great an emphasis on unemployment, physical and chemical health hazards and absenteeism, while mental illness had been of 'subsidiary interest'.[99] New research began to chart an apparent increase in cases of psychiatric illness. Authors noted that studies in the past had been hindered by a number of complicating factors, not least the 'unreliability' of diagnoses on GP certificates and confusion surrounding physical symptoms that might have an emotional cause.[100] All work that had been thus far undertaken also related to the health of workers in industry and large organizations, yet, as Albert Cherns pointed out in 1975, 60 per cent of men worked for small firms where there was no data available at all.[101] During the late 1970s and 1980s, the focus of attention shifted to the well-being of executive workers, in part framed by the political context and Thatcher's free-market economics. It was also energized by the theories of the cardiologists Meyer Friedman (1910–2001) and Ray Rosenman on Type A personalities, which heightened anxieties about the impact of work-related stress on executives – a concern that was largely focused on men.[102]

Conclusion

Despite considerable interest in the associations between the stress of life and sickness, during the post-war period a form of 'collective silence' continued to surround the ways in which men coped with emotions and associated factors such as alcoholism and psychosomatic symptoms. In the workplace and during leisure activities, ideas about the degree to which it was seen as appropriate to admit to emotional difficulties discouraged men from seeking help for problems both at work and at home. Men appeared unable or unwilling to reflect on the causes of their problems. Leaders in industry were reluctant to acknowledge alcoholism or mental illness in the workforce, due to fears that the stigma might adversely affect the standing of their business. GPs and hospital physicians were poorly trained in psychological medicine and, until the late 1970s, were usually male and therefore affected by the same difficulties when challenged to be reflective or emotionally expressive. Many unwittingly colluded with stereotypical views about femininity and masculinity, providing psychiatric diagnoses for women and somatic diagnoses for men. Quite often, both the male patient and doctor were satisfied with a somatic diagnosis and looked no further.

During the 1970s, when concern was eventually raised about female alcoholism, research questions were constructed around a completely different framework, one less focused on aspects of treatment and diagnosis and more on what it might be about the female role that caused women to abuse alcohol. Betsy Thom has argued that the feminist movement of the 1960s was instrumental in this respect, since it had begun to frame women's health issues in political, social and economic terms. It thus provided the ideological motivation for explanations of women's use and misuse of alcohol, emphasizing the social and psychological context of drinking.[103] For men, there was no corresponding initiative that questioned aspects of the male role that might impact on their well-being and ability to cope. This was compounded by the dominance of the disease theory during the 1950s and 1960s which assumed the alcoholic to be in the minority, diverting attention away from broader consumption levels and social factors in causation. According to Thom, a shift away from the disease theory towards a public health model of prevention did not come until the 1980s.[104] The problem was exacerbated further by the fact that manufacturers of alcoholic beverages directly targeted men in their advertising campaigns which promoted drinking as not only a pleasurable pastime, but also increasingly as a way to relieve stress.[105] These advertisements appeared widely in daily newspapers, but also in publications directed exclusively at men such as *Lilliput* and *Men Only*. As Lemle and Mishkind noted in 1989, through the second half of the twentieth century, social drinking increasingly became a primary cultural symbol of 'manliness'.[106] Heavy drinking symbolized greater masculinity than lighter drinking and the more a man tolerated his alcohol, the more manly he was deemed.[107] Accounts from a Mass Observation investigation into public houses and drinking confirm indeed that working-class men were inclined to drink to appear 'tough' and to fit in with their peers. Beer-drinking was also widely associated with increased sexual performance.[108]

In his discussion of male emotional illness, Mark Micale notes of the Victorian era that, 'the homogeneously male medical community contrived to ignore an entire field of potential study'.[109] Of present times, he is more optimistic, suggesting that Western medicine no longer plays a commanding role in producing the dominant fictions of masculinity. We now live, Micale argues, in 'a fundamentally new environment for viewing and discussing gender and masculinity'. However, he notes that 'it would be foolish to contend that this process is complete'.[110] He is right to be cautious since, as this chapter has shown, during the decades following the Second World War, there were few formal discussions about psychological illness and coping in men, despite evidence that many male cases existed either undiagnosed in the community, or presenting in primary care complicated by psychosomatic symptoms. In contrast, a gendered landscape that assumed that women were more likely to experience mental illness provided fertile ground for academics, clinicians and social commentators alike. Recent research indicates that the number of men experiencing common mental disorders is still underestimated, a problem exacerbated when practitioners rely on their male patients' ability to volunteer information about mental health concerns.[111] Suicide statistics from the mid-twentieth century continue to show that men are persistently more likely to end their own lives; perhaps a consequence of their failure to seek help for psychological disorders.[112] It is clear from these recent studies that social and cultural factors continue to influence ideas about masculinity, femininity, vulnerability to stress and ways of coping, just as they did in the decades after the Second World War.

Acknowledgements

This research was funded by the Wellcome Trust, grant number WT091661MA. I would like to thank the Trust for their continued support. I would also like to thank the fifteen retired general practitioners who were interviewed for this project.

4 WORKING TOO HARD: EXPERIENCES OF WORRY AND STRESS IN POST-WAR BRITAIN

Jill Kirby

> I was working, well I was working three, four nights a week, weekends I was, just couldn't keep up with it ... I was violently sick going home in the car, for no apparent reason ... and then on another occasion the same sort of thing happened, just out of the blue for no reason at all, and er anyway I went in for a check-up and they reckoned it was nerves or something was affecting my stomach. It was actually overwork and stress and stuff like that.[1]

Stress is ubiquitous in twenty-first century Britain, responsible for millions of lost working days and the focus of a whole industry designed to help us avoid it.[2] It was not always thus. This chapter explores how people such as James Lyon, quoted above talking about his work in the oil industry in the 1970s, experienced 'stress and stuff like that' in the period between the Second World War and the 1980s, and in particular stress related to their work. By tracing peoples' shifting attitudes towards stressful experiences, examining how they explained those experiences and analyzing the reactions of others to them, this chapter will highlight three key areas of discussion. Firstly, it examines the complex interplay of factors such as status, identity and gender in shaping attempts to make sense of stress. Secondly, it explores continuities and discontinuities in understandings of mental health problems among both sufferers and colleagues across a forty year period. Finally, it reflects on what appears to be a surprising lack of popular awareness of stress in the 1970s despite the work of Hans Selye, Richard Lazarus and others to popularize the concept from the 1950s, and an increasingly prominent discourse around stress within the popular print media.[3]

Adults experiencing stress in the post-war period were of a generation that grew up without the benefit of the National Health Service (NHS), at a time when, for many, levels of income made the purchase of medical help rare or even unattainable. Amongst this generation, attitudes towards health, whether mental or physical, were largely driven by values arising from a necessary pragmatism. The poor, working-class women surveyed by Marjory Spring-Rice (1887–1970) in 1939 demonstrated clearly a 'grim and tacit acceptance' of low standards of health, such that, despite a huge variety of ailments ranging from constant headaches to anaemia and gynaecological problems, many of them felt justified in answering 'yes' to the question of whether they generally felt fit and well.[4] Their norm of good health was in many cases a state of chronic ill-health, according to Innes Pearce and George Scott Williamson, the founders of the pioneering Peckham Health Centre in South East London.[5] The absence of serious debilitating illness *was* good health for such women and their families and, although working men had more access to professional medicine via panel doctors, men's health was often little better.[6]

Against such a background, working- and middle-class attitudes toward health and sickness tended towards the stoic and the pragmatic. As one man born in the inter-war years told Mass Observation (MO) in 1997, 'the state of our health wasn't something we ever talked about as far as I remember'.[7] Such a view was supported by popular contemporary household medical manuals, which warned against the 'unrelieved study of sickness' which did not reflect 'the attitude of all healthy people'.[8] Dwelling on ill-health was regarded as undesirable and probably indicative of an unhealthy psyche. Despite the economic imperative behind attempts to downplay ill-health, there was a strong sense that an individual's attitude towards their health made a difference and that good health was a matter of individual responsibility.[9] Another correspondent told MO in 1939 that he regarded 'illness as an acknowledgement of weakness in myself and feel ashamed of being ill'.[10] Medical self-help books of the period emphasized the importance of an appropriate 'philosophy of life' with regard to nervous ailments, one suggesting that if 'the physician has examined the patient and found no organic disease, the solution obviously rests with the patient, who then becomes his own best doctor'; the patient's achievement of 'a well-organized mind' was necessary to 'dissolve the obscure and complex tensions'.[11] People in working-class communities in particular expected (and were expected) to cope with their situation, even if that meant putting on a façade that concealed unpleasant realities.[12]

In the decades following the creation of the NHS in 1948, therefore, the population generally continued to hold attitudes towards health that were deeply coloured by their experiences before the provision of medical treatment that was free for everyone at the point of service. Indeed, there were strong continuities with the pre-war period in terms of day-to-day experiences of access to, and use of, NHS services that meant that for some there was still a strong culture of self-reliance.[13] Within this context, people's attitudes towards stress at the mid-century were consistent with an approach to health that privileged a practical, but sometimes dismissive and even brusque, view of sufferers. Such attitudes tended to be exacerbated in the case of psychological and mental suffering which, presented without the evident symptoms of a broken or diseased limb or organ, were difficult for others to understand, and were still stigmatized by fears of madness.

Seeking evidence of the kinds of experiences that we would now classify as 'stress' means accepting a wide range of contemporary synonyms for stress, such as 'nerves', 'nervous' or 'nervous breakdown', 'pressure', 'tension' and 'strain'. These terms comprised the popular language of mental distress for much of the twentieth century and, as Watkins has argued in her work on the United States, were often used interchangeably, resulting in an understanding of stress that was shaped as much by the vernacular as the professional discourse.[14] While we might now acknowledge differences between tension, anxiety, worry and pressure and the results of internal or external stressors, these examples reflect common usage at the time, which rarely distinguished between them.[15] Analysis of post-war British self-help literature, written mostly by medical professionals, reveals a deliberate use of popular terminology reflecting both the language of doctor/patient conversations and a desire to communicate effectively with a lay readership.[16] Hence titles such as *You and Your Nerves: A Simple Account of the Nature, Causes and Treatment of Nervous Illness*, *How to Live with Your Nerves and Like it* and *Peace from Nervous Suffering*.[17] The wide range of stressors identified by such authors, including the speed of modern life, brain work, heredity and over-indulgence in food and drink and sex, highlights the potential for the lexicon of stress to capture a multiplicity of experiences.

Adopting a similar flexibility of vocabulary has been key in uncovering first-hand accounts of stress. In particular the accounts presented here are based on two key types of source, both of which reflect lived experience and use of contemporary vernacular to describe it. The first is the Mass Observation Archive which was established in the 1930s as an anthropological experiment, allowing volunteers to write about their lives and the lives of those they observed. The second is oral history interviews from the British Library Sound Archive, which were recorded as life histories for themed collections, but which also happen to include accounts of stress. Both sources provide peoples' personal narratives of their experiences and, although they are thus subject to the vagaries of memory and nostalgia, they offer unique accounts of a subject that can otherwise be difficult to access. Before examining the detail of these experiences, it is relevant to reflect on contemporary attitudes to work and health and how these informed the understanding and acknowledgement of stress at work. Closer reading of several individual accounts of work and stress then reveals the ways in which the causes of stress, and the experiences of the stressed, were perceived.

Work and Health

The sources examined here can be used to illuminate how people experienced work and stress in twentieth-century Britain. Contemporary ideas about the effects of both work and unemployment on mental health referred, without exception, to male experiences of work outside the home. In the immediate post-war decades any notion that work could create mental ill-health was tied specifically to the masculine experience of work. It was only much later, with the emergence of second-phase feminism, that women's domestic activities began to be conceptualized similarly as 'work' and the psychological effects of those activities were revealed.[18]

We have relatively limited knowledge of people's attitudes to work, especially in the early twentieth century, and yet work was fundamental to a sense of identity and status, as well as often being the basis for social life.[19] That work, or the lack of work, could cause psychoneurotic illness and anxiety states was recognized in the 1930s with unemployment the subject of considerable new research.[20] Stage theories of unemployment clearly identified anxiety and mental distress as a key step in the experience, whilst Jahoda identified five latent consequences of employment which were critical to understanding the effects of unemployment, but also had relevance to debates about the function of work to the human condition.[21] Those elements focused on the importance of work for imposing a time structure on the day, shared experiences and contacts outside the family unit, links to goals and purposes beyond the individual's own aims, personal status and identity, and enforced activity. Researchers argued that these factors made work psychologically supportive and emphasized how critical to existence the function of work could be, well beyond its obvious economic necessity. This made the experience of work as damaging to health, and particularly psychological health, all the more challenging for those who suffered work-related stress.

There is a further point to make regarding the function of work and in particular its economic drivers. The importance of work as a means of survival changed across the twentieth century. A simple continuum might show the experience of work for the majority of working-class and lower middle-class people ranging from basic economic survival, at one end, to personal fulfilment and self-actualization at the other, with the balance shifting from the former to the latter across the century, particularly following the creation of the welfare state in Britain mid-century. We might contrast the stoic pragmatism of workers in the first half of the century with the increasingly individualist requirements of workers in the latter half. 'Work was life, without it you did not survive', according to one retired railway worker recalling his parents in the inter-war period, 'It came first and last, always waiting to be done'. By contrast, by the late twentieth century, it was 'essential for people to have a means of expressing their own individuality and feeling their own worth'.[22] Work had many different meanings for people, whether offering status, involving duty, providing social interaction or purpose and structure and, for many, it was a key part of their identity. Within that framework it was therefore difficult to make sense of stress in a work context without undermining and threatening those other meanings.

Improvements in people's circumstances due to the safety net of the welfare state, wider educational opportunities and greater material comfort might suggest that people began to expect more from their work as economic survival diminished as the sole purpose. However, greater expectations of work, as a means of satisfaction and self-expression, opened up the experience of work to greater scrutiny and criticism, which may well have contributed to the issue of stress and work coming to the fore by the 1980s as higher expectations bred greater disappointment. Despite physical improvements in working conditions and the fact that by the 1980s most people worked in far superior working environments to their grandparents or even their parents, people were experiencing work as psychologically more problematic than their forebears did. Changes to the ways in which people conceptualized their work and how this was reflected in society made it far easier to interpret an experience of mental distress due to work in a medicalized or psychologized way, so that, by the 1980s, although work for the majority might not be physically dangerous, it now had a greater potential to make them mentally ill.

Such suffering was not unique to the late twentieth century. Throughout the century there were people for whom the experience of work was not only a negative one, but also one which damaged their psychological well-being. As an unemployed man in his thirties told MO in 1983, 'My mother didn't work but my father did. He was an accountant. It affected our family life because the strain of my father's job was one of the factors that made him an alcoholic'.[23] The 'strain' of such work permeated the whole family. This not only reveals the nature of work-related stress, but also reinforces gendered interpretations that regarded only occupation outside the home as 'work' and therefore causative of 'strain'. The public visibility of such conditions, particularly in the mid-twentieth century, was limited and likely to be managed privately, influenced by the robustly dismissive official stance towards civilian psychological problems during the Second World War and the paucity of resources afterwards.[24] For many, it was often easier to identify their ill-health as physical and, particularly in the decades around the mid-twentieth century, of gastric origin as another MO observer commented, talking about her uncle in the 1930s:

> I have the impression that it was the responsibilities of his position which caused him to have a stomach ailment. I never knew what that was, but there were always tins of Glaxo in the house, and he ate very little of anything else.[25]

Similarly, another woman growing up during the Second World War explained that her father's work was regularly interrupted by time in bed due to an ulcer:

'He never spoke about this or theorized as to what was the cause of the illness though the doctor talked a lot about 'bottling up emotion' and being 'over-conscientious'.[26] Underlying cultural trends at the time favoured gastro-intestinal explanations of medically unexplained symptoms, as evidenced by their preponderance among servicemen during the Second World War.[27] Indeed ulcers and stress continued to be associated with each other throughout the century, even beyond the discovery of a bacterial aetiology for ulcers in the 1980s. For patients, families, colleagues and friends, physical symptoms offered a more acceptable explanation for illness than anything psychological. Mental health issues carried a stigma that prevented people from acknowledging such experiences or identifying them directly with work or an employer.

Stress at Work

How did people experience psychological or emotional problems relating to their work or to the work of colleagues and peers? The first source offering insight comes from Miss Richmond who worked as a welfare officer for the furniture and furnishings manufacturing company, Hunter and Sons and its subsidiaries, between 1943 and 1956. Her main responsibility was to follow up cases of employees absent from work; in 1944 alone, she carried out 570 visits, both to workers in hospital and to others at home across a large part of London and its suburbs. Miss Richmond recorded many of her visits to employees' homes and the conversations that she had with them about the causes of their absence. In 1949, Miss Richmond recounted the case of Mr S from south-east London, who was absent from work due to a 'breakdown':

> I had a long talk with Mr S He looks very thin and said he had lost weight because he cannot eat. He has attacks of vomiting so his doctor sent him to hospital where he was examined and X-rayed. Nothing wrong was found, the verdict being that the internal trouble is due to nervous worry. I said how sorry I was to know he was ill and asked what was the matter and then listened to his story.
>
> Mr S came to Hunters a few months ago, and was put in charge of work started by another surveyor who had left. Three orders were in a confused state and were incurring financial loss to Hunters. This worried Mr S considerably and as the financial losses increased with the progress of the work so did his worry, until it overwhelmed him and he had a nervous breakdown.[28]

She went on to explain that Mr S's employers had told him not to worry but, despite these reassurances, Mr S 'knew it was foolish but the worry had taken too great a hold of him and he was now "suffering from his nerves"'.[29]

The case of Mr S highlights several points. Firstly, there was an initial search for a physical cause for his distress partly because it manifested itself in physical ways, such as vomiting, but also because the physical symptoms were perhaps easier to diagnose and treat and preferable to the potential stigma of psychological illness. It is also interesting that the early link between Mr S's suffering and his work shifted to Mr S himself and the suggestion that it was his own fault that he had let worry take hold of him. This tells us something pertinent about perceived causations of stress and the tendency to emphasize the individual's own role in their suffering. There was a clear preference for 'blaming' the individual worker rather than the circumstances of his or her work or any other potential causative or contributory factors.[30] The idea that some people were more susceptible to psychological distress due to inherent weakness rather than external circumstance was by no means new, having been critical to deliberations about shell shock and debates about whether soldiers qualified for war pensions in the inter-war period.[31] Arguably, similar economic considerations were also at play within a work context, as it was undoubtedly preferable to see the fault as inherent in the worker, rather than the environment or structure of the workplace.

That was not necessarily the view, however, of the worker and their family, as the wife of another employee, Mr L, who had been hospitalized with 'nervous trouble' in 1954 following a similar episode two years previously, told Miss Richmond:

> she did not think it had been right because he was working under the man who had his old job and he had had an inferiority complex all the time: he is now 'just a bundle of nerves, there is nothing wrong with him physically; it is something to do with his work that has got him like this.[32]

Aside from the interesting example of a popularized psychoanalytic concept of 'inferiority complex', Mrs L's view suggests that she clearly saw the job, or the social circumstances of the job, as the cause of her husband's problem. Miss Richmond's response was to tell Mrs L that 'in the interests of both Mr L and the firm it was not possible for him to continue at his present work and they had nothing else to offer him'. Reflecting on this in her report she wrote: 'It is a sad case and I am sorry for the Ls but, after all, Shaws is not a Psychiatric Rehabilitation Centre for the employment of "nervous trouble" cases'.[33] Clearly there was a tension between Miss Richmond's human sympathy and her organizational responsibilities, but also between her perceptions of the cause of the employee's problem and the family's view.

This tension is also illustrated in Miss Richmond's report following visits to two employees absent due to 'nerves'. The vast majority of her reports show a person with considerable compassion for the workers she visited in her welfare officer role, for in many ways she functioned as a social worker, home help and confidante to Hunter's employees. However, following her visit to Mr S and another employee, absent from work for similar reasons, she submitted the following in her report:

> What a week and what an object lesson!!!!!! To listen to these two grown men telling me how their 'nerves' have gone to pieces because the 'worry of their work has got on top of them' and so on and on and on and on.

> Many illnesses, pneumonia etc cannot be helped and nobody falls and breaks a leg on purpose, but I have seen so much of this 'nervous breakdown' line and it is a thing that the individual can prevent – if taken in time. The red light is showing when you find yourself thinking about, and talking about, nothing else than your particular worry. Mental diversion is needed: people, amusements, hobbies, anything except sitting brooding and chain smoking ... To hear these 'nerve' people talk one would think it was a question of life or death confronting them. They are quite out of focus with reality. It is no use talking to cases like these two I have seen this week. They are too far gone.[34]

Miss Richmond evidently interpreted the problem as being due to the individual *allowing* themselves to become ill by brooding and letting worry take hold. Such a notion was not uncommon. Indeed one popular psychology book of the time suggested that 'There must be a certain pleasure in worrying or people would not indulge in it so much', while a household medical guide, drawing on Selye's ideas, sought to clarify the difference between normal worry and the usefulness of adrenalin to boost functioning, and abnormal worry which could cause physical disease.[35] Miss Richmond's response to this perceived weakness in 'two grown men' is evidently gendered, her concept of masculinity clearly not encompassing these mens' experiences of psychological suffering. She demonstrated no understanding of the experiences that these two employees were going through. This could be read as a result of her having lived and worked in London for at least part of the Second World War, when 'a question of life or death' was perhaps experienced more literally. However, her attitude also reflected the popular view at the time that individual weakness was at the heart of many work-related health problems.

Such views mirrored pre-war organizational assumptions that persisted throughout the century. During the war and in the immediate post-war period, good employees were a valuable resource and the organizational paternalism, demonstrated by the provision of welfare officers such as Miss Richmond, reflected self-interest as much as altruism or legislative compliance. Indeed concerns about the effects on industry of sickness absence due to 'nervous breakdown' were the driver behind a Medical Research Council investigation in the early 1930s, specifically focusing on concerns about employees with 'imperfect mental adaptation to conditions of work'.[36] The study covered over a thousand workers and was structured to enable researchers to identify 'recognised clinical types', with limited concern for the industrial context in which they worked.[37] This was in contrast to growing contemporary interest in psychosocial medicine, pioneered by James Halliday (1897–1983), whose work as a Regional Medical Officer adjudicating national insurance claims, in Glasgow in the 1930s, convinced him of the link between social and environmental context and psychological and physical health.[38]

However it was concerns about wartime production that largely underpinned the development of institutions such as Roffey Park Rehabilitation Centre. Created in 1943 under the auspices of the National Council for the Rehabilitation of

Industrial Workers (NCRIW), as a result of funding from a wide variety of industrial concerns, the Centre was designed to treat employees suffering from industrial neurosis or 'ill health arising from industrial fatigue, depression, nervous debility and other occupational or psychological disorders'.[39] These criteria covered a wide range of conditions and the Centre's own advisory panel recognized privately that industrial neurosis was 'a loose expression which has no medical significance ... beyond the fact that the patient has been engaged in some form of work'.[40] However, the precise terminology was of secondary importance, as the primary purpose of the Centre was simply to restore workers to sufficient health to return to work. The Centre claimed that 82 per cent of its cases returned to 'normal full-time employment, usually in their original capacity'.[41] Miss Richmond's experience and opinions, then, might be seen as fairly common. Although there was certainly awareness of the issue of stress at work, it was seen from an institutional perspective as an issue of absence management and a problem to be overcome either by treating sick workers or avoiding the employment of those prone to stress. Within a year of opening, Roffey Park was also offering training courses to personnel and welfare officers to help them identify and deal with cases of industrial neurosis, although the focus appears to have leaned heavily towards categorizing the potentially susceptible, rather than addressing organizational shortcomings.

Positioning stress as something resulting from personal weakness was consistent with broader attitudes towards health among the immediate post-war general population. Accepting the situation, perhaps because of this personal element, appeared to be the norm. An example can be seen in the experience of Don Thompson, working for Pearl Assurance in High Holborn in the 1950s, who reported in an interview in 2006:

> Oh that was terrible, you wouldn't imagine how traumatic, that was one of my worst, working experiences I've ever had ... I went into the Fire and Compact section which dealt with traders things and there I don't know whether it was to do with the immediate managers or the manager but the pressure was intense, we seemed to have so much work and everybody was on top of you all the time and do you know in that time I got terrible eczema and I was off for about 5 weeks.[42]

Don suggested a link between ill-health and the behaviour of managers in the organization, but the focus of his interpretation reverted to his own symptoms that, in his case, were manifested in physical terms. His juxtaposition of terminology offers an interesting insight into the psychologized interpretation of such experiences. Whilst he mentioned 'pressure' as a cause of his ill-health, he described the whole experience as 'traumatic', a distinctly late-twentieth-century interpretation and indicative of the changes in popular perception of the effects of work on mental well-being. Also feeling the pressure of work in the mid-1950s was Jeff Mills, an undergraduate at Birmingham University and one of the new breed of working-class entrants to Higher Education. Jeff explained his experience in an interview in 1998:

> I knew when I got to Birmingham that I was up against some cracking students in ability and I knew I would have to work me socks off and I did but unfortunately I found it got to me and I suspect it was the first sign in me life of nervous tension. Erm it did get to me and I can remember in my last year I had to go to the doctors once or twice, I didn't realise it at the time but I wasn't sleeping particularly well, but it was all, I realise now, it was all evidence of stress.[43]

Jeff went on to surmise that much of his stress was related to 'expectations and hopes of meself' and that because his parents did not understand 'the system' he felt 'I was on my own you see'.[44] His interpretation of his symptoms when seeking medical help privileged the physical in that he sought help for sleeping difficulties and, as he acknowledged, it was only retrospectively that he tied his symptoms together with the overall experience of the stress of studying.

It is interesting to note that, despite Jeff's experiences as an undergraduate, by the 1970s, when the stress concept was largely accepted among the medical profession at least, there was still rather more continuity than change in his experiences of mental distress relating to work. In his interview Jeff explained that he had worked as a Deputy Head in a school in the Bolton area in the early 1970s. At that time he was recently promoted and ambitious. However, he started to experience unfamiliar symptoms:

> I suddenly discovered I wouldn't go into shops. I didn't want to go anywhere where there were people and yet I would go into school where there were lots of people ... we'd go to Bolton on a Saturday and I would sit in the car rather than go in a shop. Um, don't ask me what it was I just had feelings of terror, me mind would go blank, it was almost a fear I suppose. And this was really getting to me and I thought, 'I don't understand this', and at the time I still thought it was physical.[45]

Although Jeff experienced his symptoms as both sudden and psychological, he attributed them to a physical cause. On another occasion his experience was completely different:

> I was riding towards the traffic lights coming home one night in a place called Moses Gate and I got pains in my arms and I thought was in my chest. And I stopped the car and the lights were on red and I just opened the passenger door to ask a woman to get me an ambulance to get me some help I didn't feel well at all.[46]

Rather than ask for help, Jeff shut the door and broke the speed limit hurrying home, but reported: 'I thought about it and then over the next three or four weeks I started to have all sorts of symptoms ... the usual ones: couldn't sleep, bad eyes, bad head'. He kept going to work and believed that he was still doing his job adequately, but retrospectively came to see:

> what I didn't realise was I was working too hard I realise it now, but it's taken a long time. I was working so hard it was unbelievable … I was almost running the school and I was obviously trying to impress and I wanted to be a Head and I was doing all sorts of courses and I did virtually everything, the school discipline, timetable, day to day cover and all this sort of business.[47]

The persistence of his symptoms and his growing distress eventually led Jeff to get a second opinion, after his own general practitioner (GP) prescribed medication that made his headaches worse. The second doctor diagnosed him with what he referred to as 'complete nervous exhaustion and stress, nothing but', prescribed tablets and told him to take a fortnight off work. Jeff summed up his experience, commenting: 'I don't think the people at work ever knew. I don't think I ever showed it at work I just coped, but out of work things were just falling apart and I got through it thank God'.[48]

Jeff's inclination to explain his symptoms in physical terms reflected the ways in which his body reacted to distress, but it also highlights the privileging of physical, over psychological, explanations at this point in time. It did not occur to Jeff that his work might be affecting his health, in spite of the fact that by the early 1970s there was a growing popular discourse of stress and work, evident for example in the *Daily Mirror*'s feature on the 'Seven Ages of Stress' in October 1972 and in a case reported in *The Guardian* two years later, in which stress was used as a defence in a murder trial, entitled 'Man "Broken by Stress"'.[49] However, as Jeff's experience suggests, popular awareness had not yet reached the point where people applied the concept to themselves. Nor was stress organizationally institutionalized. Although Jeff did not think that his stress showed at work, it seems likely that there could have been some indication, but his employers apparently were either not aware or, in keeping with ideas about personal responsibility, left it to Jeff as his problem rather than theirs. The suggestion that he was 'working too hard' was something that he found difficult to assimilate. There was a reluctance to ascribe his problem to his work.

Elsewhere in his life story, Jeff demonstrated an underlying sense of the world as a competitive place and this perhaps underscored his reluctance to admit that he could not keep up. It is suggestive also perhaps of the extent to which his work contributed to his self-worth and masculine identity. Jeff was a member of the post-war generation that Roper has identified as living with the 'necessity to deny stress' and disavow anything 'soft'.[50] Jeff's account also illuminates the ways in which his experience with his GP suggests that institutional and professional discourses on stress were being framed within the context of pharmaceutical treatments, which in his case made him feel worse, not better. Certainly the early 1970s was a period in which the prescribing of minor tranquilizers for the treatment of 'mild to moderate emotional symptoms in primary care' was reaching astonishing proportions.[51]

This reflected the fact that pharmaceutical companies were now marketing the conditions their drugs purported to treat, as much as the drugs themselves.[52]

Jeff's reluctance or inability to relate his illness to his work tells us something interesting about attitudes to work. His fears were not about economic survival and he was not afraid of losing his job in terms of survival: he was university-educated and was in a relatively stable profession. However, his work was clearly important to him, to the extent that its meaning could blind him to the effects it was having on him. The meaning of work for Jeff, although never expressed concretely, centred on his own sense of purpose, identity and status coupled with a sense of duty and loyalty.

A different example of the experience of stress comes from Peter Allen, born in 1950 in Yorkshire. Like Jeff Mills, Peter was taking on his first managerial role in the early 1970s.

> When I was about 23/24 I was first put in charge of a lot of people and I actually had a nervous breakdown which in those days was quite a traumatic experience 'cos nobody really understood mental health very much.[53]

Peter's use of language is pertinent: despite the growing popular discourse of 'stress', he referred to his 'nervous breakdown'. It is also notable that he categorized this as 'traumatic', as Don Thompson did, using a term which was perhaps more common in the popular lexicon of the late 1990s when he was talking, than in the 1970s when he actually had the experience. However, the other key point is the lack of apparent understanding from other people – 'nobody really understood mental health very much'.[54]

Peter was put in charge of sixty local authority gardeners and tried to base his management on that of his boss, whose style was to order people about and 'shout at them'. This did not work for Peter, as he explained:

> I went off, I just collapsed one day. I just keeled over one day and I went home and I was taken home and the doctor said 'oh you've had a nervous breakdown'. I didn't know what it was, there wasn't anything broken or twisted or anything, your lungs weren't bad it was a nervous breakdown.[55]

Peter's experiences were physical, but he was given a psychological diagnosis, which he himself did not understand. His framework for understanding illness was based around symptoms that were visible and this left him poorly equipped to make sense of what was happening to him. Peter's GP prescribed Valium which, when he did return to work, had a detrimental effect on him as it interfered with his short term memory: 'I had to write everything down because any time you thought of anything it was wiped off the blackboard ... so that took a lot of getting over that'.[56] Although Peter did not explicitly say so, he hinted that treatment was potentially as bad, if not worse, than the condition that it was designed to alleviate, something which some psychologists were beginning to argue at the time.[57]

Like many others, Peter found that other people did not really understand what had happened to him:

> In those days well people just used to say 'he's had a nervous breakdown' and for the first two hours they were very sympathetic, but after that it was, you know, it's not like a broken leg if you can't see it, if it's not manifest then people, if it's in your head, can't quite understand it.[58]

Peter's return to work may have been made more difficult by the contemporary lack of understanding. Ten years later, a widespread familiarity with the concept of 'stress' might have made that return easier. However, speaking in 1998, Peter made another comment regarding the reactions of others:

> I hear these days people say he's gone off with his, what do we call it now we call it pressure, stress that's it stress, gone off with stress, and people say well I don't know why he's stressed, he don't do anything. You know that sort of thing. But people don't realise that stress is brought on by a lot of different things.[59]

His comments suggest that even by the end of the century and two decades in which stress had become legally recognized within the framework of Health and Safety legislation, with the Health and Safety Executive suggesting in the 1990s that 5 million working days were being lost to stress each year, people generally were still suspicious of it.[60] Such suspicions confirm Peter's earlier comments about the visibility of symptoms, since those which could not be seen were not only hard to understand, but also more open to question. Peter implied that people had only a limited perception of stress as something resulting simply from too much work, rather than as something arising from a more complex interplay of work, environment and person. Implicit also perhaps is the hint that claiming to be stressed might be a way of avoiding work or it might imply an unacceptable lack of stoicism. Also relevant in Peter's account is his attribution of his experience to 'your learning curve and part of growing up'.[61] He seems to be suggesting that his suffering was either a necessary formative stage in his career development, or simply due to his youth. He does not relate his experience to his actual work or the fact that he was suddenly given a set of challenging responsibilities for which he was ill-prepared. Echoing Miss Richmond, Peter attributed his illness to his own weakness. This provides an interesting contrast with twenty-first century notions that regard sufferers from stress as victims of their circumstances, where the tendency is to 'inflate the problem of emotional vulnerability and to minimise the ability of the person to cope with distressful episodes'.[62]

Peter and Jeff's accounts provide descriptions of specific work-related episodes of mental distress, in the context of often wide-ranging interviews which were recorded in the late 1990s at a time when the language of stress had largely been absorbed into popular culture and usage. Thus they offer insight in two ways. Firstly, they offer recall of a time when the interviewees did not have a framework in which to understand their experiences. This is highlighted by the ways in which they described what happened and also in their accounts of other people's responses. Secondly, their stories demonstrate the ways in which, by the late 1990s, when most of these interviewees were speaking, the acquired vocabulary of stress enabled them to contextualize their memories. In particular, we hear Peter searching for the 'right' word when he refers first to pressure, then stress. There is a sense of being able to put the correct label on his experience now.

Conclusion

The examination of Miss Richmond's welfare officer reports in the 1940s and the experiences of work-related stress narrated by Peter and Jeff in the 1950s to 1970s highlight a number of key issues. Firstly, despite the popularity and adoption of the stress concept following the publication of Hans Selye's *The Stress of Life*, in 1956, attitudes towards causation show powerful continuity across the post-war period.[63] It was the individual, rather than the external working environment that was pathogenic: it was the inherent weakness of workers that made them suffer, not the conditions in which they found themselves. Secondly, there was a lack of understanding amongst colleagues, friends and family and even the medical profession itself. People did not understand mental health issues and were suspicious, even in the early 1970s, of conditions that they could not see. While absence from work with a broken leg carried validity, a nervous breakdown did not. Thirdly, the tools that the medical profession had to tackle the mental distress of people like Jeff and Peter were scarcely better than those of Miss Richmond's colleagues. Pharmaceutical treatments were quite often blunt-edged tools, which created at least as much suffering, albeit in different ways, as that which they were supposed to alleviate. GPs relied on the sedative effects of sleeping pills and drugs such as Valium, both of which had negative effects for Jeff and Peter.[64] It seems that, despite the rise in popularity of various forms of psychotherapy during the 1970s, when Jeff and Peter were experiencing stress, psycho-therapeutic treatments did not appear to have reached general practice.

The 1970s was arguably the final decade before stress became the phenomenon that we understand it to be today. The experiences of those suffering from work-related stress in the 1970s bore greater similarities to experiences in the immediate post-war period than to our contemporary stress culture. Similarly the responses of others to their experiences also seem remarkably consistent across the post-war years to the 1970s. It seems likely that multiple factors were at play here, including changes to the nature of paid employment due to the mid-1970s economic slump. Coming after a 'golden age' of economic prosperity, growth, powerful trade unions, workers' rights and welfare reforms, recession paved the way for considerable reforms perceived by some as increasing demands and pressures on workers, concomitant with reducing their security and requiring greater flexibility.[65] At the same time, the introduction of the Health and Safety at Work Act in 1974 and the creation of the Health and Safety Executive to enforce its provisions placed more focus on the work environment and introduced greater organizational responsibilities for employees. The increasing proportion of women in the workforce contributed to changing attitudes towards, and experiences of, work among the general population. The 1970s was also a period when GPs found themselves better able to offer treatment for 'nervous conditions' in the form of heavily promoted minor tranquilizers such as Valium. The ability to treat effectively was positively correlated to increases in diagnosis, suggesting a tendency towards medicalizing experiences that might previously have been undiagnosed.[66] Overall the ground was being laid for considerable changes in attitudes towards work, which would begin to allow people to question the role of work and stress in dictating their mental health and to ask questions about causation which might previously have been unthinkable. Increasingly psychologized interpretations of work began to engender beliefs that experiences such as those of Jeff and Peter were due to environmental and external factors. As subsequent chapters in this volume argue, it was this process that paved the way for conceptualizing workers as 'victims' of stress.

5 INDUSTRIAL AUTOMATION AND STRESS, *c.*1945–79

Sarah Hayes

In 1946, Delmar S. Harder (1892–1973), Vice-President for Manufacturing at the Ford Motor Company in the US, introduced a new word, 'automation', into the English language. Harder coined the term as a 'nickname' to describe a production process that had been installed at the company's Detroit factory and which linked together a number of automatic machines into one integrated process.[1] The application of automatic operation to manufacturing processes was not new in the 1940s. It had been increasingly applied across the US, Europe and Britain throughout the inter-war period in a range of manufacturing contexts, including the production of textiles, cigarettes, the chemical industry and other processes where very large outputs were required. However, in the post-war period, the issue of automation and its impact, not only on the lives of individual industrial workers, but also on the psychosocial foundations of the nation as a whole, became a subject of widespread debate. Contemporary observers noted the speed and extent of change that accompanied the implementation of automated production systems within a host of new industries and raised anxieties about the possible short and long-term effects on health.

This chapter will examine both the positive and negative perspectives presented in these debates, exploring some of the key concerns around the impact of automation on the physical, mental and emotional well-being of those working in British industry in the second-half of the twentieth century. It will begin by examining public perceptions of automation, exploring the emergence of concerns around the impact of automation on worker health in the context of significant political, economic and social change in the immediate post-war period. It will highlight the polarized nature of attitudes to automation and the manner in which they shaped subsequent medical, political and industrial debates. It will argue that the growth of automation contributed to a significant shift from the long-standing concerns around physical and mental 'fatigue', which had dominated approaches towards industrial medicine in the early twentieth century and the inter-war period, to a new focus on psycho-social factors, including 'mental strain', 'nervous strain' and 'stress disorder'. Secondly, it will explore widespread concerns about the mental and physical pressures created by the introduction of Time and Motion Study practices which accompanied automation and which raised questions about the speed of technological change, the operational rates of new machinery, anxiety disorders arising from job insecurity and task re-orientation, and emotional problems arising from tasks involving the supervision of machinery, roles in which operators were simply 'waiting for nothing to happen'.[2]

Occupational health in the context of factory production has been the focus of a great deal of historical interest in the past three decades. However, much of this work has focused on the nineteenth and early twentieth centuries, with developments in the decades after the Second World War being largely ignored.[3] Studies that have examined industrial life in this specific period have concentrated predominantly on issues of industrial relations, workplace culture, and the internal politics of supervisory management practices, with particular emphasis on the development of 'Fordist' strategies in the context of industrial relations within the automobile industry.[4] The role played by automation within these developments has received limited consideration by historians. By drawing examples from three industries, namely the car manufacturing industry, the tobacco industry and the boot and shoe industry, this chapter aims to address the absence of studies in this area and to add substantially to historical understanding of debates about, and experiences of, stress and work.

Study of these industrial cases reveals two key themes. Firstly, they illustrate prominent preoccupations with the impact of modernity on mental health and emotional well-being in the post-war years. This focus particularly highlighted the notion of psychological adjustment, emphasizing the importance of the ability of individual workers to adapt mentally and physically to the rapidly changing demands of the industrial workplace. Secondly, a study of the introduction of automated processes highlights the connections between occupational health and managerial control. Concerns over workplace control emphasized the impact of automation on changing managerial strategies, worker agency and the relationship between man and machine. Central to these debates were fears that automation would result in de-humanization of the workplace, either through the removal of humans from the production processes or from workers being forced into unskilled and depersonalized roles that were controlled by technological demands.

The Growth of Automation

The term 'automation' was derived from the Greek 'automatos' (self-moving) and Harder's 1940s Fordist definition was a narrow one. His original words described automation as 'the automatic handling of materials and parts in and out of machines', with specific reference to new automated ways of moving components and materials between different stages of production. However, by the mid-1950s, the definition had been widened within industrial manufacturing to encompass three specific technical innovations: 'Transfer (Detroit) Automation', referring to the installation of automatic production lines and advanced techniques of material and product handling, and assembly; 'Control Automation', a rapid development of techniques of automatic control over manufacturing processes; and 'Computer Automation', the rapid and automatic processing of information by electronic digital computer.[5]

In Britain, the adoption of these forms of automated processes was considered the primary means of achieving the manufacturing efficiency and industrial growth needed to rebuild the economic strength of the nation in the immediate aftermath of the Second World War. With the Government actively promoting a major 'push for productivity',[6] the emphasis on ever-increasing manufacturing efficiency dominated both political and industrial approaches throughout this period in a way that had not previously been seen. Automation enabled unprecedented attainment of levels of production and profitability. According to many industrialists in the late 1940s, the potential impact of automation was of such significance that it heralded the dawn of a 'Second Industrial Revolution' and a 'New Era' of prosperity.[7]

By the mid-1950s, however, there was a growing public concern about the speed and extent of change arising from technological advancement, and about the effect that automation would have on workers' lives and on society in general. The Society for Science and the Public observed that 'at no time during automation's history has it moved so fast and so forcefully'.[8] Debates which emerged at this time were deeply polarized. Some considered automation to be an exciting, welcome, perhaps inevitable, advancement in man's harnessing of scientific and technological knowledge. From this perspective, automation was an important tool for achieving economic growth, higher standards of living, increased freedom and easier lives for all. By contrast, those who viewed automation as a potentially negative development identified ways in which automation could threaten the health and livelihoods of the nation's industrial workforce. This side of the debate foresaw a range of increasing demands, both physical and psychological, that individual workers were likely to encounter. These conflicting views of automation are evident in lectures and conference papers presented to industrialists in this period, and are neatly summarized in the title of a conference speech given to the Institute of Production Engineers in 1955 by industrialist, Sir Walter Puckey (1899–1983) who posed the question, 'The Automatic Factory: Dream or Nightmare?'[9]

In the early years of the 1950s the pessimistic view of automation as a potential 'nightmare' dominated public perceptions. In part, negativity was fuelled by images of the industrial workplace presented in contemporary popular culture, most notably, the film industry. Negative views were evident in Charlie Chaplin's 1936 film *Modern Times*, a humorous but scathing critique of the de-humanizing effects of industrialization. The film was a political statement by Chaplin on the impact of modernity on people's working lives and mental health, and resonated with a broader, long-standing notion of 'the human motor', the harnessing of human energy into industrial productivity. Anson Rabinbach has argued that, whilst this unflattering metaphor was significant in the inter-war period and persisted into the immediate post-war period, by the mid-1950s it was being replaced by a more positive perspective on automation as a means to 'liberate work from the materiality and physicality of the body'.[10] However, the visual image presented by Chaplin became an enduring representation of industrial automation, to the extent that Chaplin's film was still being publicly evoked and referenced well into the 1960s, more than twenty years after its release. In a BBC broadcast in 1964, for example, industrialist Sir Leon Bagrit (1902–79) stated:

> Most people would feel, with Charlie Chaplin in *Modern Times* at the back of their mind, that a car assembly plant represents everything they fear in the way of automatic and semi-automatic machinery.[11]

By the mid-1950s, the Government's Department of Scientific and Industrial Research (DSIR) had conceded that automation was 'whatever its faults, a word which has come to stay'.[12] The World Health Organization (WHO) noted in 1959 that the term had become 'a very real generator of anxiety reactions among workers, but even more so among the general public', adding that 'certain popular literature warns humanity against the industrial hell towards which it is inexorably moving'.[13] Debates amongst industrialists in the 1960s illustrate continuing anxieties: 'For many people, automation is a terrifying word. It conjures up visions of tyrannical machines reducing man to the status of a mere pusher of buttons or watcher of dials, abolishing the need for human thought and judgment'.[14] Psychological insecurity accompanying automation was further articulated by workers at Ford Motor Company's Dagenham factory in 1962, who stated that 'automations and all new techniques, instead of being something to be welcomed by workers, becomes something to be feared, to make us unsure of the future'.[15] However, the WHO noted the unconstructive nature of the polarized debates around automation, observing in 1959 that:

> Both at the subjective and objective level, far too many loose statements of an emotionally charged nature are being made. While some overstress the beneficial and hopeful aspects to a point where one might consider that automation is about to build a human paradise, others take the role of Cassandra and describe the changes to be expected in terms which are unduly alarming and pessimistic.[16]

In seeking to achieve an objective perspective and to examine the credibility of concerns around automation, a number of formal investigations and studies were instigated by a range of different agents, including government officials, medical professionals and social scientists. These studies presented a new perspective on inter-war pre-occupations with 'the human problems of industry'.[17] Most prominent amongst these studies were those carried out by the DSIR, the WHO, the Industrial Welfare Society, the Ergonomics Research Society, the Social Science Research Council and the London Co-operative Party. The subject was also a primary source of discussion amongst industrialists and trade unions, with a number of conferences and lecture series held by these groups specifically to explore the potential impact of automation.

The case for this quantity of research rested on the assumption that there was something special about automation which created psychosocial problems that were different from those generated by other forms of technical progress, such as mechanization.[18] An emphasis on psychosocial factors is particularly evident in a study instigated by the WHO in 1958. Focusing directly on the 'mental health problems of automation', the study aimed to examine 'the possible dangers of automation for the psychosocial foundations of human behaviour and mental health'.[19] Identifying the importance of 'psychosocial maintenance', the subsequent report called for attention to be devoted to aspects of social environment, both inside and outside the factory, for 'the protection and promotion of mental health'.[20]

The prospect of medical and scientific investigation into the effects of automation led industrialists to argue that the adoption of automated processes would create vast improvements in the working conditions of factory operatives. In their view, automation would be beneficial to health as it would result in: reduced demands for physical strength, dexterity and mental aptitude; less task-related drudgery and boredom; more remote power handling instead of close manual handling; fewer people required to operate the processes, therefore less risk to life and limb; and an improvement in processes known to be hazardous to health.[21] Representing the British motor industry, mechanical engineer Frank Woollard (1883–1957) argued, in 1955, that:

> With the aid of automation I am of the opinion that we shall enter a new phase of fine living. Automation is a means for increasing man's stature and for extending his ability to do more and more useful work; to produce in greater volume with less physical effort or mental strain – a means whereby he can bring to his fellows the fulfilment of their lawful desires and, to their homes, comfort and leisure.[22]

Observers particularly highlighted the benefits that automation would bring to the quality of life for female workers, with predictions that automation would lead to unprecedented domestic contentment. Sir Leon Bagrit, for example, observed:

> I am sure that automation is going to free both women and society from the need for routine drudgery in factories and offices. If, as a nation, we become productive enough and consequently rich enough to make the man's wage packet sufficient for the family needs, many women would prefer to go to the hairdresser rather than the factory.[23]

This statement reflected and reinforced a long-standing patriarchal belief that women would 'naturally' prefer to remain in the domestic sphere.[24] However, this rhetoric ignored the increasingly crucial role played by the female workforce in post-war industrial production. Miriam Glucksmann has argued that the advent of mass consumer production resulted in women assuming a heightened significance in the workplace, being the preferred source of semi-skilled labour for many employers.[25] Automation therefore provided greater opportunities for women to gain employment, although the roles and tasks they were assigned were restricted within gendered boundaries. Elisabeth Hagen and Jane Jenson have further argued that there was a change in the broader relationship between women and work, with their attachment to employment becoming more permanent.[26] Debbie Palmer, however, has noted higher rates of sickness absence amongst women employees than men.[27] Contemporary sociologists Alva Myrdal (1902–86) and Viola Klein (1908–73) concluded that 'conflicts of loyalty' between work and domestic responsibilities resulted in higher levels of stress for women, leading to ill-health.[28] Interviews with female operators working in the shoe industry in the 1960s highlight the significance of social relationships as a key factor in the maintenance of mental health in the workplace. Their accounts suggest that emotional support from fellow workers was important in aiding their individual abilities to balance the demands of work and domestic lives, and to adapt psychologically to technological or structural change in the workplace.[29]

Medical studies also supported the possibility that automation could be a beneficial development for certain aspects of worker health. The WHO report stated that:

> In fact, while automation is often thought to be 'de-humanising' the production process, it is considered on the other hand to relieve humanity from a great deal of drudgery and strain such as resulted from the introduction of earlier types of mechanisation, particularly those in which hard physical effort was replaced by the repetitive work of the assembly line.[30]

However, the report also concluded that:

> automation must be considered both as a source of possible improvements in mental health and as a source of new types of strain which will require full consideration and fully planned preventative action.[31]

The 'new types of strain' identified by the WHO, and its call for preventative action, resonated with other studies which warned that different forms of automation could give rise to specific problems that would affect particular groups of workers in varying ways. They highlighted issues relating to three specific groups: assembly line workers, staff employed to monitor computerized systems and office workers. The studies predicted problems relating to two key issues: psychological adjustment and managerial control.

Psychological Adjustment and Adaptation

It was widely recognized that automation meant change. As several contemporaries argued, it was fundamentally a process which sought to remove human labour from the industrial process in the name of efficiency.[32] It involved changes to the production processes on the factory floor, the types of machines used, the placement and location of machines, the numbers of workers needed to operate and oversee the machines and the types of tasks and operations that workers would be required to do. Several prominent studies highlighted the potential for mental and emotional stress arising from these specific changes. Primarily, this included the loss of long-established jobs as humans were replaced by machines, the reallocation of tasks, the 'de-skilling' of the workforce, the monotony of tasks created by automated processes, the physical isolation of workers and the increased demands and physical strains of shift work.

Identifying the significant impact that such changes could have on mental and emotional health, from the mid-1950s onwards medical professionals began to link automation with a newly emergent medical model of adaptation and 'stress', conceptualized and popularized by Walter B. Cannon (1871–1945) and Hans Selye (1907–82).[33] The extent to which an individual worker might be affected by stress in the newly automated workplace was seen to be determined by their ability to adapt to change, with studies underlining the need for workers to be psychologically prepared for change, and to be flexible and open to the likelihood that the arrival of automation in their factories would result in them being assigned different tasks to those for which they had been trained or had grown accustomed to performing. The 1959 World Health Organization (WHO) report particularly highlighted the role played by individual adaptation and adjustment in the maintenance of good mental health:

> The adaptability of human beings is great, and most individuals maintain themselves in adequate mental health by an active search for the minimum social and emotional requirements necessary for this purpose and by active adaptation to changes in their social situation within the household or family, within the working group, and within the one or more recreational groups of which most people are members.[34]

Revealing a theoretical approach framed around well-established psychological notions of individual differences, it observed that 'change requires a certain adaptation and the capacity for this varies from one individual to another', emphasizing that 'the extent of adaptive effort required is likely to show considerable differences between individuals'.[35] The WHO went on to conclude that the introduction of automation had several potential psychological repercussions that could result in 'reactions affecting mental health'. These could be emotional reactions, arising from the anticipation of the possible consequences of new technological methods, or reactions of persons exposed to actual physiological and psychological strain.[36] It stated:

> Where the adaptive effort is beyond the resources of the individual the minimum level of social requirements for mental health will not be reached and a clinically recognizable state of ill health will appear.[37]

One of the primary adaptations noted was adjustment to changes in staffing and employment levels that would accompany automation. The greatest fear expressed in many debates was that it would lead to a diminution of labour requirements and widespread unemployment; humans would be replaced by machines. Labour MPs representing the Co-operative Society built this prospect into their official definition of automation, pronouncing in 1957 that 'automation can be simply defined as the move towards production without human labour towards the factory without workers'.[38] The WHO noted the prominence of this argument in 1959, observing that 'even quite responsible authors have been known to state that "it is perfectly clear that this [automation] will produce an unemployment situation in comparison with which the depression of the thirties will seem an unpleasant joke"'.[39]

Much of the fear over unemployment amongst British workers arose from observing the spread of automation in the US Reports which cited instances in the automobile industry where a workforce of 23,000 was reduced to 10,000 following automation, or a radio assembly line, where two workers now did the job of 200.[40] Archival sources indicate that British fears linking automation to unemployment were perhaps well-grounded. Trade union documents relating to employment tribunal disputes within the tobacco industry reveal that, since 1938, a gradual introduction of new types of automated machinery and new methods of production had resulted in 8,000 fewer workers employed in the industry by the mid-1950s. This trend was verified by figures published in the *Ministry of Labour Gazette* which identified a continuing reduction of 1,600 male and 4,500 female workers employed in the industry between 1950 and 1956.[41]

It was noted, however, that despite a reduction in the labour force of approximately 23 per cent since 1948, productivity had actually increased by 20 per cent between 1947 and 1952. Evidence presented in industrial tribunals argued that, whilst technological improvements could be considered one possible factor in this increase, this phenomenon had mostly resulted from 'a greater concentration of effort, both physical and mental, on the part of a smaller number of operatives'.[42] This implied that automation provided employers with the opportunity to reduce the size of their workforce, but that the reduced workforce was subsequently placed under significant pressure to meet ever-increasing production targets. Evidence to support this trend was also presented by trade union shop stewards at Ford, who highlighted how tensions arising from fluctuations in car sales were used as an opportunity by management to reduce the number of workers on the automated production lines:

> If 100 men are producing 100 cars and the number required dropped to ninety, then ten men would be taken off. But when the schedule went back up to 100 jobs again, only seven men would be put back. Thus ninety-seven men would now be doing work previously done by 100. With the schedule of vehicles fluctuating daily this device led to many clashes.[43]

A reduction in the numbers of operatives and line workers per unit area could impact on emotional well-being in other ways. Several studies highlighted the negative effects, on psychological health, of isolation and solitude experienced by many workers in the industrial workplace. The WHO noted that this problem frequently affected assembly-line workers in instances where worker numbers had been significantly reduced and machines repositioned to prevent social contact.[44] Deliberate prevention of social contact between workers as a planned management strategy has been recorded as the source of emotional stress in sociological studies of the car industry in this period.[45] The WHO observed the 'depressing effects which excessive isolation may produce' as 'the absence of social contacts is something which, by his very nature, man cannot endure for long'.[46] However, a survey conducted by the Department of Scientific and Industrial Research (DSIR) in 1960 concluded that physical isolation did not necessarily equate to social isolation, and that operators may have had the freedom to leave smooth–running machines for brief periods. The WHO subsequently concluded that isolation occurred most often in situations of 'insufficient automation', and that increased automation would actually reduce the problem.[47] Both surveys did, however, acknowledge that social isolation could occur in workplace situations where the noise of machinery was so excessive that workers could not talk intelligibly to each other, even at close quarters. They noted that this problem was most likely to arise in workshops with smaller automated machines, such as automatic looms.[48]

Debates emphasizing the negative impact on mental health and emotional well-being created by the experience and reality of redundancy and unemployment also highlighted the significant levels of anxiety created by imagined fears around job insecurity. Anxieties created by job insecurity reinforced a theory presented by psychiatrist Harold G. Woolf (1898–1962) in 1953 that new emotional tensions, or 'loss of anchorage', occurred in the post-war period as a result of rapid social change and political instability in the context of a changing world order and the emergent Cold War.[49] Drawing on Selye's work, Woolf argued that 'man's sensitivity to his place in society, his status in the eyes of other men, is central to the problem of stress'.[50] Further psychiatric debates emphasized the important role that work played in creating and reinforcing personal status in society, individual social identities and positive mental health. Exploring the role of industry in the aetiology of stress disorder in 1966, psychiatrist J. D. Sutherland (1906–91) observed that 'work activities give man a part of his very identity', warning that 'a threat to his own individual contribution can prove extremely disturbing'.[51] Automation provided such a threat in its requirement for individual adaptation to changes in long-established and highly-skilled work activities, which previously had required many years of training and experience to master. Many of the negative expectations about automation, therefore, centred on worries about the changing nature of work activities and tasks, particularly fears around the replacement of skilled jobs with semi-skilled or unskilled work.

De-skilling of the workplace had serious implication for the psychological self-esteem and economic potential of workers where existing training and experience were no longer of use or value to employers. The relationship between skilled work and psychological health was emphasized in industrial health literature at the time. For example, one psychology text-book published in 1950 stated:

> What are the psychological and social factors in modern life which produce an attitude of mind amongst so many persons, which prevent them from working to the best of their capabilities? In most individuals it can be ascribed to an absence of the natural joy of craftsmanship arising from skilled labour.[52]

As well as a loss of status and psychological self-esteem, the re-categorization of workers from 'skilled' to 'semi-skilled' or 'unskilled' had significant implications for earning potential as less skilled work resulted in lower pay grades. Further fears centred on the assumption that re-assignment to unskilled tasks would increase 'drudgery' in the workplace and workers would become little more than robotic components of the machinery, as foreseen in Chaplin's *Modern Times*. This fear is evident in a range of literature produced by contemporary worker organizations, which regarded automation as a process of depersonalization and dehumanization. Several arguments were presented by industrialists and politicians in attempts to dispel this perception. For example, the DSIR stated in 1956 that: 'automation will not make robots of us all. On the contrary, it will demand wider knowledge, greater ability and a higher degree of skill from worker and manager alike'[53] According to Alastair Reid, previous historical analysis has been similarly framed by an assumption that technological innovation would inevitably lead to de-skilling, neglecting the requirement for new or different skills.[54] In order to promote a positive message, the DSIR produced a pamphlet in 1960, which set out a detailed description of the range of new skills, particularly amongst technicians and managers, that would be required in each field of automated processes.[55] One specific area where higher degrees of skill would be needed was identified as 'Control Automation'.

Control Automation involved the overseeing and supervision of machines, demanding adaptation from manual work to perceptual activities. These were the sitting-down, dial-watching jobs, where, in the words of R. C. Browne, Professor of Industrial Health at the University of Newcastle, staff were often passively 'waiting for nothing to happen'.[56] In these jobs, knowledge and skills would only be needed if something went wrong. Industrialists argued that this form of task could bring major benefits to some workers. Presenting a paper to a symposium on 'The Changing Demands of Modern Work and Control', held in Bristol in 1957, Chris Jones of the Metropolitan-Vickers Electrical Company created an image of a new industrial utopia, arguing that the emergence of these types of jobs would create a new category of 'brain-worker', or 'mental-craftsman', who, between periods of 'on-call' work, would spend most of their time at home. Drawing on nostalgic images of a pre-industrial rural idyll, he argued that the home and factory would come together 'as in the heyday of the (pre-industrial) crafts'.[57]

Vicky Long has argued that the mixing of industrial and domestic as a psychological tool for increased productivity was a feature of the establishment of new 'model factories' in the inter-war period.[58] However, whilst this tactic was successfully embraced in the earlier period, the idealized notion presented by industrialists in the 1950s was strongly challenged by contemporaries. Several medical studies, for example, warned that, in reality, the unseen demands of these jobs could actually result in high levels of mental strain and anxiety. The WHO suggested that these jobs entailed greater responsibility, as workers had to ensure the smooth running of large and extremely costly machines around which whole processes, even whole factories, operated, and which resulted in major economic repercussions if things did go wrong. They argued that, contrary to the belief that operators sat all day doing nothing, these types of tasks required a high degree of attention, accompanied by the need to keep alert for many hours every day in order to react instantaneously to alarm signals which might vary in perceptibility and only rarely went off. The study found that this perceptual burden resulted in particularly 'heavy nervous strain', as the operator was not able to offset his vigilance by any other motor activity. The need for constant attention could also be accompanied by unrecognized subliminal attention, preventing rest and resulting in muscular and psychological fatigue. It was argued that this could produce 'strain on the total personality and even permanent "tension states" which could provoke neurotic and psycho-neurotic disorders'.[59]

In addition to psychological problems, medical professionals writing in *The British Medical Journal* warned of the physical consequences of this type of work, stating, in 1957, that 'long periods of muscular inactivity, with greater responsibility, and too little physical and too much mental stress' might lead to an increase in degenerative vascular disease, noting that this was a development that was already apparent in the US.[60] Accounts from other industries highlighted the physical fatigue and emotional stress experienced by operatives working on production lines centred on conveyor belt systems. One operator in the car component industry recalled:

> The pressure was constant; it ensured a high level of production for the firm but it took its toll on us. At the end of the day we were all 'jaded', but which limbs ached the most depended on the particular job you'd been doing. The jobs were hard on the eyes – concentrating so hard all the time ... made your head buzz.[61]

Increased levels of physical and emotional stress arising from automation were used by trade union representatives as a bargaining tool for demanding reductions in working hours. In a dispute involving a worker at the Wills Tobacco factory in Bristol in 1956, for example, representatives from the Tobacco Workers' Union argued:

> with machine speeds higher now than ever before, and with 80% of the processes consisting of a repetitive nature, the present nine hour day is too long ... Whilst the employers may rightly claim that the increases in production were due largely to the introduction of new types of expensive machinery, it was also true that those machines had increased the mental strain of the workers concerned and the monotony of the work to be performed by those workers.[62]

In this case, the tribunal supported the evidence presented by the employer, thus providing a legal validation for industrialists' arguments that automation did not negatively impact on physical or mental health. Despite the warning presented by medical professionals and worker representatives, examination of debates between industrialists indicates that concerns over the ability of the workforce to adapt to these types of change were readily dismissed. The President of the Institution of Production Engineers, for example, stated at an industry conference in 1955 that:

> the impact of automation on the mass of working people is not, in my view, very likely to bring them new worries. The great expansion in mechanisation is conditioning men to accept change.[63]

Archival evidence suggests that anxiety and psychological pressure arose as much from the expectation and fear of change as from the actual experience and reality. Browne argued that the prospect of automation might give rise to a 'transient feeling of tension in the early months' which would disappear once workers had got used to the new machines.[64] A study carried out by the Industrial Working Party for the Boot and Shoe Industry in 1946 supported this theory, noting that once workers had become familiar with new automated systems, they did ultimately acknowledge the changes as an improvement in their working conditions. Their report states that, at one factory where automation had been newly introduced, the alteration 'was not well liked at first', but workers 'soon adapted themselves to the new arrangement and found they were less fatigued at the end of the day's work'.[65] There was, however, one issue which dominated worker concerns above all other throughout this period, and which had featured prominently in public conceptions of automation. If the nature of post-war industrial work was to be determined by the demands of new technology, then who was in control: management or worker; man or machine?

Controlling the Line: The Impact of Time and Motion Study

The issue of control in the maintenance of mental health is a crucial but highly complex one. In terms of health in the workplace, 'control' was defined as the freedom of individuals to make decisions affecting their immediate working environment. This included such factors as the pace and rhythm of work, the choice of working position, the allocation of tasks and adjustment of the temperature or humidity of the workplace. It was also framed around a complex interplay between different agents, including management hierarchies, trades unions, independent consultants, politicians and individual workers. The subject of workplace control and its impact on industrial relations and economic performance in post-war British industry has been the subject of historical investigation.[66] However, the relationship between production control and worker health has been less fully explored. In the context of post-war industrial production, the key factor which dominated debates about the impact of automation on health was the setting of the speeds at which automated production lines would run.

Decisions over machine speed were framed by the theories and methodologies of 'Time and Motion Study', an idea introduced by Frederick Winslow Taylor (1856–1915), in the US in 1911.[67] Presented as a form of 'scientific management' widely referred to as 'Taylorism', this system ensured that every aspect of a task was broken down into an individual action. The time that each action took to complete was then measured and recorded with a stop-watch. When the actions of several workers were measured, an average time for the production task could be calculated, providing the basis for the settings of each machine in a production line.[68] Taylor's original approach was later adapted by his student Frank Bunker Gilbreth (1868–1924) to include the filming of actions by motion camera, and it was this system that was widely adopted in British factories throughout the 1950s.[69] A founding member of the Society for the Promotion of Scientific Management, Gilbreth and his wife Lillian (1878–1972) developed an adaptation of Taylorism that attempted to encompass the human element as well as the technical. Gilbreth devised a technique of work measurement called 'micro-motion study', employing a motion picture camera to record the performance of a worker on a job, with a clock calibrated in hundredths of a minute placed in viewing range.[70] This technique enabled an analysis of the motions, time and condition surrounding the job. The operating speed of the automated production lines would subsequently be set at the 'Standard Time' pace identified by Time and Motion consultants.

In his study of Taylorism and scientific management in the inter-war period, Rabinbach has noted that, whilst embraced by industrialists seeking ways of increasing individual worker efficiency, Taylor's system was criticized by those who warned that it jeopardized the health and safety of workers through a blatant disregard for workers' health and well-being. He has particularly highlighted French opposition to the system, where the approach was condemned by trade union leaders as 'ferocious', 'barbaric' and 'the organisation of exhaustion'.[71] He has also argued that Taylor's system shifted effective control from the shop floor to management, a development that had significant implications for worker health.[72]

Historical analysis of Taylorism in the post-war period validates this conclusion. Studies have focused on the application of these strategies predominantly in the context of the Ford Motor Company, an adaptation referred to as 'Fordism'. Studies have emphasized the ways in which 'Fordism' became synonymous with a management approach based on surveillance, supervision and discipline, particularly in consideration of the establishment of a new British factory at Halewood, Merseyside, in 1963.[73] Authoritarian surveillance, together with the intensification of productivity through accelerated processes and increased competition, heightened physiological and psychological pressure on workers, reinforcing the potential for physical, mental and emotional problems. Whilst the application of scientific management at Ford was, as historians acknowledge, an exceptional case within British industry, it served to provide a model for manufacturing efficiency that other companies sought to emulate. Consequently, Time and Motion practices were adopted across many different industries in Britain in the years immediately following the Second World War.

The widespread adoption of Time and Motion Study methodologies meant that many production line workers were carrying out specific tasks at a constant speed that was dependant on a range of variable factors, such as the targets of a particular factory or department, the demands of specific customer orders, the level of urgency of completion of orders or the judgements of individual foremen or supervisors. The necessity for workers to keep pace with pre-set production lines resulted in both physical and emotional problems. Physical strain could occur, for example, from the repetitive nature of the task. One movement might have to be repeated several thousand times in each shift, causing problems with repetitive strain injuries and muscle pain, particularly in the hands, arms, neck and shoulders. Physical pain was exacerbated in instances where operators were new to specific tasks or where established tasks were altered. Contemporary sociological surveys of production line work illustrated these problems. One operator recalled the unrelenting nature of this type of work:

> I was completely exhausted. I had terrible pains in my neck and back, and found it hard to keep up with the speed of the line – but the trays kept coming so I just had to carry on.[74]

Problems arose particularly in situations where the calculations produced by Time and Motion Study experts severely underestimated the time that workers would take to carry out tasks effectively. An indication of the emotional pressure arising from this type of problem was presented by the Joint Shop Stewards' Committee at the Ford Motor Company in 1962:

> An estimated timing is laid out before a new model is built and as the time allowed is too short there is constant pressure by the company to get the man to do the job in the estimated time. A man may be told that he should do a job in two minutes when in fact he needs five minutes. Then the company will continually 'chase up' to get the job done in two minutes.[75]

Conscientious employers built in specific periods of time to allow for certain necessary actions outside of the immediate production demands. At Somerset shoe manufacturer C. & J. Clark, a pioneering advocate of Time and Motion Study in Britain from 1946 onwards, additional allowance was built into the 'Standard Rate' to cover two ten minute periods for 'attention to personal needs, fatigue and numerous small happenings such as waiting for work, minor machine breakdowns, obtaining instructions and repairing faults'.[76] However, accounts from other factories indicate that this allowance time was not always included. In setting out his vision for Time and Motion practice at Ford, Henry Ford stated in 1922 that 'a man must have every second necessary, but not a single unnecessary second'.[77] This view appeared to frame the approaches of some employers in the post-war period, with one worker on a car component line recalling:

> We couldn't do the things you would normally not think twice about, like blowing your nose or flicking hair out of your eye; that cost valuable seconds and no time was allowed for it ... If you couldn't keep up with the line, you were out.[78]

Problems arising from working to controlled speeds were highlighted in the annual report of the Chief Inspector of Factories in 1963, which stated that: 'When fatigue does occur in persons working at their own speed, a simple deterioration of performance occurs, but in work at controlled speeds, hurried actions and judgements result, quickly leading to a disruption of performance'.[79] He went on to highlight the link between control and mental health, observing that 'one example of the latter might be over-activity exhibited by individuals who find they cannot control a situation, or who anticipate that they will not be able to control it. As fatigue develops, over activity may be replaced by inertia'.[80]

One of the key problems with Time and Motion Study was that the implementation of timings and calculations was open to abuse by employers. These occurrences are illustrated in disputes over 'speed-up'. Machines would be set at an agreed rate at the beginning of a shift but the speed would be increased as the shift progressed. Workers at Ford's Dagenham factory, for example, highlighted the way in which the managers would increase the workload on the line by 'gradually increasing the line speed with more cars going down per hour without any increase in the labour force'.[81] This problem was also noted in a paper on Time and Motion Study commissioned by the Trades Unions' Congress (TUC) in 1949. It stated that 'to many union members the terms are synonymous with "speed-up" and involve further breaking down of craft and "inhuman standardization"'.[82]

The mental and emotional stress arising from 'speed-up' was most clearly demonstrated in Hew Beynon's sociological survey of workers at Ford's Halewood Factory conducted in the late 1960s. Interviewing workers about their experience of controlled production lines, Beynon's study emphasized an extreme lack of consideration for the physical and mental well-being of workers by the Halewood management. One worker recalled, for example, the refusal of managers to stop the line if a worker was injured or taken ill:

> They wouldn't stop the fucking line. You could be dying and they wouldn't stop it. If someone was hurt the first thing the supervisor thought about was filling the job. He'd start doing the work before he made sure the bloke was all right. I tell you he could have been dying and they wouldn't have bothered.[83]

The reluctance to stop the line in these circumstances is also indicative of the high levels of pressure within management hierarchies to meet production targets. Beynon provides the most graphic example of the ways in which the application of Time and Motion Study was taken to extreme at Halewood, as one worker recalled the refusal of management to stop the line after a worker had suffered a heart attack:

> He collapsed ... y' know flat on the floor. His face was an awful grey colour. We all rushed round him like and the buzzer went. The line started. The foreman came running across shouting 'get to work ... get on the line'. And there we were sticking things on the cars and he was lying there. He must have been lying there ten minutes ... dead.[84]

Beynon's study provided a controversial account of the application of scientific management practices at Ford and was criticized at the time of its initial publication as being biased towards the militant trade unions.[85] Whilst there is clearly scope for further comparative studies into worker experience at Ford and other companies to gain a more balanced view of the implementation of Time and Motion Study methodologies, archival evidence indicates that significant anxieties arose from the anticipation of Time and Motion Study. Concerns are evident in letters sent to the TUC in the late 1940s from union representatives working in industries where these methods were being newly introduced. One letter from the Leicester and District Trades Council urged the TUC to 'take firm action against the introduction of Time and Motion methods in industry ... as it can be very detrimental to the operatives concerned'.[86] Recognizing the inevitability of the adoption of motion study throughout industry, the TUC sought a greater understanding of the methods, commissioning, in 1949, surveys by the Work Measurement Research Unit at the University of Birmingham and the National Production Advisory Council.[87] International conferences on work study and automation were also held at Transport House, London, in November 1954 and May 1956. The TUC concluded that 'much of the hostility to motion and time study is not directed to the methods themselves, but to the ways in which they have been used'.[88] Consequently, a series of training courses for shop stewards was instigated to familiarize them with the methodologies, thus placing them in a stronger position for negotiations with management over speed rates.[89] Confident that this would enable a degree of joint control, the TUC subsequently urged their members to co-operate with the process and support employers wishing to implement the systems.

Sources indicate, however, that neither the employers nor the unions gave any consideration to the possible negative impact on health of Time and Motion Studies, a position that was also evident in government-funded studies. Whilst accepting that 'automation is likely to create serious problems', a DSIR report on *Automation* published in 1956 emphasized the potential benefits of automation and failed to make any specific reference to health.[90] For employers, the overwhelming argument in favour of automation was that it frequently resulted in new wage structures, predominantly payment by piece-work, which replaced existing systems of payment by hourly rate.[91] Employers argued that automation therefore presented an unprecedented opportunity for workers to increase their earning potential, whilst also benefitting from reduced working hours. Tolliday has highlighted the successful role of incentivized piece-rates in ensuring worker co-operation and efficient continuous production throughout the 1950s and 60s.[92] However, the balance between pay and working conditions was a delicate one which could be easily upset by changes implemented by management through Time and Motion Study.

Despite the incentive of greater earning potential and the support of the trade unions, Time and Motion Study continued to be regarded with suspicion by the workforce in many factories and experts employed to assess and implement the timings were viewed as feared agents of the management, perceived by operatives as being 'on the other side'.[93] At Clarks's factory in Street, Somerset, the management was forced to concede in 1958 that the Motion Study Department was 'the most maligned department in the organisation'.[94] A series of articles promoting the department appeared in the company's staff magazine, *Clarks Courier*, in an attempt to improve the tense relationship between the 'motion study men' and the workers.[95] In addition, evidence from other factories indicates the emergence of worker agency in the development of strategies to mitigate the unrelenting demands of the assembly lines and to regain some degree of personal control. Common ploys were for operators to cause mechanical breakdowns on the lines so that additional rest periods could be taken whilst the machines were repaired.[96] Workers at Ford's Dagenham factory revealed further strategies:

> When new machinery is being brought into operation, and a section of the plant is speeded up, workers respond by sending half-finished cars down the line and refusing to co-operate in the speed-up or in getting the machine to work properly.[97]

The strategies of worker sabotage recorded in sociological studies imply that tensions between management and production workers around the implementation of Time and Motions Study played a more significant role in the decline of British industry in the second half of the twentieth century than has been previously acknowledged. Historical analysis of post-war British industrial decline indicates that, by the 1970s, employers had been unable to maintain direct control over the production processes on the shop floor.[98] There is scope for further historical analysis and comparative studies to gain greater insight into the experiences of individual workers subject to these methodologies and to the role played by the psychosocial changes arising from automation in the breakdown of industrial relations in this later period.

Conclusion

The implications of automated production processes for physical, mental and emotional health were clearly a cause of major concern throughout Britain in the second half of the twentieth century. Doctors focusing on the psychosocial health of the nation raised awareness of a range of potential factors that could have significant repercussions on worker health. They particularly emphasized factors that could impact on mental and psychological health, shifting concerns away from the emphasis on physical factors and issues of physiological fatigue which had dominated the inter-war period. The instigation of Time and Motion

Study practices accompanying automation had the potential to aid both the working conditions and earning potential of industrial workers, but the positive effects of scientific management greatly depended on the maintenance of a delicate balance between the demands of economic production targets and the physical abilities, limitations and emotional needs of individual operatives.

The conflicting nature of the evidence and the polarized opinions of scientists and medical professionals presented industrial employers with the opportunity to ignore the health implications of automated processes and draw on a range of scientifically validated studies and opinions which concluded that 'there is little evidence that automation really causes ill-health'.[99] They were consequently able to exploit the positive features of automation presented in these studies, notably, the potential for relieving the 'drudgery' and physical demands of industrial tasks and the opportunity for greater earning potential presented by new wage systems based around 'piece-work'. This position ignored a wealth of evidence which suggested that, far from providing opportunities for new categories of 'brain workers' to sit around 'waiting for nothing to happen', automation presented all workers with a range of new challenges and demands which could impact significantly on physical, mental and emotional well-being. Significant reductions in the numbers of workers needed to carry out automated tasks and a transformation in the nature and level of skills required meant that workers had to be able to adapt, both physically and psychologically, to rapidly advancing technological change in ways that were historically unprecedented.

Contemporary sources suggest that the greatest levels of psychological stress and anxiety arose as much from the fear and anticipation of potential changes brought about by automation as from the reality and experience of change. Similar fears about the stress induced by the acceleration of new industrial and communication technologies were evident in the writings of the American journalist Alvin Toffler (b.1938) and others.[100] Worker resistance to the widespread adoption of Time and Motion Study throughout British industry in the second half of the twentieth century therefore reflected wider social fears around the impact of modernity on everyday life at a time of immense social change, reinforcing concerns that the future nature of working life would be increasingly determined by the demands of machines and 'the tyranny of time'.[101]

6 CULTURAL CHANGE, STRESS AND CIVIL SERVANTS' OCCUPATIONAL HEALTH, *c.*1967–85

Debbie Palmer

In the 1960s, high levels of sickness absence and stress-related illnesses among civil servants prompted interest in occupational stress. Alarmed at the rising cost to the public purse, in 1962 the Civil Service set up a three-year study into sickness absence.[1] Interpreting the findings, the Service's Chief Medical Advisor, Sir Daniel Thomson (1912–76), argued that stress levels had risen because some employees had failed to adapt to rapid cultural change during the 1950s. The survey showed a social gradient with employees in the lowest grades having much higher absence rates than their senior colleagues. Thomson set out to determine what underlay this gradient but his report was suppressed and did not have a long-term impact. This chapter explores continuity and change in stress discourse between the 1960s and the 1980s by comparing Thomson's report with the Whitehall II study, which was set up by Sir Michael Marmot (1945–) in 1985 to investigate the importance of social class for health by following a cohort of office-based civil servants. I shall argue that, although both Thomson's and Marmot's research related a steep inverse social gradient to stress-related diseases, the accounts of stress mobilized by the two studies were different.

While we have a growing historical literature on the physiology of stress in the twentieth century, we know little about how theories of stress impacted on the health and performance of workers and organizations. Recent studies on occupational stress have begun to address its changing forms. Elianne Riska has suggested that although coronary-prone American middle-class white men, subsequently labeled Type A by Meyer Friedman and Ray Rosenman, occupied positions of control in the 1950s, they felt that responsibility at work to be an emotional burden. By the 1980s, these men were expected to cope with the stresses of work.[2] Anne Harrington, Charles Rosenberg and Kristian Pollock have considered cultural change as central to the ways in which stress emerged as a twentieth-century phenomenon, noting how the concept of stress became associated with the increasing pace of modern life leading to consequences for an individual's health.[3] The narrative of disease as a consequence of social and economic growth was powerful, Rosenberg explains, because it could be used 'in a variety of contexts with a variety of social motives'.[4] Its ability to be used selectively to support different views meant that it could locate the source of stress-related illness not only as the individual's responsibility and his or her failure to adapt to change, but also as the product of a 'pathogenic social structure'.[5] Thus the language of stress functioned, as Pollock argues, as a means of organizing ideas about social order.

The notion of cultural change also influenced 'scientific' conceptions of stress. Mark Jackson reveals how the science of stress was shaped by a wide range of socio-political and cultural, as well as biological, factors. The 1950s, Jackson argues, marked an important shift in the meaning of stress as far as laboratory science and medicine was concerned. Hans Selye (1907–82) and others began to employ the term stress 'to denote either the internal physiological processes generated by environmental pressures or the dynamic interaction between organisms and their environment'.[6] By extending these issues into the workplace, this chapter comprises three main sections: the first discusses the inter-related histories of stress and absenteeism; the second examines Thomson's study of sickness absence and stress in detail; and the final main section analyses Marmot's understanding of the relationship between stress, work and health.

Histories of Stress and Absenteeism

Occupational stress research in Britain began after the First World War with the establishment of the Industrial Fatigue Research Board, which developed into the Industrial Health Research Board under the Medical Research Council. Alongside the National Institute of Industrial Psychology, this group sponsored a large number of studies into stress and absenteeism, which were supplemented by the work of various personnel research committees during the Second World War.[7] By the mid-twentieth century, work was increasingly a focal point for concerns about the stress of life. Commentators attempted to determine the extent to which sickness absence rates had risen because of the ways in which individuals were unable to moderate stress. John Hill and Eric Trist (1909–93), for example, linked the rise in sickness absence at a steel works and a coalmine with individual personality characteristics. Drawing on Freudian ideas of illness as a form of escape, Hill and Trist concluded that sickness absence provided individuals with a way of temporarily withdrawing from the stress of work rather than leaving altogether. The 'accident-absence addicted minority' were, they argued, 'prone to paranoid hostility and apt to disown responsibility for what they do'. Poor relationships with employers were interpreted as the result of bad relationships with one's own super-ego.[8] Hill and Trist were criticized for focusing too exclusively on individual motivations and ignoring the social meaning of absences.[9]

James Lorimer Halliday (1897–1983), Regional Medical Officer for the Department of Health for Scotland, explained an increase in insurance incapacity claims between 1931 and 1936 in terms of the ways in which Western society was making modern populations sick. High sickness and absenteeism rates were expressions of 'neurosis', according to Halliday, indices of a 'sick society' caused by changes in the ways people lived and worked. A breakdown in traditional family and community relationships were two of the factors Halliday considered responsible for a decline in communities' health.[10] Halliday viewed psychosomatic illness within a Freudian framework, as a form of dependent regression.[11]

Halliday's work is significant because it suggested that changes in emotional life could be mapped through insurance claims rather than through individual case histories and that different social groups bore different mental costs in terms of stress and strain.[12] The surveillance of normal populations emerged in the Second World War as a way of remapping the spaces of illness, according to David Armstrong. Capturing illness as an experience rather than a lesion, surveillance of health problematized normality as it located illness outside the body. Symptoms and signs of illness were re-read as risk factors, opening up a space of future illness potential.[13] Epidemiological surveillance of the relationship between social class and health was also an integral aspect of the mid-twentieth-century social medicine movement. Concerns about social conditions and health, prompted by studies by James Spence (1892–1954) and John Boyd Orr (1880–1971), recognized the importance of poverty in the causation of disease, leading to a renewed emphasis on environmental causes of disease.[14]

Concern about high levels of absenteeism prompted the Medical Research Council's Social Medicine Research Unit to set up a study into sickness absence under the leadership of its director, Jerry Morris (1910–2009).[15] Morris's influence on post-Second World War public health and social medicine was profound.[16] His work with Richard Titmuss (1907–73) on the epidemiology of peptic ulcer mapped how social and material conditions were related to health outcomes.[17] As well as social factors, Morris's conceptualization of social medicine included ideas about lifestyle and modifying individual behaviour with respect to diet, physical exercise and smoking. The rise in sickness absence, Morris argued, was due to social change and its impact on individual attitudes to work.

Morris examined sickness benefit claims from 1949–64 and reported his findings at a meeting of the Section of Occupational Medicine of the Royal Society of Medicine chaired by Austin Bradford Hill (1897–1991). Despite 'advancing medical knowledge' and 'improving standards of living', Morris argued, claims for sickness benefit had rapidly increased between 1951–60, caused by 'a social revolution' in the mid-1950s. As society became more affluent, demonstrated by a marked increase in consumer expenditure and a growth in national insurance benefits and sick-pay schemes, so attitudes towards health and sickness, work and leisure had changed.[18] Capacity for work, Morris suggested, was 'far more than a medical problem, it is physical, mental and social – reflecting group behaviour, the mood of the time and a multitude of pressures'.[19]

The notion of cultural change not only played an important part in shaping contemporary ideas about stress, but also influenced explanations of men's and women's health. By the late 1960s a body of research agreed that women employees had much higher rates of sickness absence than men.[20] Contemporary commentators, including Alva Myrdal (1902–86) and Viola Klein (1908–73), linked the problem to domestic responsibilities, which, they argued, still rested on women, producing 'conflicts of loyalty' between work and family life.[21] Despite the challenge of juggling two roles, Myrdal and Klein concluded that married women employees were in better mental health than married women who did not work.[22] Stephen Taylor (1910–88), assistant editor of *The Lancet* and a rising medical politician, confirmed in 1938 that young suburban housewives were prone to a new type of neurosis that resulted from modern civilization frustrating instinctive desires and from the failure to achieve emotional balance.[23] Other contemporary explanations of women's high absence rates emphasized the characteristics of women's work, particularly the fact that women generally held low-status, low-paid and repetitive jobs.[24] In her recent historical studies, Ali Haggett suggests that women's higher rates of illness can be attributed in in part to the fact that they were more likely to report symptoms. She also questions feminist critiques of the traditional domestic role by arguing that many women in the 1950s and 1960s found great satisfaction in domestic roles and that mental illness was more likely to be caused by relationship breakdown.[25]

By the 1950s, both stress and rising sickness absence were linked to individual personality characteristics as well as to broader group responses to rapid social change. While Freudian ideas were influential in both cases, epidemiological studies also identified a relationship between social class and health and the importance of environment in disease, but had yet to focus on explanations of the social gradient of stress-related ill-health. It was against this background that Thomson interpreted the causes of rising sickness absence among civil servants.

Daniel Thomson's *Sickness Absence Report*, 1967

The idea that sickness absence could be managed by improved epidemiological studies began to attract government interest in the mid-twentieth century. Pressure for civil service reform increased in the late 1960s partly because of a shift towards a managerial view of government, which involved transferring ideas about management techniques developed in private sector management into public sector organizations.[26] Led by Harold Wilson (1916–95), the Labour Party came to power in 1964 on a new deal of modernizing Britain through the application of science, technology and best management practices in a revised version of the pre-First World War campaign for 'national efficiency'.[27] Britain's sluggish economic performance together with the post-Suez problem of its changing place in the world, provided a context of self-doubt and questioning, prompting debates about what was wrong with Britain in the late 1950s and 1960s.[28] The Civil Service came under scrutiny following accusations that it was outdated and attached too little importance to management techniques.[29] Studies found that most top grade civil servants lacked management training, had largely irrelevant educational backgrounds and were becoming more socially exclusive.[30] According to John Garrett, the public and parliament 'suddenly vilified [the civil service] for being too well paid, too well pensioned and too luxuriously staffed'.[31]

One problem was that the concept of a job for life made it difficult to remove inefficient members of staff. Tensions developed between doctors and managers about how to remove poorly performing employees. Doctors complained that managers preferred to use medical retirement, with its more generous pension, than the complicated and long-winded formal procedures for dismissal of unproductive staff.[32] In the early 1960s, personnel officers (or 'establishment officers', as they were known in the Civil Service) began to discuss the problem of irregular attenders whose absence was attributed to ill-health.[33] Policy at this time involved a welfare officer either visiting the employee at home or interviewing them at work; if no improvement followed, the employee was referred to the Treasury Medical Adviser and retired on medical grounds. [34]

In 1965, the subject of attendance was raised again when establishment officers complained of a small minority who took frequent absences because of minor ailments that did not justify medical retirement but caused significant management problems.[35] Doctors argued that cases of medical retirement were often more about inefficiency, that departments relied on them to make management rather than medical decisions and that they were forced 'into phony decisions'.[36] Departments were instructed to treat all frequent absences as inefficiency.[37] Guidelines defined unacceptable amounts of sick leave and a study into sickness absence was set up by Sir Walter Chiesman (1900–73), Thomson's predecessor, partly in response to union pressure criticizing the Medical Service for being too detached and impersonal.[38]

In 1966, Harold Wilson's concern about a lack of professionalism in the Service prompted the Committee on the Civil Service, under the chairmanship of Lord John Fulton (1902–86), to examine its structure, recruitment, training and management. For political historians, the Fulton Committee is remembered because it is seen as a major landmark in the historical development of the Civil Service.[39] In the present context, however, its importance lies in its impact on the reorganization of Thomson's occupational health service. Of particular interest in this regard, is the Committee's criticism of the very small number of civil servants dismissed for inefficiency. Efficiency was the report's driving force and it condemned the fact that only twenty-three civil servants on average were dismissed annually for misconduct or inefficiency out of a total workforce of 450,000.[40]

The Fulton Report recommended that management of the Civil Service be taken away from the Treasury and located in a new Civil Service Department (CSD), which was established on 1 November 1968 and included Thomson's Medical Advisory Service (MAS). Thomson's role was to reorganize the MAS to improve control of sickness absence, and, although he wrote of his determination to end management's practice of using medical retirement as a way of removing incompetent employees, the structure of the new MAS was shaped around ways of helping management to identify the inefficient, a term that Thomson closely associated with 'stress'.[41]

Thomson set up a surveillance service, which used employees' medical records to help identify the 'inefficient', particularly those with 'poor sickness records' or those who demonstrated evidence of 'chronic physical or mental illness'.[42] As an epidemiologist, Thomson had previously researched tuberculosis and poliomyelitis,[43] but in 1965 he switched his focus from infectious to chronic disease. Reflecting Halliday's and Morris's thinking that social change had a detrimental impact on the general population's health, Thomson used his inaugural presidential address to the Royal Society of Medicine's Section of Epidemiology and Preventive Medicine to argue that epidemiological research should focus on the rising levels of chronic disease caused by 'patterns of social change'. Mental health, he argued, was gaining importance because epidemiology was now concerned with quality of life rather than longevity.[44]

Thomson's reorganization plans also included providing a more personal clinical service, with doctors regularly attending departments to see employees on a one-to-one basis, to identify 'the stressed and inefficient at work'.[45] As I will show later, Thomson understood stress as an individual rather than a social problem that was mediated through internal psychological resources rather than external social structures. This explains why he wanted to provide individual medical care. The MAS already provided one-to-one clinics in several departments giving advice about 'work conditions, sickness absence and inefficiency'.[46] Thomson was critical of the ways that GPs dealt with sickness absence, alleging that they handed out sickness absence certificates too easily, sometimes 'at the patients' whim'.[47] He wanted to provide a clinical service run by hospital consultants.[48] But his views about the best way to structure occupational health care differed from many Civil Service doctors who advocated a more radical approach along the lines set out by the British Medical Association (BMA) in its 1961 report *The Future of Occupational Health Services.*[49] The BMA prioritized preventative measures and recommended that services should include health education, prevention and treatment of accidents and support following illness.[50] Thomson was determined to resist civil service doctors' demands to change the framework of occupational health care in this way, and his ability to do so may have been reinforced by the government's reluctance to legislate a national occupational health policy, despite pressure from the BMA and the Trades Union Congress.[51]

The creation of the CSD and its review of medical services forced Thomson to justify his plans for the MAS. Drawing on his epidemiological background, he turned to statistical evidence to support his case, arguing that the department's contribution to the drive for efficiency would be to control sickness absence. He set out his interpretation of the sickness absence data in an introduction to *The Sickness Absence Report*. Establishment officers suppressed Thomson's introduction and the report was published without his contribution in January 1970, eighteen months after *The Fulton Report*.[52] Thomson's ideas reflected the interest of the organization rather than the employees, for whom he showed little sympathy. He was particularly critical of the personal shortcomings of lower grade civil servants. Establishment officers may have been anxious that, if widely known, his ideas would have exacerbated rising tensions among civil servants, which culminated in strike action in 1973.

The study was based on a 5 per cent random sample of sick leave records for 450,000 non-industrial civil servants. These were mainly desk-based workers and were divided into four main categories stratified according to grade and status: an administrative category of about 2,500 mostly university graduates; a professional class; an executive officers class; and a category of clerical officers, typists and messengers. The study measured the amount of certificated and uncertificated sick leave taken in each staff group to establish the general level of sickness, its frequency and duration and the pattern of cause of leave.[53] It found that only 5 to 10 per cent of employees were responsible for half the number of sickness absence episodes. Lower-grade civil servants experienced the highest incidence of illness in all eight of the disease categories studied.[54] Administrators took an average of 1.8 certificated days sick compared to the 12.7 taken by the lowest grade, male messengers. Causes of absence were coded by the fourteen main headings of the short list of the Eighth Revision of the International Classification of Diseases.[55] The eight disease categories chosen suggest that Thomson understood psychosomatic illnesses largely as stress related. A number of leading figures active in the field of stress research and psychosomatic medicine were interested in the organic consequences of stress reactions. Thomson's list included influenza and bronchitis; coronary thrombosis; angina; other circulatory disorders; digestive disorders; mental disorders; injuries; musculoskeletal disorder and pregnancy. Although there were significant differences, such as Thomson's omission of inflammatory, allergic and metabolic disorders, the conditions identified as stress-related causes of sickness absence clearly resembled Hans Selye's chronic 'diseases of adaptation' and the psychosomatic diseases studied by Franz Alexander (1891–1964) and his colleagues.[56]

Like many earlier advocates of social and psychosomatic medicine, Thomson understood the rise in psychosomatic illness as the product of rapid cultural change. The problem of sickness absence, he argued, was 'much more than a "medical" one', and reflected, 'group behaviour, molded by the mood of the times and a variety of social pressures'.[57] It was a 'manifestation of a malaise affecting modern society', one caused largely by changes in the nature of environmental stressors.[58] Shifting social patterns such as the extended family's loss of influence and the disappearance of small working units had changed employees' attitude to illness.[59] Furthermore, Thomson argued that modern living lowered a person's threshold to stress and this, he explained, was why 'the wide assortment of illnesses associated with stress [was] increasing'.[60]

Thomson attempted to combine social ideas about stress with the psychoanalysis of Freud. His model of stress disease was much closer to the Freudian idea of illness as a form of escape, rather than the alarm reaction or role adjustment proposed by Selye and Robert Kahn respectively.[61] Stress, according to Thomson, was mediated through internal psychological resources:

> If we are subjected to over-much stress, we will often react quite subconsciously against it by developing symptoms which will deliver us from the need to go on dealing with our life situation – we become ill or diseased.[62]

Thomson also used Freudian analysis to interpret the inverted gradient in sickness absence. Lower-grade employees, Thomson argued, lacked the capacity for hard work and were reluctant to take on responsibility. These grades, Thomson explained, attracted people who found security in working in large groups because of:

> an undesirable regression to childhood dependency; the group being the natural environment to the child. Frequently those who choose to work in large groups are self-selected since for them individual responsibility and freedom are repellent.[63]

Thomson considered 'insufficient responsibility' and lack of opportunity to be causes of physical and mental ill-health that could be treated by increasing responsibility and promotion.[64] Those who failed to achieve promotion were advised to avoid future stress by accepting their place in the natural physical and mental hierarchy. Thomson instructed them to 'accept without a feeling of jealousy or grievance at other people's rather better luck', arguing that some people have 'inherent great attributes' making them 'natural pace-makers and out-runners'.[65] Not only were lower-grade employees considered more likely to regress when stressed, but Thomson also noted that they often sub-consciously learned to repress their personalities in order to fit into the civil service culture of restraint.

This had disastrous effects on mental health, he added, and 'frequently culminated in a depressive breakdown between the ages of 45 and 55 when the psychic isolation [had] become unbearable'.[66] He recommended that civil servants detach themselves 'from the emotional pressure that people and organisations bring'.[67]

Thomson also considered the monotonous nature of civil service work detrimental, suggesting that 'mental illness was a product of coping with the dreary governmental treadmill' rather than pursuing 'the spirited adventure which evolution-wise life was intended to be'.[68] He perceived stress to be the consequence of failure to adapt to the modern work environment. Modern men and women, including civil servants, he argued, were 'finding it hard to escape from [their] biological past'. He understood the body in terms of mechanisms created in response to past environmental concerns, arguing that there was a poor fit between the repetitive nature of office work and humankind's genetic heritage shaped by centuries of hunting and gathering. Echoing Cannon's formulation of the flight or fight response, Thomson considered that what was once an appropriate instinctive response was no longer suitable to the modern age. This biological explanation facilitated an individualization of stress in so far that responsibility was placed on the biological individual who could do little to change his situation except for trying to modify outmoded instincts.

Administrators' resilient constitutions, as well as their capacity for and 'dedication to relatively interesting and responsible work', explained their resistance to stress.[69] Top grade civil servants had different, and superior, physical characteristics, Thomson argued, revealed to him by his experience of physical examinations over the years. Their exceptional fitness, he mooted, was a reflection of 'hereditary, environmental and intellectual factors' and their sickness record an example of 'how resilient the human constitution is and how it can thrive on hard work'.[70] Thomson's references to administrators as male was not accidental, but reflected the realities of work and promotion opportunities: there were only 236 women compared to 2,453 men in this grade in 1970.[71]

Thomson highlighted two key aspects of contemporary debate about work and health in the 1960s: gender and class. In 1967, women formed 40 per cent of the non-industrial workforce with the majority employed in the lower grades as clerical officers and assistants.[72] The belief that women were better at detailed and repetitive civil service work was regarded as justification for the fact that they populated the lowest paid and least rewarding grades.[73] Thomson's sickness absence study found that women had much higher rates of certificated and uncertificated sick leave than men and that their patterns of absence differed in so far that women took shorter and more frequent absences. The average annual number of certificated days for women was 9.8 days compared to men's 6.6.[74] Women took 70 per cent more sick leave than men mostly for minor complaints.[75] Gender also influenced the type of illnesses affecting civil servants. For example, women had higher rates of mental disorders than men, and mental disorder was the most common cause of female retirements compared to cardiovascular disease for men.[76] Men had longer periods of sick leave, but Thomson explained this by arguing that women's depressive illnesses were mostly related to the menopause and middle age and therefore more likely to respond to drug therapy.[77] He considered men's depression to be more serious and more insidious.

Married women's sickness absence rates were higher than those of single women and married and single men, a pattern explained by Thomson in terms of their 'divided loyalties'.[78] Although he considered the impact of other aspects of women's work, such as frequent job transfers, and the monotonous nature of work, he claimed that women used sick leave to cope with everyday life and family crises.[79] In the case of pregnancy, women were entitled to two months maternity leave, but according to Thomson, 'quite often the time off duty [was] extended on account of minor medical conditions' so that 'many doctors, both inside and outside the service, believe there is a certain amount of abuse'.[80] Rather than attempting to overhaul the maternity system, Thomson blamed individuals, interpreting sickness as a sign of personal weakness rather than a symptom of an inadequate system. However, in the case of female clerical staff absence he argued that the problem 'went beyond the strictly medical into the broadly psychological field' and that improvements were 'as much in the power of management and welfare services as in that of the medical'.[81] The crux of the matter was whether those women with a history of absence due to domestic crises were inefficient employees. For Thomson, the challenge was to separate management decisions about inefficiency from doctors' decisions about medical retirement.

A key aspect of Thomson's work focused on individual characteristics rather than the situational or environmental causes of stress. But in the 1970s, a radically different, and clearly international, approach to the phenomenon of work stress was emerging. Issues relating to work-related stress and its impact on individual health had been discussed in Sweden for many decades. Bertil Gardell (1927–87), professor of work psychology at Stockholm University, was one of the first to suggest that jobs that entailed relatively little worker autonomy or skill tended to be associated with poor mental health.[82] Researchers such as the American Robert Karasek and the Swede Thores Theorell investigated the association between work characteristics and mental health throughout the 1970s and 1980s.[83] Their conceptualization of stress in terms of demand and control was developed further by Jeffrey Johnson and Ellen Hall, who demonstrated that the degree of social support at work further influenced the onset of illness.[84] The British impact of this research agenda was clear. Michael Marmot (1945–) spent three months working with Theorell at the Karolinska Institute in Stockholm in 1984 and he credited this experience with forming the framework of his ideas for the Whitehall II study.[85]

Michael Marmot and the Whitehall II Study

Unlike the sickness absence study, which was set up and interpreted by civil servant doctors, the Whitehall II study was established by the independent epidemiologist Michael Marmot, from University College London. The study of 10,308 office-based civil servants aged between 38 and 65 years was funded by a series of small grants from the Medical Research Council (MRC), the National Heart, Lung and Blood Institute in the USA and the Health and Safety Executive.[86] The first Whitehall study had been set up in 1965 by epidemiologists Donald Reid (1914–77) and Geoffrey Rose (1926–93) from the London School of Hygiene and Tropical Medicine. Civil servants were chosen because of their large numbers, their ease of accessibility and the fact that Reid had close connections with Thomson.[87] The prevalent view, according to Marmot, was that poor people developed diseases of material deprivation and that rich people suffered from heart disease and peptic ulcer. The first Whitehall study showed this was not so: there was an inverse social gradient of mortality from virtually all causes, with lower grade of civil servants exhibiting a higher risk of death.[88]

Interest in inequalities in health developed in the 1980s following evidence that the gap was widening despite growing prosperity. Although health inequalities were much discussed in the pre-Second World War period, the advent of the National Health Service (NHS) promised a fresh start.[89] There was little discussion of inequalities in the early 1950s when relative poverty and unemployment were reduced to a fraction of pre-Second World War levels. But from then on unemployment levels rose at a gradually accelerating rate and health inequalities widened.[90] Dorothy Porter suggests there was a significant shift after the Second World War as researchers turned to social behaviour rather than social structural inequalities to explain disease.[91] In 1977, the Labour government appointed Sir Douglas Black (1913–2002) to chair a working group to review information on inequalities in health and suggest policy. This report confirmed that health inequalities were deepening and recommended that broad social policy change was necessary to improve the situation.[92] Published on an August bank holiday in 1980 with 260 copies available, this politically-sensitive report caused a media furore. Because of the moment and manner of its publication, its impact was greater, leading to a growth in research in health and inequality.[93]

Marmot had already developed an interest in health gradients during his doctoral dissertation on heart disease in Japanese immigrants to the USA, in 1975 at the University of California. Most epidemiologists at the time attributed Japanese longevity to their low-fat diet, but Marmot explained their low rates of heart disease in terms of the degree to which they were able to maintain their traditional culture, which provided a close-knit community with stress-reducing emotional and social support.[94] Social cohesion, Marmot argued, had a protective effect on health and this finding shaped his approach to the Whitehall II studies. Arriving in London after his PhD, Marmot was asked by Rose and Reid to consider Whitehall I findings from a social perspective. Marmot decided that it was not so much poverty but status that had a profound effect on people's health. 'What I think Whitehall I led me towards', he argued, 'was what goes on in the mind is very important for what goes on in the rest of the body. So we talk about psychosocial processes – how social influences affect the mind and how that in turn affects other parts of the body to change risk of disease'.[95] One of the key aims of the Whitehall II study was to identify the psychosocial processes responsible for inequalities in health.

Marmot also drew on studies of non-human primates for insights into the possible mechanisms linking social status to health. He relied heavily on the evolutionary psychological models proposed by Robert Sapolsky (1957–), who showed that in baboon populations lower status animals had higher levels of cortisol secretion.[96] Reflecting dominant theories of the biology of stress, Marmot argued that animal studies suggested that it was not smoking, lack of exercise or inadequate medical care that led to the social gradient in humans; rather predictability, control, threat to status, the presence or absence of social supports and the possibility of having outlets were the five key characteristics of potentially stressful situations.[97]

Marmot had a different perspective of civil servants' stress to Thomson. According to Marmot, stress was mediated through external social structures. His focus was measuring work and social life characteristics rather than the personal attributes of the worker. The individual was of interest but only in terms of his or her interface with society and the effects of structural factors on health. Differences that arose from the social environment and their impact on the causes of illness were, Marmot argued, more likely to emerge in the form of group differences. Previously trained as a medical practitioner, Marmot had spoken of his initial struggle to move away from investigating individual differences and towards relating patterns and rates of disease to the characteristics of particular societies.[98] The contrast between studying individuals and groups caused tension and controversy, particularly with psychologists whose core concern was with the former. For example, Richard Lazarus (1922–2002) and Susan Folkman,(1938–) amongst others, proposed a model that illustrated the role of psychological factors in mediating the relationship between work, the employee's personal attributes, the appraisal of threats and the ability to cope.[99]

The original research aim of the Whitehall II study was to investigate social and occupational influences on health and illness. The study included 3,413 women and 6,895 men. Participants were from clerical and office support grades, middle-ranking executive grades and senior administrative grades.[100] It adopted a different methodology to Thomson's study because of its interest in the association between stress and work characteristics. Like the earlier study it measured sickness absence but to assess the work environment it supplemented these statistics with self-reported questionnaire data, personnel managers' ratings of participants' jobs, assessment of work characteristics and a range of physiological tests. The first phase of data was completed in 1988, since when there have been a further six phases of data collection. Its findings have suggested that the lower the grade of employee, the higher the morbidity and mortality rates in a range of diseases including coronary heart disease, diabetes and metabolic syndrome.

In searching for the causes of the social gradient, the Whitehall II study noted that social gradients in health could change.[101] This challenged Thomson's view that psychosomatic illness was caused by genetic profile and therefore fixed, that high-grade civil servants were genetically predisposed to both good health and achieving high social position, and that clerical officers were predisposed to worse health and work with little responsibility. The fact that the gap in life expectancy between men in the top and bottom social classes had increased between 1972 and 1996, from 5.5 years to 5.7 years, Marmot argued, was evidence that its causes were social.[102]

Marmot used two models to devise a conceptual framework for thinking about psychosocial disease. The first was Karasek and Theorell's demands-control-support model (DCS), which developed from Gardell's work and focused exclusively on work characteristics. The DCS model predicted that job strain was likely to occur when a worker faced high job demands in combination with low job control and low social support from colleagues and/or managers. It presupposed a mismatch or imbalance between the psychological demands of work and the resources of the individual. The study found that the combination of high demand and low control influenced various biological pathways. Thus, lower grade civil servants had higher rates of sickness absence, mental illness, heart disease, diabetes and lower back pain.[103] The association between low levels of control and an increased risk of heart disease was independent of a range of individual personal characteristics.[104]

One of the problems with this model was that it failed to grasp the role of consciousness in mediating the relationship between work characteristics and health. Whilst it explained why certain working environments were stressful, it did not account for why some people had the ability to withstand job strain. Its dependence on self-reported assessments was criticized for not taking into account whether these reports were influenced by factors independent of the workplace, which might have affected an individual's state of mind leading to pessimistic assessments of work characteristics and health.[105] This criticism was perhaps unfounded because the Whitehall II study did acknowledge the importance of individual perception. For example, susceptibility to psychiatric disorder related to work was recognized as inseparable from how the person perceived, interacted with and reacted to working conditions.[106]

The notion that employees' response to work stress might entail both a subjective and social dimension was partially recognized by the study's adoption of Johannes Siegrist's (1943–) effort-reward imbalance model.[107] This attempted to extend the epidemiological approach of the DCS model by incorporating subjective assessments and interpretations expressed by workers. It suggested that mental distress and its health consequences arose when a high degree of effort was not reciprocated with adequate rewards in the form of pay, status and opportunities for advancement.[108] A distinction was drawn between extrinsic effort (situational factors which made work more demanding) and intrinsic effort (personal factors such as motivation). The Whitehall II study claimed that an effort-reward imbalance was associated with increased risk of alcohol dependence, mental distress, sickness absence and heart disease.[109] The strength of this model was that it began to account for the ways in which subjective dimensions of work characteristics were experienced and interpreted by workers. But its dependence on self-report data raised difficulties of identifying the degree to which perceived lack of reciprocity in effort and rewards was determined by work-related factors, factors outside work or the personality traits of the worker.

Like earlier sickness absence studies, the Whitehall II study revealed a higher rate of minor morbidity among women but more serious rates of morbidity and mortality amongst men. Marmot and his colleagues concluded that this may have been the result of women's position in the employment grade structure, which remained comparatively poor. 50 per cent of women taking part in the study were employed in the clerical and office support grades compared to 9 per cent of men.[110] The study also suggested that women's high mild morbidity rates were either because 'the health effects of the work/family interface are greater for women' or 'the work/family interface may be the actual reason for the absence but a subjective medical reason may be given because it is considered more acceptable'.[111] According to Feeney, this explained women's higher rates of headache, migraine and neurosis.[112]

For Thomson, this relationship between stress, work and domesticity was to be understood in terms of the individual civil servant who had to deal with 'the nagging wife' or 'the domineering boss' at home.[113] By contrast, Marmot and other Whitehall II researchers explained the stress of the work/home interface using the demands-control-support model. Similar to the negative effects of having low control at work, women who reported low control at home had higher risks of heart disease. However, in contrast to Thomson, Whitehall II found that the stress of conflict between work and family life affected the health of men as well as women.[114] The crucial factor appeared to be the degree of control over one's life.[115] Being from a lower household social position was a significant predictor of low control at home among women. It was this group of women, the study tentatively suggested, that lacked the material and psychological resources to cope with excessive household demands and family responsibilities.[116]

Conclusion

In 2011, British employees took 131 million days off sick. Sickness absence rates remain a problem for employers who pay nine billion pounds annually in sick pay and employees who suffer through loss of income as well as from the illness itself. Although overall absence rates have fallen by 25 per cent since 1993, the rate attributed to stress/anxiety/depression appears to be rising, from 11.8 million in 2010 to 13.3 million in 2011.[117] Interpreting this rise is complicated but it suggests that we still do not fully understand, and are not able to provide solutions to, the problems of workplace stress. Marmot's seminal work on health inequalities now informs government policy discussions, but his outstanding theoretical contributions to understandings of work stress have yet to be translated into policy or practice.

This chapter has argued that understandings of work stress have been historically specific and shaped by structural, political, scientific and cultural conditions that change across time. How stress at work was understood changed significantly from the late 1960s to the 1980s. For Thompson, the changing focus of epidemiology from infectious to chronic diseases, reactions to rapid social and cultural change during the 1950s and civil service reform all shaped his interpretation of the relationship between stress and work. For Marmot, Scandinavian accounts of work stress as the product of external work characteristics, primate studies and evidence of a widening gap in health inequalities in the 1970s together provided the conceptual and experimental basis for his ideas.

The chapter has also shown how understandings of work stress shifted in the late twentieth century away from emphasizing the importance of the role of individual personality characteristics towards stressing external social structures. Although Marmot attempted to redress this balance by including the effort-reward imbalance model and self-report data, critics argue that Whitehall II studies have not paid enough attention to the personality traits of the worker.[118] Organizational factors are now seen to be better predictors of sickness absence than individual psychological correlates, yet stress management is most often aimed at individuals rather than organizational change. In 2006, a team of researchers from six European countries concluded that 'managers still seem to think stress and mental health problems are a sign of "weakness" of the individual rather than something the organisation needs to change'.[119] It appears that, in spite of Marmot's contributions, individual weakness and personal responsibility have not disappeared from narratives of stress at work.

7 MEN AND WOMEN UNDER STRESS: NEUROPSYCHIATRIC MODELS OF RESILIENCE DURING AND AFTER THE SECOND WORLD WAR

Mark Jackson

In 1945, two American psychiatrists working for the US Army Air Forces published an influential study of the impact of stress on human behaviour. Having examined and treated several thousand airmen suffering from some form of psychological or psychosomatic illness during the Second World War, Roy R. Grinker (1900–90) and John P. Spiegel (1911–91) claimed that neurotic reactions to warfare were triggered not primarily by individual weakness or failure, as was often assumed, but by the 'harsh reality' of combat: the 'stress of war', they argued in the first line of the book, 'tries men as no other test that they have encountered in civilized life'. Grinker and Spiegel's explicit emphasis on men in their opening statement was not accidental. Although they sometimes referred generically to 'individuals' or 'humans' suffering from stress-related symptoms, their analysis focused exclusively on the manner in which male Air Force personnel experienced and manifested the stress of combat, either during active service overseas or following repatriation.[1]

Grinker and Spiegel's interest in the reactions of male pilots reflected the contemporary reality of warfare, and the military and political significance of returning ill and injured servicemen to the front line or to productive work as rapidly as possible. The exclusion of women from combat and the primacy of concerns about identifying vulnerable aircrew and reducing the impact of neuroses on operational efficiency, led perhaps inevitably to an emphasis on the psychology of men under stress. But the investigative framework adopted by Grinker and Spiegel also neglected a reality. Women did serve in the armed forces, particularly in the air force but also in navies and armies, on both sides of the Atlantic and they were routinely exposed, like their male counterparts, to the dangers of bombardment and anxieties associated with separation. In addition, wartime diaries reveal the manner in which women played active roles in promoting civilian morale, social cohesion and industrial productivity in the face of imminent death and destruction.[2] However, the commonality of men's and women's experiences during combat was neatly elided in contemporary studies of stress, which, by focusing on 'valiant men', tended to reinforce the subsidiary, and mainly passive role played by women in maintaining or restoring social stability. In Grinker and Spiegel's analysis on the impact of battle stress, women figured only in terms of their capacity to facilitate or hinder the domestic and sexual rehabilitation of husbands and fathers returning home from the war.[3]

Military preoccupations with men under stress were replicated elsewhere during and after the Second World War, particularly in North America but also in Britain. Studies of the mental and physical health of soldiers in the Korean and Vietnam conflicts, psychological experiments exploring the behaviour of college students under pressure, investigations into the effects of fatigue and stress on commercial pilots and clinical accounts of stress-related illnesses amongst workers focused almost exclusively on men and downplayed the effects of stress on women.[4] Even studies that acknowledged that personality, emotional responsiveness and cultural identity were key variables in determining an individual's capacity to withstand stress, such as the investigations carried out by American psychologist Richard S. Lazarus (1922–2002) and his colleagues, tended to treat men and women together as 'a homogeneous group' and to rely on men as exemplary experimental subjects.[5] Although some studies of occupational stress and sickness absence foregrounded women's vulnerability to domestic and workplace pressures,[6] when women were considered separately in post-war reflections on the determinants and consequences of stress, it was more usually in terms of their propensity to induce (or less often mitigate) anger and emotional disturbances in men.[7]

The relative absence of clinical interest in the behaviour of women under stress or in investigating the similarities and differences between men and women is striking, given the strong tradition on both sides of the Atlantic of regarding psychological vulnerability as a feminine attribute. Framed by assumptions about the appropriate roles of men and women at work and in the home, late nineteenth-century studies of insanity and neurasthenia suggested a greater tendency for women, particularly amongst the upper classes, to suffer from nervous fatigue and exhaustion in response to the pace and pressure of modern lives.[8] In the early twentieth century, the boredom and loneliness of life in the suburbs were thought to be responsible for inducing anxiety in emotionally labile middle-class housewives: according to the English physician Stephen Taylor (1910–88), the suburban neurotic was created by a combination of constitutional susceptibility, the transformation of domestic responsibilities and expectations, and the growth of certain forms of leisure and popular entertainment.[9] Although post-Second World War feminist writers, such as Betty Friedan

(1921–2006), Germaine Greer (b.1939) and Ann Oakley (b.1944), attempted to reconfigure neuroses in women as the products of patriarchal oppression and culturally-determined constraints, rather than biological difference, accounts of mental illness continued to be coloured by a persistent belief in the greater emotional and psychological instability of women.[10]

Historians of stress, like their scientific and clinical predecessors and peers, have tended to overlook the significance of gender. While historians of psychiatry have constructively analysed the impact of gender on the manifestations and representation of neuroses and other forms of mental illness, comparable studies of stress have largely ignored the place of gender in shaping scientific theories of stress, clinical debates about patterns of stress-related diseases and the manifestations and experiences of stress. Critical focus on the impact of contemporary notions of masculinity and femininity on the prescription and consumption of tranquillizers, evident in studies on both sides of the Atlantic,[11] has rarely been replicated in historical accounts of stress and health. Often working within, rather than challenging, the intellectual frameworks constructed by stress theorists, scholarly studies of the history of stress have persistently disregarded gendered disparities in personal experiences, clinical models and treatment modalities.[12] It is only recently that historians and sociologists have begun to pay greater attention to gender as a key determinant of scientific accounts and subjective experiences of stress.[13]

In part, the relative absence of nuanced historical analyses of gender and stress reflects on-going political interest in the significance of shell shock, combat stress and post-traumatic stress disorder, a spectrum of complaints that continue to be identified solely with the male theatre of war.[14] Military fixations with damaged soldiers have been reproduced by historians of stress, who have also regarded war neurosis, in all its guises, as the archetypal modern stress reaction. Yet the decision to exclude gender from historical studies of stress threatens to distort analysis in key ways. It tends not only to marginalize women's experiences of stress, but also, in the present context, to artificially detach women's experiences of war from those of men. As Carol Acton has pointed out in her provocative study of the correspondence between Vera Brittain and Roland Leighton during the First World War, the exclusion of women from histories of war, which has its origins in their 'exclusion from combat', operates to reinforce assumptions about the passivity of women in relation to men and to emphasize the separation, rather than connectedness or interdependence, of men's and women's stories and memories of war. For Acton, historians should be contesting, not reinforcing, the 'polarisation of men and women, home and front, that has become a conventional trope of war'.[15]

By exploring the evolution and reception of neuropsychiatric models of men's and women's responses to stress during and after the Second World War, this chapter aims to invigorate, and more closely connect, historical studies of gender, stress and warfare. The first section analyses the manner in which military medical officers understood what came to be known as 'flying stress' (or sometimes 'aeroneurosis') in terms of non-specific physiological and psychological reactions to the dangers and fatigue associated with prolonged aerial combat. Borrowing from both biological and psychoanalytical models of emotional adjustment to hardship, this formulation established men as the clinical norm for investigating and understanding stress reactions and reinforced prescribed standards of heroic masculine, and, by inference, timid feminine behaviour in the face of fear. Analysis of wartime and post-war discussions of flying stress suggests that experiences of shell shock in the First World War did not challenge hegemonic notions of masculinity to the extent suggested by some historians: participants in debates about the pressures on pilots continued to adhere to traditional Victorian principles of masculine resilience in the face of danger at least into the third quarter of the twentieth century.[16]

The second section of this chapter focuses on a singular study of stress amongst female British air force personnel, carried out by two psychiatrists working at a Royal Air Force centre for neuropsychiatric patients during the mid-1940s. Although they acknowledged that women serving in the Women's Auxiliary Air Force were exposed, like their male counterparts, to extremely stressful situations, the authors of this investigation emphasized the primary role of women's character and temperament in determining psychological health. In doing so, they betrayed and bolstered contemporary assumptions about the emotional immaturity and psychological vulnerability of women. Fashioned by traditional discourses about the domestic responsibilities of mothers and wives and by contemporary concerns about rising levels of mental illness, wartime and post-war studies of stressed women, like those of stressed male pilots, served only to consolidate normative notions of masculine strength and feminine frailty: norms that were precisely what was at stake in contemporary analyses of combat stress. In spite of evidence that all air force personnel and civilians suffered in similar ways from much the same traumas during and after the war, well-entrenched cultural norms served to highlight differences, rather than similarities, between the experiences and resilience of women and men under stress.

The Human Response to Flying Stress

The concept of flying stress was introduced by the British physician James L. Birley (1884–1934). Having qualified in both physiology and medicine, Birley spent most of his working life as a physician at St Thomas's Hospital and the National Hospital of Nervous Diseases in London and became renowned, according to his obituary, for his attempts during the First World War to describe the reactions of 'the normal individual to the stress and strain of an entirely strange and exacting environment'.[17] It was as Chief Medical Officer to the Royal Air Force that Birley observed at first hand the impact of nervous breakdowns amongst pilots during the battle of the Somme, when large numbers of healthy young men had struggled to cope with the demands of 'an unnatural and dangerous occupation'.[18] Like its terrestrial counterpart shell shock, flying stress was thought to be largely a product of mental strain, sleeplessness, fatigue and fear, generated in this instance by the psychological strain of flying at altitude, oxygen deprivation and the proximity of death.[19] When a pilot's psychological defences were weakened by 'shock or prolonged strain', Birley argued in his Goulstonian lectures in 1920, he began to experience a lack of confidence and a range of physical symptoms such as palpitations and shortness of breath. If not managed effectively, this stage of what pilots referred to as 'wind up' often progressed to a more debilitating state of anxiety: 'He becomes irritable, unsociable, morose, losing his inspiring personality, and adopting a black outlook on things in general'.[20] Turning increasingly, but unsuccessfully, to smoking and alcohol to maintain his composure, the stressed pilot eventually surrendered to his emotions, leading to the inevitable termination of his flying career.

Although he emphasized the situational determinants of flying stress, Birley recognized the prominent role of temperament and emotional reactivity in shaping men's ability to fly and their resilience under pressure. His formulation of the integrated psychological and physical reactions triggered by flying was based not only on his observations of pilots, but also on his reading of the work of Sigmund Freud (1856–1939) on instinct, W. H. R. Rivers (1864–1922) on mental reactions to the environment and Walter B. Cannon (1871–1945) on the physiology of emotions.[21] Like many of his clinical colleagues, Birley occupied an ambiguous position within the armed forces. Employed to protect the mental and physical health of recruits, military doctors were also commissioned to bolster the forces' commitment to operational efficiency, which demanded the identification of temperamentally unfit or malingering soldiers, the elimination of manpower wastage and the restoration of personnel to the front line as rapidly and effectively as possible.[22] In contrast to some of his contemporaries, however, Birley refused to condemn the distressed pilot and maintained that techniques for accurately identifying the physical and psychological characteristics of the ideal pilot or soldier remained inadequate. According to Birley, flying stress was a 'perfectly normal reaction to a very abnormal environment'.[23] The blame for rising rates of nervous breakdown during the later stages of the war, he argued, lay primarily with the policy of recruiting younger and less experienced men to the service, rather than with the lack of courage of the pilots.

Birley's articulation of flying stress became influential within the Royal Air Force, but his sympathy for stressed military personnel was disputed by his peers. Many of the witnesses giving evidence to the War Office Committee of Enquiry into 'Shell-shock', of which Birley was a member, emphasized the importance of a soldier's 'neuropathic predisposition', rather than the force of circumstances, in the aetiology of shock and condoned a clear distinction between deserving wounded soldiers and their undeserving neurotic compatriots.[24] As several historians have suggested, this differentiation was not only based on contemporary notions of masculinity, which demanded male courage and fortitude at times of stress, but was also shaped by military and economic expediency.[25] In order to deter soldiers from malingering and avoiding active engagement (thereby threatening conventional notions of manliness) and to reduce the financial burden of the war, shell-shocked soldiers could be executed for cowardice and desertion and those suffering from neuroses were not entitled to a war pension.

Military attempts to prevent breakdown and to promote morale in the armed forces through better recruitment, training and leadership gained momentum during the inter-war years as the personal and domestic consequences of demobilization became apparent, economic conditions deteriorated and another global conflict approached. After the First World War, shell-shocked war veterans and their families had struggled to cope with the psychological and physical effects of emotional distress and unemployment.[26] During the recession of the 1920s and 1930s, clinical interest in the capacity for stressful circumstances to trigger psychosomatic illness was further encouraged by an apparent increase in functional disorders, including hypertension, dyspepsia and asthma, and by rising levels of sickness absence through chronic disease.[27] Alarmed at rising rates of absenteeism, delinquency, mental illness, criminality and alcoholism, proponents of a more holistic form of psychosocial medicine, such as the Scottish physician James Lorimer Halliday (1898–1983) or the American pioneer of constitutional medicine George Draper (1880–1959), began to link chronic illness not primarily to personal inadequacy, but to the 'deprivation, frustration, upset, strain, or difficulty' of modern lives.[28]

The continuing military significance of these patterns of illness was evident in sporadic inter-war reports of medical emergencies while flying, including the case of a Royal Air Force corporal who suffered a perforated duodenal ulcer, and in a 1927 study by the Cambridge psychologist, Frederic C. Bartlett (1886–1969), who subsequently became a founder member of the Flying Personnel Research Committee. Bartlett's inter-war investigations led him to conclude that the failure to adapt to military life was caused by temperamental weakness, a position that continued to dictate Air Ministry advice to medical officers responsible for the health and fitness of pilots.[29] It was during the Second World War, however, that flying stress emerged once more as a military priority amidst concerns that cases of combat stress were adversely affecting the discipline, competence and morale of the armed forces. Attempts to limit the impact of fear and fatigue varied. While men and women in the air force used alcohol, cigarettes and sex to subdue their anxieties, as well as drugs such as Benzedrine to enhance mood and performance and to maintain energy for both flying and recreational activities,[30] official treatment protocols initially involved encouragement, reassurance and sedation.[31] The spectre of execution for cowardice and desertion had receded, but the penalties for being unable to conquer fear and resume active service remained stringent. Introduced in response to the high numbers of psychiatric casualties amongst air-crews during the early months of the war and employed as a critical alternative to the more benign concept of flying stress, a diagnosis of 'lack of moral fibre' led to loss of rank, discharge and the forfeiture of an entitlement to a pension.[32]

One of the most influential formulations of flying stress during the later years of the Second World War was elaborated by the neurologist Charles P. Symonds (1890–1978). Having completed his medical training after the First World War, during which he had served with the Royal Flying Corps, in 1934 Symonds was engaged as a civilian consultant to the Royal Air Force. At the outbreak of the Second World War, he was appointed initially as a group captain before being promoted first to Air Commodore and, subsequently, Air Vice-Marshal. Symonds analysed 2,000 cases of neuroses amongst pilots and interviewed 200 station and squadron commanders and medical officers. Acknowledging, but also challenging, some of Birley's work, Symonds insisted that the term flying stress should be applied only 'to denote the load which air-crews have to carry', rather than the state of anxiety or depression induced by combat. Like earlier accounts of shell shock and insanity, Symonds's depiction of pilots under stress highlighted the reciprocal relationship between external pressure and predisposition. In the psychologically unstable and those with domestic anxieties, relatively non-stressful flying duties could precipitate neurotic reactions. As the level of stress increased, however, even men with no predisposition to neurosis would eventually break down.[33] Symonds explained the capacity to cope with flying stress in biological terms. Although he referred to the psychological or behavioural attributes of masculinity, such as fear, courage and heroism, to explain both resilience and collapse, his conceptual model was primarily a physiological one: the promotion or depletion of fearlessness and confidence were analogous to the processes of neurological excitation and inhibition. Pilots' responses to fear and danger could be conditioned, he intimated, in much the same way that Pavlov's dogs had been conditioned to salivate in response to a stimulus.[34] Evident also in contemporary studies of fear and courage, it was this formulation of combat stress as a conditioned response that underscored beliefs that more effective recruitment, training, discipline and leadership would mitigate the effects of stress in war.[35]

Symonds's interest in the parallels between physiological and psychological processes was not unusual in this period. Inter-war accounts of 'wind up' in air-crews; wartime investigations of anxiety states in the navy; the formulation of 'physio-neurosis' by the American psychoanalyst Abram Kardiner (1891–1981); and studies of the distribution and symptoms of psychosomatic conditions emphasized not only the similarities between physical and mental reaction patterns, but also the role of physiological processes in determining the manifestations of emotional distress.[36] According to one study of anxious sailors, published in 1943, reactions to stress proceeded in stages driven primarily by changing physiological responses. The initial stress of separation from home and family, combined with the physical discomfort, danger and monotony of service life, led to the rising heart rate, blurred vision and muscle tension associated with the adrenaline-driven 'fight or flight' reaction described by Walter Cannon in the 1920s. On prolonged exposure to stress, sailors developed not only psychological disturbances but also physical symptoms of anxiety, including palpitations, tremors, sweating, dyspepsia and high blood pressure, followed by exhaustion and the inability to perform duties.[37]

Awareness of the physiological dimensions of stress reactions did not preclude more pejorative appraisals of an individual's incapacity to cope. Although Winston Churchill's physician, Lord Moran (1882–1977), acknowledged the effects of fatigue, strain and anoxia (or 'air hunger') on the bodies and minds of pilots and recognized the role of the adrenal glands in mediating adaptation to stressful circumstances, he nevertheless continued to argue that two-thirds of pilots who had broken down during the Second World War had done so because of an 'inborn' flaw: 'the way a man is made', he suggested in 1950, 'matters more than the risks he runs'.[38] Moran's formula was probably derived from the most significant post-war study of psychological disorders in flying personnel, published by the Air Ministry in 1947 and written largely by Charles Symonds and his colleague Wing Commander Denis J. Williams, who had both worked with Bomber Command.[39] According to Symonds and Williams, 67.7 per cent of pilots suffering from flying stress demonstrated a predisposition to psychological breakdown. Many of these pilots were stressed not solely by flying duties, but also by other factors such as marital difficulties and financial worries. For Moran and his contemporaries, anxiety, depression and hysteria were caused by the failure of weak men to cope with the stress of life.

While they often conceded the possibility that even 'men of the toughest fibre' might break down,[40] the authors of many studies of stress amongst pilots and soldiers, during and after the war, believed that it was primarily flawed temperaments that undermined resilience and that measures of emotional immaturity could be used to predict psychological collapse. In 1943, the Scottish psychiatrist and psychoanalyst W. Ronald D. Fairbairn (1889–1964) suggested that soldiers who had broken down displayed an infantile dependence on their mothers and a form of separation-anxiety that could not easily be erased by enhancing group morale. In contrast to memories of his loving parents, the neurotic soldier supposedly regarded the armed forces as 'an angry father' and 'heartless mother', leading to resistance to authority, a desire to return home and psychological breakdown.[41] A man's failure to adapt to service life, like a civilian's tendency to be overwhelmed by fear of bombardment, was regarded as the product of a volatile combination of constitutional timidity, emotional immaturity and intellectual inferiority.[42] At a time when psychoanalytical theories were supposedly losing purchase within British psychiatry, Fairbairn's analysis was explicitly Freudian: like disordered family and social relationships, neurotic reactions to war were the product of unresolved emotional conflicts generated during childhood.[43]

Whether framed primarily in physiological or in psychoanalytical terms, post-war discussions of flying stress did not consider the potential similarities or differences between men and women. Many investigators recognized that men who were not involved in flying duties also suffered from stress and that women in the air force worked in similar non-combat roles to men at home and abroad, but post-war studies continued to focus exclusively on the experiences and behaviour of male air crew and assumed that stress responses were generic or universal in nature, differing only according to individual character and constitution. Men provided the model for exploring and explaining what Symonds had referred to in 1943 as the 'human response to flying stress'.[44] This normative approach was not only determined by military exigency but also borrowed heavily from the practices and perspectives adopted by prominent stress researchers. In the influential physiological studies of stress and adaptation carried out during the 1930s, 1940s and 1950s by Hans Selye (1907–82) and his colleagues, stress constituted a non-specific response to external stressors. Selye's insistence on non-specificity and his uncritical use of laboratory animals to demonstrate the effects of stress in humans served to flatten differences between species, sexes and, to some extent, individuals.[45]

Appropriating Selye's scheme, most researchers investigating flying stress believed that different forms of physical hardship and emotional pressure disturbed biological equilibrium and distorted behaviour through the activation of a shared, and broadly predictable, system of organismic responses. According to squadron leader and statistician D. D. Reid in his 1948 study of sickness and stress in operational flying, while the specific physical conditions of battle and industrial work might change, the general 'principles of action in human behaviour' remained.[46] Subsequent reflections on combat stress were even more directly shaped by a formulaic physiological model of adaptation. In a brief study of stress and aviation presented to the Society for Psychosomatic Research in 1958, Group Captain and consultant psychiatrist V. H. Tompkins suggested that military life could 'upset the balance of the organism', particularly in 'human material' predisposed to breakdown.[47] Organismic instability and adaptive failure were evident not only in psychological and psychosomatic symptoms, but also in physiological indicators: the stress of service life led to the increased excretion of 17-ketosteroids and higher levels of adrenaline, features of stress that were being used by military doctors to develop improved measures of a soldier's suitability for service and were subsequently employed to assess resistance to fatigue amongst both civilian and naval pilots.[48]

Post-war theorists of psychological stress similarly avoided any explicit comparison between men and women in their attempts to generate what Roy Grinker referred to in 1956 as a 'unified theory of human behavior', which drew direct parallels between psychological, social and physiological systems.[49] The most influential psychological studies of stress and coping during the 1950s, 1960s and 1970s were carried out by Richard Lazarus, who exclusively selected men for his studies and entirely conflated any differences between men and women. While Lazarus recognized the role of personality and emotionality in dictating performance under stress and, occasionally, referred to the impact of 'male and female roles' on behaviour, his account of the mechanisms of psychological adjustment reflected contemporary preoccupations with the common neuroendocrine pathways of stress, as well as concerns about the capacity of individual 'subjects' to adapt to their domestic and working environments.[50]

Psychologists, psychiatrists and neurologists on both sides of the Atlantic tended to follow much the same course, emphasizing the integration of physiological and psychological processes and investigating stress responses primarily in male athletes, students and workers. In a 1957 study of factors that determined the capacity to master stress, Daniel H. Funkenstein and his colleagues at Harvard investigated only the reactions of 'college men' exposed to various 'stress-inducing situations', mapping their ability to control acute and chronic stress against various personality measures.[51] In Funkenstein's studies, women appeared only as mothers responsible for shaping their sons' tendencies to exhibit anxiety under pressure.[52] British publications adopted a similar conceptual and analytical framework. In the proceedings from an Oxford conference on mental health research in 1960, contributors drew largely on physiological, psychological and ethological studies of adaptation in order to establish precisely how individual personality factors determined the extent to which stress led to the 'disorganization of behaviour' and disease.[53] This is not to say that psychologists were unaware of the biological and cultural factors that dictated the variable responses of men and women to social tensions and military conflict.[54] Rather, it demonstrates the extent to which, within the community of stress researchers, men were considered to be the prototypical or normative human subjects.

Women at War

Given the tendency for physiologists and psychologists to disregard biological and cultural differences between men and women as variables that might shape performance under stress and for military authorities to focus on male fitness to fight, it is perhaps not surprising that most post-war reflections on flying stress avoided overt references to biological sex or gender, preferring instead to concentrate on the presence or absence of courage only amongst what the British historian Lord David Cecil (1902–86) had referred to, in 1942, as the 'Englishmen of history'.[55] Yet, as many historical accounts have shown, discussions of traumatic neuroses in both war and peace were laden with assumptions about gender differences in personality, vulnerability and social responsibility. Echoing earlier and parallel formulations of shell shock and combat stress, most investigators of flying stress believed that pilots in the Second World War had broken down because they exhibited feminine character traits, such as emotional immaturity, or were overly dependent on their mothers leading to separation-anxiety.[56] Gender stereotypes appeared in other guises. Some men collapsed or developed psychosomatic symptoms apparently because they were troubled not predominantly by the extreme trauma of conflict, but by accumulated domestic, marital and financial problems, which were magnified by the time available for 'brooding and bitterness'.[57] Suspicions that wives had 'sought companionship' elsewhere fuelled fears of rejection, even amongst pilots who had themselves been unfaithful while overseas,[58] but they also reflected the force of contemporary expectations that women's primary responsibilities were for making and maintaining homes and marriages and for helping to rehabilitate returning veterans socially and sexually. In most accounts of the causes and management of flying stress, women appeared not as stressed but as stressors.

Dominated by critical attention to the construction and preservation of masculinity, historical studies of flying stress, and indeed of war more generally, have largely replicated the contemporary neglect of women under stress. Women have not been entirely excluded from historical studies, but their experiences have been marginalized both in heroic, sometimes autobiographical, narratives of the 'Brylcreem boys' and in more scholarly studies of the experiences of pilots in the Allied air forces.[59] Even in Martin Francis's more detailed analysis of British culture and the Royal Air Force during the war, the experiences and contributions of members of the Women's Auxiliary Air Force are reduced to their role in boosting the morale of male pilots and severely wounded servicemen,[60] reflecting a tendency (now as then) to value women more for their domestic and erotic potential than for their direct contributions to the war effort. As Carol Acton has pointed out in relation to the Great War, women have been seen as incidental to the history of combat in other ways. While men have been associated with action, women have often been caricatured as passive 'waiting wives', thereby perpetuating wartime and post-war preoccupations with male fortitude under stress.[61]

Memoirs written by members of the Women's Auxiliary Air Force make clear, however, that British women contributed equally to the war effort both abroad and at home, not merely in supporting roles incidental to combat, but as Squadron Leaders and Section Officers, as radio operators, mechanics, electricians, nurses and meteorologists, and in some cases as pilots.[62] In one of the few historical accounts to foreground the work of female pilots, Giles Whittell has exposed the extent to which 'Spitfire women' of the civilian Air Transport Auxiliary were responsible for flying injured soldiers, service personnel, new and damaged planes, and medical supplies to and from the frontline. These women endured conditions no less hazardous than their male counterparts but, flying unarmed, they were unable to retaliate in response to enemy fire. Fifteen of the 164 auxiliary women pilots died in action during the war, including Amy Johnson (1903–41) whose military exploits were memorialized in the 1942 film *They Flew Alone*.[63] Although the personal recollections of air force women might be regarded as idealized or romanticized, much like those written by their male counterparts, they testify both to the 'outstanding courage [of women] under stress' and to the shared, rather than disconnected, nature of men's and women's wartime experiences.[64] As one of the female Section Officers in Bomber Command, Grace 'Archie' Hall, insisted in a compilation of reminiscences from her peers, 'We, Also, Were There'.[65]

The routine and symbolic integration of men and women in the air force, in terms of shared responsibilities and comparable uniforms, did not preclude the perpetuation of gender stereotypes. Although members of the Women's Auxiliary Air Force, the Women's Royal Naval Service and the US Women's Army corps were regarded, and often regarded themselves, as equal to men, they were also frequently relegated to supporting roles or considered unfeminine. Military advice to service women to eat healthily and exercise sufficiently was 'based on a direct appeal to female vanity': women were expected to be concerned primarily with their shape and appearance.[66] There is some evidence to suggest that women in the air force shared men's preoccupations with women conforming to normative configurations of beauty, but the memoirs of service women also reveal that they exploited opportunities to individualize their uniforms and to highlight the importance of their contributions to achieving military objectives.

It is possible to evaluate further the force and consequences of clichéd understandings of women's capacity to conform to, and cope with, military life by focusing on accounts of women who exhibited psychological difficulties while in service. Very few studies of stress in the armed forces, or indeed in civilian contexts, considered the experiences of women directly. But on-going investigations by two physicians and squadron leaders in the Royal Air Force are particularly instructive. In 1944, S. I. Ballard and H. G. Miller published the results of their initial analysis of 2,000 cases of psychoneurosis, psychosis and psychopathic conduct disorder observed in air force personnel attending a specialist neuropsychiatry centre located in a Royal Air Force station. The study evaluated the frequency, causes and categories of psychological and psychosomatic conditions, as well as the distribution of psychological illness by sex and the efficacy of various treatment and convalescence protocols.[67]

The majority of service personnel (1,366) treated by Ballard and Miller were classified as suffering from neuroses, including affective disorders such as anxiety, depression and fatigue (739), hysteria (330), psychopathic states (290) and obsessive and compulsive disorders (7). 439 patients demonstrated organic nervous disorders, 62 were diagnosed as mentally defective, 45 were suffering from psychotic conditions such as schizophrenia, manic-depression and paranoia, 2 were thought to be malingering and the remaining 86 were either diagnosed with another medical condition or showed no evidence of a significant disorder. Of particular significance in the present context is Ballard and Miller's conclusion that 80 per cent of 250 cases selected at random for retrospective analysis indicated a strong individual predisposition to neurosis or a positive family history of psychological disorder, a broken home, poor work record and 'educational backwardness', all of which were presumed to increase the likelihood of psychological collapse while in service. In this sense, Ballard and Miller's conclusions replicated contemporary beliefs that constitutional and domestic factors were more significant causes of nervous breakdown under stress than 'real or anticipated exposure to physical danger'.[68]

Unusually for studies of stress-related conditions, Ballard and Miller compared the distribution of psychological disorders amongst men and women and their subsequent military trajectory. Of the 2,000 patients, 1,765 were men and 235 women. However, according to Ballard and Miller the most significant feature of their study was not the crude rates of breakdown amongst men and women, but the fact that women were far more likely to be invalided out of the service than men: 48 per cent of women suffering from functional disorders left the service as opposed to only 10 per cent of men suffering from similar conditions. The explanation for this distinction lay in men and women's differing susceptibility and resilience to stress. For Ballard and Miller, women were less able to adapt to service life as a result of an 'appreciably higher degree of constitutional emotional instability and neurotic predisposition'. This argument was based not on clinical or experimental evidence, but on the presence, amongst these women, of a number of circumstantial and constitutional factors assumed to be associated with psychological vulnerability:

> This is shown particularly in such factors as broken homes, unduly strong attachments to home and parents, and previous evidence of lack of persistence and of social adaptation. Many are solitary, shy individuals, living at home, with few external interests, addicted to knitting and sewing, and dependent on maternal decisions. A considerable proportion have never had a civilian job. This group is a particularly unfavourable one, and tends to break down readily under conditions of community regimentation.[69]

Ballard and Miller's explanation of psychological breakdown in terms of temperamental predisposition and the tendency for women to form strong emotional attachments borrowed directly from parallel discussions of flying stress amongst men, as well as from contemporary psychoanalytical theories about the impact of childhood trauma and clinical accounts of civilian neuroses. Given their emphasis on the constitutional and situational determinants of neuropsychiatric conditions and the force of their underlying assumptions about female weakness, it is not surprising that Ballard and Miller regarded remedial approaches as ineffectual in women, leading to their frequent discharge from service: 'it is useless', they wrote, 'to return such women to duties, whereas men can and frequently do make a satisfactory adaptation'.[70]

Highlighting the lack of previous investigations into women suffering from war neuroses, Ballard and Miller subsequently pursued the question of psychiatric casualties amongst service women in more detail. Their justification for focusing on women was not only (or perhaps not primarily) the mental health of their patients, but the potential for such a study to address the socio-economic aspects of neurotic breakdowns and to illuminate debates about war neuroses more generally. Throughout the war, psychiatrists had debated the impact of conflict on the psychological health of civilians. Opinions as to the relative contributions of constitution and circumstances and the comparative resilience of men and women in the face of wartime adversities differed. For many researchers, it was impossible to discern obvious differences between the prevalence of traumatic neuroses in men and women. According to the Russian-born psychiatrist and asylum superintendent Isaac Atkin (1900–93), cases were evenly distributed between the sexes. Although it sometimes appeared as if women were more easily affected by the stress of air raids, the reasons for this lay solely in their greater propensity to display emotions rather than in their inherent psychological vulnerability.[71] Like other commentators during and after the war, Atkin suggested that the major factors determining resistance to stress were to be found in personality traits and domestic circumstances shared by women and men alike. Childhood experiences, low intelligence, a neurotic or timid predisposition, an unhappy marriage, alcoholism, an unsatisfactory job and sexual difficulties were more important than the fear of impending death.[72]

In contrast to Ballard and Miller, some clinicians suggested that women were less vulnerable to stress than men. During the war, Felix Brown, a psychiatrist in the Emergency Medical Service, concluded his discussion of civilian psychiatric casualties by insisting that women were 'by no means a weakening element in the general population, in fact the male cases of emotional shock and psychoneurosis seen resulting from air-raids outnumber the females in the ratio 30 to 18'.[73] This distribution was not always interpreted in a favourable way for women. Some years after the war, I. McD. G. Stewart, a physician in Bristol, suggested that women were 'almost immune' from stress. However, the reason lay not in their increased resilience but in their unsuitability for, and exclusion from, the worlds of intellect and commerce: stress belonged 'to the office and the technician's bench, not to the kitchen or the Labour Exchange'. Like 'primitive races' and the lower social classes, Stewart insisted, women were overly preoccupied with more mundane matters and less likely to be troubled by modern stressful circumstances.[74]

Ballard and Miller's second contribution to this debate, published in 1945, was more empirical than many contemporary studies, but no less laden with cultural preconceptions. Although women exhibited many of the same psychoneurotic signs as men, they tended to display fewer somatic symptoms. Nervous dyspepsia, for example, was rarely evident in women, a factor explained in terms of the 'socially acknowledged and permitted emotionalism of women', in contrast to the 'sterner emotional code' that forced men to somaticize their distress.[75] Similarly, while hereditary predisposition to breakdown was an important factor in both sexes, it was more commonly present in women and more likely to interfere with military duties and result in discharge from service. According to Ballard and Miller, this trend was the product of both the temperamental instability of women and the manner in which service in the armed forces subordinated the 'traditional female values and primary biological functions' of women.[76] Although anxieties about child-bearing and domestic expectations may have understandably influenced some women's capacity to cope with separation from home and the demands of service, Ballard and Miller's formulation also revealed a pervasive and discriminatory vision of women as emotionally unstable, psychosexually immature, intellectually inferior and incapable of adapting effectively to the stress of life. Such preconceptions were reinforced by the tendency for military authorities and civilian commentators to regard men who broke down under stress as feminine and inadequate in comparison with their more resilient and more masculine counterparts.[77]

Not all post-war commentators fully accepted or adopted the framework for understanding the causes, manifestations and consequences of neuroses in either women or men proposed by Ballard and Miller. On both sides of the Atlantic, opinions continued to differ as to the relative impact of heredity and environmental circumstances on the appearance of neuroses. According to the American psychiatrist and Brigadier General William C. Menninger (1899–1966), men broke down because of the stress of war rather than because of any personality disorder, an interpretation that led him to advocate greater attention to 'social psychiatry' and, like many British military physicians, to promote the consolidation of group cohesion and morale through effective leadership and training.[78] By contrast, other physicians mobilized psychoanalytical theories to emphasize the role of personality or childhood experiences, such as parental divorce and death, in shaping the capacity to cope with the traumas of war, the personal and family challenges of repatriation, and the stresses of everyday domestic and working life.[79] Some of these accounts appreciated the inter-connectedness of the wartime experiences of men and women by recognizing similarities between the isolation of servicemen and the loneliness of their wives at home.[80] In addition, they sometimes acknowledged the cultural, political and demographic, rather than merely biological, determinants of women's contributions in peace and war.[81]

It is striking, however, that in many post-war discussions of the impact of stress on psychological health Ballard and Miller's construction of women as biologically fragile, emotionally labile and mentally vulnerable, and their sharp differentiation between male and female temperaments, remained largely intact. Studies of men and the few studies of women under stress continued to betray similar gendered assumptions. Inter-war and wartime beliefs that menstruation, lactation and the menopause might determine women's responses to stress, evident in advertisements suggesting that menopausal women suffered more during air raids, continued to influence post-war accounts of anxiety neuroses.[82] Studies of workers' health and sickness absence perpetuated a separation between the capacities of men and women to cope with stress and located the cause of women's vulnerability not in the nature of the work, but in the nature of the individual.[83] And men who broke down during combat continued to be regarded as timid, emotionally unstable and sometimes intellectually inferior, a set of qualities more commonly used to characterize women who had struggled to cope with the demands of conflict and the threat of bombardment, or who appeared to break down after the war under the strain of domestic life.

The enduring popularity of contrasting evaluations of the capacity of men and women to cope with stress can be traced to contemporary concerns with returning men to the workplace and restoring social stability, as well as to growing anxieties about the personal, political and economic burden of rising levels of mental illness in post-war communities. As a number of historians have argued, during the post-war period even women who had served in the war were expected to return happily to domestic duties and be content to organize the home, rear children and provide a stable family environment for returning soldiers and working husbands: women's wartime work had been only a temporary interruption to established duties and expectations.[84] As wives and mothers, women in the late 1940s and 1950s were valued primarily for their ability to safeguard the health and welfare of men and children, a role that carried considerable responsibilities but also served to restrict women to domestic chores. The restoration of male productivity and national prosperity required the 'perfect wife' to create an 'ideal home'. In circular fashion, these assumptions and expectations generated the conditions for the exclusion of women from the workplace and the perpetuation of distress from fatigue and loneliness. The portrayal of women by military psychiatrists as emotionally immature and psychologically vulnerable not only legitimated beliefs that women were inadequate and ill-equipped for work, but also bolstered post-war welfare policies designed to reinvigorate family life and restore national economic and political stability through the domestic labour of wives and mothers. In spite of the efforts of feminist authors as diverse as Alva Myrdal (1902–86), Viola Klein (1908–73), Simone de Beauvoir (1908–86), Betty Friedan and Hannah Gavron (1936–65) to forge 'a new cultural identity for women' and to resist the reactionary forces that appeared to be curtailing women's freedoms and opportunities,[85] the contributions of women in the armed forces and their psychological needs at home were overshadowed by preoccupations with masculine norms and with the heroic exploits of men at war and work.

Conclusion

In 1941, an editorial in *The Lancet* claimed that the Second World War constituted 'a great emotional unifier', leading people to have 'a new confidence in each other'. Rather than breaking down established social relations or precipitating widespread psychological distress, the war appeared to encourage 'spontaneous emotional solidarity' and to heighten morale and resilience in the face of death and material destruction.[86] From a contemporary wartime perspective, stress and anxiety were the exclusive preserve of neither men nor women, neither the old nor the young, and neither the lower nor the middle classes. Some historians have expressed hopes that scholarly studies of war will reveal the shared, rather than disparate, nature of wartime experiences and, in the process, serve to recover the previously hidden histories of women and the manner in which women's mental health was as strongly governed as that of men by economic, situational and occupational contexts, rather than merely individual psychological frailty. Carol Acton's study of the First World War and Tessa Stone's account of gendered military identity during the Second World War have both drawn attention to the opportunity that the history of warfare offers to reappraise the experiences and contributions of women and men during and after periods of stress.[87]

Occasional contemporary appeals to explore more directly the differences and similarities between the emotions and behaviour of men and women under stress, or appreciate women's capacity to cope, proved ineffective. During the post-war decades, investigations of physiological and psychological reactions to stressful circumstances continued to focus on male stress, to regard male responses as the norm and to downplay the depth and significance of stress in women.[88] Evocative examples of the tendency to relegate women to the clinical shadows and to denigrate the severity or significance of their stress are not difficult to identify. In 1956, a popular British self-help guide to 'healthy minds and bodies' highlighted the greater frequency and importance of stress-related ulcers in men.[89] In an even more unrestrained commentary that drew heavily on Hans Selye's physiological formulation of stress responses, the Canadian journalist Fred Kerner compared the inevitable competition and tension felt by working men forced to 'live up to a picture of masculinity' with the less demanding role of 'homemaker'. Men suffered more heart disease not because they were 'weaker', but because they were faced with 'more stress in their daily lives than women':

> While nobody underestimates the job of being a housewife and mother, it has been found that men especially seem to have ailments which can most often be traced to prolonged tension. It seems that in spite of the many responsibilities involved, a woman's work at home apparently does not entail the same type of strain which most men undergo from day to day while working.[90]

Preoccupations with the occupational pressures encountered by men reflected the lived experiences of post-war generations. Studies of the association between cardiovascular disease and Type A personality carried out by Meyer Friedman (1910–2001) and Ray H. Rosenman from the late 1950s, or subsequent studies of male executive stress on both sides of the Atlantic, reflected the overwhelming preponderance of middle-class men in leadership positions in commerce and industry.[91] If Grinker and Spiegel's wartime focus on male pilots under stress was the product of an exclusively male fighting force, so too were post-war investigations of the psychiatric strengths and weaknesses of 'typical air force pilots', who were also almost exclusively men. In these on-going studies of military personnel, attention to the role of women was restricted to an assessment of their contribution to the satisfactory social and sexual adjustment of their husbands or to their impact as mothers on their pilot sons' emotional stability.[92] During the 1960s and 1970s, when stress and fatigue also emerged as possible determinants of commercial pilot error and when airline safety and working conditions were becoming prominent political issues for trade unions, airline companies, governments, travellers and the media, only 0.027 per cent of American airline pilots were women, resulting in a continuing emphasis on men's ability to cope with the stress of flying and on training the 'right type of man'.[93] The effects of flying on women's health were considered primarily in terms of the energy expended by stewardesses, in comparison with shop assistants or housewives, or in terms of the impact of flying on menstrual cycles.[94]

Yet, the predominance of men in military and civil aviation after the war was itself determined by gendered evaluations of capacity and fitness and by the re-confinement of women to the home. Interpretations of the findings from post-war investigations reflected and consolidated long-standing gendered assumptions about the greater emotional immaturity and psychological vulnerability of women. At a time when larger numbers of women were entering the workforce, psychoanalytical theory, clinical practice and pharmaceutical marketing strategies not only continued to focus on women as less robust than men and unable to cope even with domestic duties, but also blamed nervous breakdown in women on individual susceptibility rather than social circumstances or occupational demands. During the 1950s, 1960s and 1970s, attempts to challenge assumptions about women's coping strategies or to emancipate women from domestic and occupational drudgery were impeded by persistent and prejudicial assessments of women's resilience under stress, assessments that had been forged particularly strongly by wartime and post-war commentators on stress in service.

Historical attempts to reconceptualize the responses of men and women to stressful circumstances during either war or peace have similarly faltered. In spite of Carol Acton's emphasis on the inadequacy of any history that separates, rather than connects, the experiences of men and women during the stress of war, we still have few historical studies that effectively confront past and present assumptions about the capacity of men and women to cope with stressful life events. Like their clinical predecessors, historians of stress have tended to reinforce the dominant paradigm: most historical accounts have ignored gender as a major determinant of scientific theories of stress and have largely overlooked or underestimated the contributions and experiences of women in coping with the stress of separation, combat, bombardment, repatriation, occupational reintegration and domestic rehabilitation during and after the war. Closer interrogation of the ideological climate within which clinical studies of stress were devised, and clearer engagement with personal accounts of coping, will allow us to see beyond clichéd and formulaic assumptions about masculine strength and feminine frailty and to develop a more inclusive historical account that marries, rather than divorces, the stories of women and men under stress.

Acknowledgements

The research on which this chapter is based was generously supported by the Wellcome Trust, Grant No. 082834/Z07/Z.

8 STOMACH FOR THE PEACE: PSYCHOSOMATIC DISORDERS IN UK VETERANS AND CIVILIANS, 1945–55

Edgar Jones

'Peptic ulcers are much rarer now than they used to be', observed Dr Frank Assinder, a general practitioner (GP) in Carshalton Beeches, Surrey, when he was asked to recall the early days of the National Health Service (NHS), adding that 'nervous dyspepsia was a common diagnosis'.[1] In the aftermath of the Second World War, family doctors became increasingly concerned by the apparent spread of ailments such as indigestion, rheumatism and skin rashes throughout the population.[2] Few of these symptoms could be ignored because they might indicate the presence of serious or developing pathology. Indeed, stomach disorders rose up the health agenda of the late 1940s and early 1950s as health officials identified an epidemic of peptic ulcer. Evidence of perforation from post-mortem studies confirmed that this was, in part, the outcome of a verifiable disease process.[3]

Given that men of working age seemed particularly vulnerable to peptic ulcers, the Medical Research Council commissioned a report from Richard Doll (1912–2005) and Francis Avery Jones (1910–98) into *Occupational Factors in the Aetiology of Gastric and Duodenal Ulcers*.[4] Published in 1951, this authoritative study ruled out social class as a causal variable but concluded that those in jobs with responsibilities for others were at elevated risk. Doll and Jones were undecided whether it was the nature of the work itself or the personality of the employee that was the determining factor. In the pre-war period, Walter Cannon (1871–1945) had provided a physiological account of the relationship between emotion and physical states, while from the mid-1950s the burgeoning concept of stress was supported by endocrinological evidence from Hans Selye (1907–82).[5] A growing number of doctors with an interest in psychosomatic medicine believed that changes to the environment, or ways that individuals interacted with it, played an important part in the spread of gastrointestinal disorders. The 'day-to-day experience of the consulting room and surgery tells its own story', reported a team of family doctors. Their study of six general practices led them to conclude that the role played by stress 'as an important contributory cause of disease' was beyond doubt.[6]

Historians such as Paul Addison and David Kynaston have explored the cultural impact of the Second World War on British society, evoking a nation coming to terms with the material and psychological effects of the conflict, but also seeking to adapt its institutions and economy to a new world order.[7] Considerable research has also been conducted into the post-war design and development of public health systems, together with the impact of state welfare on families during this period.[8] Alan Allport has analyzed the demobilization of conscripted servicemen, many of whom encountered problems adjusting from an adventurous or high-risk lifestyle to the mundane disciplines of office and factory employment.[9] Although much has been learned about stressors affecting civilians and soldiers during the conflict itself,[10] less has been written on the mechanisms that individuals employed to cope with the memories of terrifying experiences whilst returning to peacetime routines of work and recreation.[11] This raises questions about the extent to which ailments seen in primary care were a product of processes of adjustment and rehabilitation. The changing culture of somatization has become a central question for historians as they seek to understand the relationship between psychological and physical elements in common illnesses.[12] Following Gerald Grob's historical survey of peptic ulcer in America, medical historians have taken an increasing interest in stomach disorders.[13] Ian Miller in particular has studied the British experience of stomach illnesses from the nineteenth century to 1945, identifying a series of factors that led to the adoption of stress as a causative mechanism.[14]

Building on these studies, this chapter explores the apparent spread of stomach disorders throughout Britain in the aftermath of the Second World War. It explores how the conflict itself had both focused attention on psychosomatic illnesses and also provided a range of causal explanations. The part played by the NHS in attempting to treat and quantify this ill-health is also analyzed. The 1950s witnessed the increasing identification of stress as both a physiological and a psychological phenomenon tied to modern living. Armed with a new scientific model for functional symptoms (that is those without demonstrable organic basis), doctors who had a research interest in psychosomatic medicine increasingly sought to explain duodenal ulcer and nervous dyspepsia in terms of worry and workplace pressures. Finally, the chapter investigates why gastrointestinal complaints appeared so common and the extent to which they were interpreted as bodily manifestations of traumatic memories.

Wartime Context

The need to conscript a mass citizen army had brought stomach disorders to the top of the health agenda. In December 1940, an editorial in the *British Medical Journal* noted that peptic ulcer had become a significant cause of invalidity from the British Expeditionary Force,[15] such that the military authorities feared for the fighting strength of the army. Urgent study was undertaken not only of servicemen invalided from France but also of those hospitalized in the UK during training and anti-invasion duties. Many of the hypotheses explored in 1940–1 continued to frame post-war debates. For example, the heavier nature and high meat content of army food was proposed as a cause of stomach disorders, together with the fact that soldiers on exercise had irregular mealtimes.[16] A further causal hypothesis was excessive smoking by servicemen, encouraged by the free issue of cigarettes. Yet there was a serious and compelling objection to these hypotheses. Sir Henry Tidy (1877–1960), a physician with a special interest in ulcer, discounted active duty and army food as causal factors because 'peptic ulcer and all dyspeptic disturbances were noticeably rare' during the First World War when similar stresses had operated and when a similar diet had been served.[17] Population data supported his case: only 709 soldiers had been discharged from the British army by the end of 1915 with peptic ulcer compared with 23,574 at the end of 1941.[18] This observation, and the failure to establish a statistical association with smoking,[19] encouraged physicians to explore the idea that particular personality types were vulnerable to stomach disorders.

In the pre-war period, Daniel T. Davies, a physician at the Royal Free Hospital, and A. Macbeth Wilson, a psychiatrist at the Tavistock Clinic, collaborated to investigate the personal histories of ulcer patients.[20] They found that in 84 per cent of cases an anxiety-provoking event, such as change of job, the death of a close relative or unemployment, had preceded the illness. In a follow-up study of patients who had suffered internal bleeding or perforation, Davies and Wilson concluded that 'unusual emotional tension' was associated with these medical emergencies and that patients had been 'harassed and worried by their responsibilities and by environmental changes'.[21] After the outbreak of war, personality became increasingly implicated in peptic ulceration as studies of particular groups of servicemen showed different rates of stomach illness. Submariners, for example, appeared almost immune to peptic ulcer, an observation explained by a selection programme designed to identify the fittest and most robust sailors.[22]

Of particular significance for the post-war period was a study conducted by J. N. Morris (1910–2009), a physician, and Richard Titmuss (1907–73), an expert in social policy, which reported an association between employment rates and the incidence of stomach disorder.[23] They found that deaths from perforated ulcer had fallen during the early 1930s in areas with high unemployment.

However, as the economy recovered, bringing new jobs, ulcer mortality rose, apparently as a consequence of the return to work. Industrial and commercial employment was thought to be associated with stress, to which the ulcer personality was considered vulnerable. Morris and Titmuss concluded that 'it is hard to resist the conclusion that urban life nowadays is an ideal soil for the flowering of the ulcer temperament'.[24] A richer diet and greater consumption of cigarettes and alcohol associated with a return to work were thought to be secondary to personality. According to Morris and Titmuss, the significant rise in ulcer mortality for males between 1939 and 1941 was a consequence of 'heavy air attacks'. However, women in urban areas had been exposed to the same dangers as men and yet their mortality from ulcer fell over the same period.[25] Interpretations of these trends continued to vary. Sir Arthur Hurst (1879–1944), who had founded the Gastroenterology Club in 1937 as a vehicle for specialists to exchange information,[26] concluded that worry in conjunction with rising alcohol and cigarette consumption lay at the heart of the epidemic: 'the constant anxiety of the years between the two great wars, which led to the steady rise in the incidence of gastric disorders, can be fully realized only by those whose memories go back to the care-free days before 1914'.[27] Based in a British army hospital, Major C. A. Hinds Howell argued conversely that servicemen who broke down with an ulcer possessed a 'constitutional weakness'; in civilian life they were 'only just able to accommodate themselves to their home environment', but they lacked the resources to cope with the extra demands of a military lifestyle.[28]

In 1942 a Rockefeller Foundation-funded, US study of eighty randomly selected patients with peptic ulcer appeared to show that pathological changes and symptoms were correlated with strong emotions, chiefly fear and anxiety. The study's author, George Draper (1880–1959), who was a key figure in the growing field of constitutional medicine, argued that 'lesions of peptic ulcer are associated with psychic traumata as definitely as inappropriate food'.[29] Having concluded that dietary factors were secondary, Draper recommended that treatment pay less attention to the lesion itself and focus more on psychological re-education to wean the patient from 'the mother principle and re-establish his self respect'.[30] Draper and his colleague Abraham Myerson (1881–1948) believed that chronic diseases, such as peptic ulcer, hypertension, rheumatoid arthritis and asthma, were either a consequence of maladaptation to modern industrial life or illnesses in which homeostatic attempts to adapt to environmental stress had disturbed the stability of mind and body.[31] Similarly, Hans Selye drew on wartime reports of peptic ulcer to support his account of the 'general adaptation syndrome'.[32] The reported increase in the incidence of perforation after air-raids, he believed, could be explained in terms of an adreno-cortical defence reaction, comparable to that produced in animals 'by exposure to stress'.[33] By creating episodes of intense emotion, the Second World War offered doctors with an interest in psychosomatic medicine regular opportunities to study the impact of stress on health and well-being.

The conflict also established a strong cultural association between stomach disorders and combat. 'Guts' was a popular term for courage, while the phrase 'no stomach for the fight' meant cowardice. The US Air Force, when stationed in the UK, had coined the term 'lack of intestinal fortitude' as an official euphemism for loss of will power.[34] Suspected ulcer was also recognized as an escape route for servicemen wishing to avoid hazardous duties and it was popularly, but erroneously, believed that swallowing chewing gum before a barium meal X-ray would simulate ulceration.[35] Thus, by 1945 the connection between the stomach, military service and emotion had found an established place in British medical and popular culture, while ulcer, a painful disorder and potential cause of death without an effective treatment, was a source of apprehension and dread throughout the population.

The Clinical Picture

Yet, when Britain again found itself at peace and the stresses of conflict had ceased, stomach disorders continued to spread and deaths from perforated ulcer rose until the mid-1950s.[36] Reports by family doctors from the post-war period suggested that patients were often troubled by indigestion and abdominal pains. Dr John Fry (1922–94), a Beckenham GP, systematically collected data from every patient contact and found that the most common presentations in the period 1952 to 1956 were digestive disorders (12 per cent), skin disorders (10 per cent) and psychoneuroses (8.5 per cent).[37] In addition, Fry reported an increased incidence of peptic ulcer in men over 30 and under 60, but believed that the illness was over-diagnosed because only 21 per cent went on to have surgical treatment; most patients, he observed, 'manage quite well' with alkalis and diet. More puzzling still was the fact that patients seemed to recover naturally with time. Fry proposed that the natural history of duodenal ulcer includes 'a natural and spontaneous cure with advancing age'.[38] Given the unreliability of the various tests for duodenal ulcer (barium meal, occult bloods and fractional test meal), it was surprising that Fry did not speculate whether such cases were false positives. Fry also found that women reported only marginally lower levels of digestive symptoms,[39] despite the fact that the incidence of peptic ulcer, established by post-mortem studies, was significantly lower in females.[40] This finding was supported by the national morbidity survey of 1956–7, which suggested that gender was a powerful predictor of ulcer but not disorders of stomach function.[41] Smoking was considered a crucial factor, partly because it was believed that worried men were more like to smoke heavily: a 1949 survey showed that 79 per cent of males smoked compared with 38 per cent of women, who on average smoked only half as many cigarettes as men.[42] In contrast to psychoneuroses, indigestion and abdominal pain were culturally acceptable symptoms for men, not least because multiple interpretations were possible including stress, poor diet and over-work.[43]

Not only did individual doctors identify patterns of illness, but the developing science of statistics and the need to monitor a state-funded health service also encouraged national surveys of morbidity. In 1950 Dr William Logan, chief medical statistician of the General Register Office, had recruited ten English GPs for a three-year pilot study. This revealed 'wide differences between practices' and demonstrated the need for a large representative survey.[44] With the co-operation of Dr R. J. F. H. Pinsent, chairman of the research committee of the College of General Practitioners, Logan recruited family doctors in England and Wales to collect patient data in a standardized manner. Reliant on volunteers, who received no extra payment for the additional work involved, Logan encountered difficulties assembling a geographically representative sample.[45] Initially, 176 GPs based at 110 practices were recruited but when Logan identified gaps in Lancashire and the extreme north, the composition of the sample was modified.[46] In the event, 108 practices (representing 410,000 patients) agreed to collect standardized data to provide an overview of 'communal ill-health' in the English and Welsh populations.[47]

Over twelve months in 1955–6, GPs recorded every consultation by diagnosis on pre-printed cards which were then posted to the General Register Office at Somerset House for analysis.[48] Without efficient computers, the data collection and analysis was laborious. Not until April 1957 had the data been punched manually into 650,000 machine-readable cards and calculations of rates could begin.[49] The first report of symptom and diagnostic statistics took two years to collate. Additional reports followed at two-yearly intervals.[50] Among the most common presentations were: abdominal pain and disorders (2.6 per cent), dyspepsia (0.9 per cent) and peptic ulcer (0.8 per cent), compared with psychoneurotic disorders (5.1 per cent) and skin disorders (6.5 per cent). Although significant regional variation was recorded for 'disorders of the function of the stomach' (from 6.8 per cent in the East and West Ridings, 5.9 per cent in London and the southeast to only 2.9 per centin the south of England) there was no clear explanation for these differences.[51] Geographical variation was also reported for 'psycho-somatic disorders' by region but with no explicable pattern: northern (4.2 per cent), London and the southeast (2.8 per cent) and Wales (0.9 per cent).[52] It is possible that these variations reflected underlying population factors, such as income, patterns of employment and age distribution.

How did contemporaries interpret these patterns of illness? Desmond O'Neill, a psychiatrist at St Mary's Hospital, Paddington, and a key mover in the Society for Psychosomatic Research, believed that dyspepsia was in the main a 'stress disorder',[53] that is a disorder caused by an emotional interaction precipitated by a crisis in the patient's life. The symptoms would resolve, O'Neill argued, 'when the situation changes for the better, or the patient learns to adapt to it without undue tension'.[54] He was less persuasive in explaining how a psychological conflict was translated into physical symptoms ('a response-complex'), but suggested that the area of the body unconsciously 'chosen' to express this conflict was in part determined by family history: 'dyspepsia often seems to run in families ... it is always difficult, however, to separate the influence of inheritance from that of family environment'.[55] Apart from pointing to unhealthy eating habits, O'Neill was unable to explain why so many stress disorders focused on the stomach, rather than other areas of the body.[56] In popular culture, indigestion was associated with stress in situations where emotions could not be expressed openly. For example, Joe Lampton, the principal figure in the best-selling novel *Room at the Top* (1957), observed, 'there was a bad taste in my mouth, the indigestion which always attacks me when I'm angry'.[57]

Arthur Hurst believed that a 'constitutional tendency', based on both physiology and personality, predisposed individuals to ulcers.[58] Treatment, he argued, had to effect a significant change in the 'conditions of life'. In essence, this required a rigid adherence to a prescribed diet: no longer than two hours between meals, only foods that could be chewed into a mush, no more than six cigarettes a day, and avoidance of alcohol. During periods of overwork or 'mental stress', Hurst recommended, 'one day or half-day a week should be spent resting in bed or on a couch', whilst any minor infection should be addressed by remaining in 'bed on a light diet' until completely recovered.[59] Today, this programme reads like a hypochondriac's charter, but it pre-dated the therapeutic revolution and the discovery of effective medicines that accelerated recovery times. It was, nevertheless, a regime that appealed to anxious or neurasthenic patients seeking to avoid stressful situations.

The need to ration basic foodstuffs during the Second World War had exerted a major impact on the nation's diet and in the post-war period restrictions tightened still further. A balance of payments crisis that limited the ability of the UK to purchase imported foodstuffs led to cuts in summer and autumn 1947 and the introduction of potato rationing. Although bread rationing ended in July 1948, the milk ration was cut to 2.5 pints a week in September 1949.[60] Significantly, the regular consumption of milk along with biscuits between main meals was a key recommendation for the management of duodenal ulcer,[61] whilst one of the most popular over-the-counter medicines to treat indigestion was 'Milk of Magnesia'. Through these processes, both rationing and stomach disorders came to occupy a central place in British post-war culture.

National Health Service: Clinical Context and Policy

The epidemic of stomach disorders, indeed of psychosomatic illnesses in general, may have been the result of changes to the provision and funding of state health and welfare facilities: new ways of recording medical data; the creation of a heath service free at the point of delivery; and a general public encouraged to demand treatments as a reward for enduring six years of war. In June 1938, the Ministry of Health had been tasked with setting up an Emergency Medical Service to provide free hospital and out-patient treatment for civilians injured or sick as a result of air-raids.[62] The private health service lacked the capacity to cope with the expected rush of casualties and large buildings were commandeered to serve as hospitals, while nurses and ancillary staff were recruited to create a nationwide service.[63] In November 1942, Sir William Beveridge (1879–1963) published his report on the welfare of Britain and set an agenda for a more interventionist state. Designed to address 'want, disease, ignorance, squalor and idleness',[64] proposals for reconstruction and reform in the post-war period included a unified system of compulsory social insurance that would fund unemployment, injury, maternity and sickness benefit.[65] Speaking for the government in the Commons in February 1943, Sir John Anderson announced the acceptance of a 'comprehensive health service to ensure that for every citizen there is available whatever medical treatment he needs in whatever form he needs it' offered without charge or a means test.[66] The promise of welfare reform was proposed in part to maintain the fighting spirit but also because the plan met with popular support. Moreover, government funding directed at improving acute and casualty services, provided by the Emergency Medical Service, offered a tangible model for a more broadly-based National Health Service.[67] Once the war was over, people felt entitled to make full use of free medical facilities and both family doctors and hospital out-patient clinics struggled to cope with rising numbers of patients seeking advice and treatment, creating long waiting lists.[68] Titmuss believed that these changes, together with a general erosion of deference to authority, also fostered a more 'questioning and critical attitude to medical care' among patients.[69]

Despite a lack of capacity, surveys conducted in the mid-1950s found that the NHS was well-regarded and GPs were trusted. However, this goodwill allowed successive governments to neglect the health service and chronic under-funding and regional inequalities were allowed to persist.[70] Over-worked family doctors often had little time for each patient. Most did not offer an appointment system leading to queues and a potential barrier to attendance.[71] GPs tended to avoid psychological issues. In 1951–2 supported by the Nuffield Provincial Hospitals Trust, Stephen Taylor (1910–88) conducted a qualitative survey of ninety-four family doctors in thirty practices.[72] The study had been prompted by trenchant criticisms of British general practice published in *The Lancet* by J. S. Collings, a visiting Australian doctor.[73] In the published version of his report, Taylor revealed a curious mistrust of psychiatric diagnosis in primary care, arguing that 'there is substantial truth in the hypothesis that the better the clinician, the less often does he diagnose neurosis'.[74] This implied that a patient who presented with a physical symptom, and one that might indicate serious illness, was much more likely to gain the attention of his GP than one who reported low mood or general anxiety. Persistent and painful dyspepsia could imply an ulcer and a family doctor would risk a charge of negligence if he dismissed a patient without an investigation and follow-up appointment. Furthermore, patients were routinely asked about their bowel habits. It was believed, though without foundation, that constipation or the retention of products had toxic side effects.[75] This preoccupation with gastrointestinal function sent a powerful message to patients that abdominal pains would be taken seriously. Indeed, a patient suffering from severe indigestion probably believed that this merited a day or so off work and needed the doctor's official sanction.

Referral to a hospital out-patient department was unlikely to have offered the dyspeptic patient a more nuanced explanation of their symptoms. Fyfe Robertson, a reporter for the *Picture Post*, observed in 1954 that 'too many patients feel that to too many out-patient doctors they are not *people* at all, but card numbers and diseases'.[76] 'Autocratic behaviour among hospital staffs', Titmuss believed, 'with behind them a long tradition deriving from military discipline ... is thereby strengthened by the invasion of scientific techniques, by increasing specialisation and the growth of professional solidarities'.[77] The birth of the NHS also coincided with the dawn of a golden age of high-technology medicine. Notable advances included the growing availability of natural and synthetic antibiotics, anticoagulants, reliable blood transfusion, innovations in anaesthesia, diagnostic X-radiology and electrocardiography, as well as more refined techniques of pathological investigation and mechanization in the operating theatre. Such innovations transformed the capacities of hospital medicine and created conditions for the proliferation of medical and surgical specialties.[78] New science-based treatments scarcely promoted a listening culture of empathy. The growth of specialist departments in district general hospitals, hailed as one of the achievements of the early NHS,[79] also hindered the development of psychosomatic medicine. The increasing number of focused expert opinions discouraged holistic assessments of a patient's health and often led to a sequence of referrals as each consultant could find no recognizable pathology within their sub-speciality.

Psychosomatic Interpretations

In 1941 Arthur Hurst argued that the increased incidence of duodenal ulcer was in part a function of improved investigative techniques: 'the deformity of the bulb in duodenal ulcer was not recognized with the X-rays before 1920, and even the clinical diagnosis dated only from about 1908'.[80] This suggests that the apparent epidemic of psychosomatic illness was, in part, a reflection of new ways of thinking about disease. In a 1943 paper to the *The Lancet*, James Lorimer Halliday (1898–1983), a Scottish regional medical officer, defined psychosomatic illness as 'a bodily disorder whose nature can be appreciated only when emotional disturbances are investigated in addition to physical disturbances'.[81] Halliday believed that British populations had undergone a 'psychosomatic transition': illnesses formerly characteristic of the middle-aged and elderly were spreading into a younger population and disorders once characteristic of women were becoming increasingly common in men.[82] Diseases showing an upward trend, he argued, were precipitated by 'upsetting events' and suggested that the psychological effects of a changed environment were the cause. He identified a wide variety of common disorders to which this interpretation applied and believed that psychological factors could not only precipitate an illness but also have an impact on its course and duration. Whilst Halliday made no overt reference to war, he acknowledged that 'an emotionally upsetting external event or a period of abnormal stress' could act as a trigger.[83] The psychosomatic transition was of concern because it was identified as a significant and growing cause of sickness absence.[84] Halliday believed that the health and fertility of the nation was in terminal decline because 'psychosomatic affections' (such as asthma, rheumatism and peptic ulcer) were rising inexorably because people were increasingly consumed by anxiety and other pathological emotions.[85]

Whilst the explanation proposed by Halliday did not meet with broad approval, it did reflect a growing interest in the relationship between emotions and bodily states. This, in turn, followed the foundation of departments of psychological medicine in leading universities, drawing psychiatrists into the education of medical students and multi-disciplinary research projects.[86] The psychoanalyst John Rickman argued that these developments added 'a new dimension to the medical interview'.[87] The problem for most doctors, however, was a lack of clinical time to implement this approach. In addition, financial constraints imposed on the newly-formed NHS prevented the expansion of psychiatric services in the post-war period, leaving the detection and initial treatment of psychosomatic illness to family doctors.[88]

Responses to these patterns of illness and the managerial and economic problems that they created varied. Set up in January 1955 under the presidency of Dr John Hambling, a Canterbury physician, the Society for Psychosomatic Research sought to bring clinicians together from a wide range of disciplines to understand 'the human organism in health and disease'.[89] In the 1958 edition of *A Textbook of Psychiatry*, David Henderson observed that 'psycho-somatic medicine' was both 'a method of clinical approach to all patients' and a way of interpreting 'a group of physical diseases or syndromes'.[90] War, he argued, not only increased the incidence of such disorders but also developed understanding of 'these principles' because fear and anxiety 'are among the commonest causes of the physical discomforts for which medical advice is sought'.[91] Henderson illustrated the change in clinical practice that these ideas prompted: 'in the past it has commonly happened that symptoms referred to by the patient as indigestion were accepted as such by the doctor and labelled as "dyspepsia" which was then treated as a disease *sui generis*'.[92] Now, if the doctor had time, he would explore whether an emotional conflict had triggered the pain and attempt to resolve the underlying cause rather than merely treat the symptom.

These ideas found expression in the Medical Research Council report from Richard Doll (1912–2005) and Francis Avery Jones (1910–98) into *The Aetiology of Gastric and Duodenal Ulcers* published in 1951. Their survey of 6,047 men and women found that social class could not explain why some people with dyspepsia developed ulcers while others did not. Doll and Avery Jones believed that occupation was a significant risk factor. Jobs associated with a high incidence included doctors, foremen and business executives ('responsible positions in industry'), while farm workers, clerical and administrative staff were at low risk. Although 'anxiety over work was complained of more frequently by men with proved ulcers than by men without symptoms of dyspepsia', the authors remained uncertain whether stress was the primary aetiological factor or whether symptoms were the product of a particular personality type, one prone to diligence and worry.[93] They developed the pre-war hypothesis that individual characteristics explained differences in rates:

> The duodenal ulcer subject has frequently been described as an over-conscientious, hard-working, ambitious type of man, and it is reasonable to assume that it is this type who would most readily complain of anxiety from over work, and who would tend to become appointed to positions of responsibility. It is considered ... that men with this conscientious type of personality are particularly prone to develop duodenal ulcers.[94]

Although the 1958 edition of Henderson and Gillespie's *Textbook of Psychiatry* placed duodenal ulcer in the category of physical illness, the authors added 'emotional factors are believed to be of decisive importance'.[95] In 1959, two American cardiologists, Meyer Friedman (1910–2001) and Ray H. Rosenman, applied this model to explain variations in rates of cardiovascular disease. Men with Type A personality, characterized by ambition and competitive drive, were considered to be at particular risk.[96] Thus, as notions of constitutional medicine spread, an individual's innate qualities and patterns of behaviour were associated with a range of significant health hazards.

Impact of the War

Official histories have argued that the transition from war to peace was managed successfully, avoiding the large number of war-pension claims for shell shock that followed the First World War. 'Up to the end of 1948', Titmuss concluded, 'no evidence was forthcoming to suggest that there had been any dramatic increase in neurotic illnesses or mental disorders in Britain'.[97] Planned demobilization, full employment, advances in psychological treatment and an interventionist government have been cited as reasons for the containment of traumatic memory. However, during the conflict itself, a number of psychiatrists had argued that the health effects of the conflict might not be revealed until the return of peace. Employed by the government to survey the psychological impact of air raids, Aubrey Lewis warned that the full effect of 'war-related stress' might be delayed and that 'the evil harvest may be reaped afterwards'.[98] Equally, a national survey conducted in 1943 by Dr C. P. Blacker (1895–1975) found that many directors of psychiatric clinics believed a 'latent neurosis' existed in the civilian population. Whether this developed into overt psychological or psychosomatic disorder after the war was dependent on 'the social and economic conditions ... and the moral atmosphere which prevailed'.[99] One hypothesis considered by contemporaries to explain the epidemic of stomach disorders was that the offer of financial compensation through the war pension system and the creation of a free health service encouraged people to exaggerate their symptoms. In 1943, the burden of proof had been reversed in favour of the claimant, with the increasing likelihood that an application to the Ministry of Pensions would be successful.[100] Whilst the majority of individuals presenting to their GP with dyspepsia or a suspected duodenal ulcer were not in receipt of a war pension, they may nevertheless have felt entitled to officially-sanctioned time off work or other state benefits.

Joanna Bourke has proposed an alternative hypothesis to explain the apparent epidemic of psychosomatic illness in the immediate post-war period. She has argued that the decline of tangible external threats after 1945, together with the therapeutic revolution, contributed to the rise of generalized anxiety in British society.[101] Whereas in the past a frightened individual might turn to the community or a religious institution for advice and support, emotion became increasingly focused on individuals rather than groups. No longer threatened by invasion or aerial assault and with a small but growing range of effective medicines supplied free of charge, a culture of anxiety developed in post-war Britain which found expression in psychosomatic illnesses. The 1950s occupied a transitional position: traumatic experience remained fresh in the memory and former members of the armed forces and emergency services often struggled to adjust to routine peacetime roles. To what extent, then, were indigestion and stomach pain bodily expressions of emotional conflicts? This is, of course, an unanswerable question but it is instructive to try to assess popular responses to the war.

The government was concerned about the health of some returning soldiers and in particular those who had been prisoners-of-war. During the course of 1943, British military authorities had become increasingly aware of problems with repatriated officers. Although returned to duty, high rates of invalidity and disciplinary incidents in men with excellent military records suggested that imprisonment had adverse consequences.[102] In the summer of 1945, the government unveiled a national rehabilitation programme. Re-education and employment were the focus of the twenty 'Civil Resettlement Units' (CRUs) set up by the War Office,[103] while the Royal Air Force opened a number of 'Resettlement Training Centres'. Brigadier H. A. Sandiford, director of army psychiatry, believed that 'resocialisation' was the aim and that 'finding a suitable job' was the most form of important therapy.[104] CRU courses lasted a month but could be extended. They included factory visits and social activities to bring the former prisoner-of-war into contact with 'institutions, individuals and situations towards which he was often burdened with feelings of mistrust and suspicion'.[105] Week-end leave was designed to bridge the gap between army and home life. The intention of providing each unit with a resident psychiatrist was not met due to staff shortages. Symptoms and changed behaviour were interpreted as a consequence of poor nutrition and confinement, together with insufficient time to adapt to widespread social and cultural changes that had occurred during their imprisonment.[106]

Anecdotal reports from the post-war years offered evidence of demoralization amongst the civilian population. Visiting Britain during the winter freeze of 1946–7, Christopher Isherwood wrote that Londoners 'didn't seem depressed or sullen' though 'their faces were still wartime faces, lined and tired'.[107] Accounts in Mass Observation diaries provide conflicting evidence: Edie Rutherford, a Sheffield housewife and clerk, wrote in May 1947, 'folk are not in a despairing mind, in spite of all', while a month earlier Maggie Blunt, a publicity officer in Slough, recorded 'our nerves are on edge, our anxieties and depressions enormous'.[108] The problem for the historian is that anecdotes can be found to support any hypothesis and without representative population studies it is impossible to know how widespread demoralization was or whether it was sufficiently deep to impact on mental and physical health. That the government funded schemes designed to lift the morale of the nation (such as the 1948 Olympic Games and the 1951 Festival of Britain), at a time when these were scarcely affordable, suggests that the mood of the people was generally downbeat after the euphoria of victory had passed. As many contemporaries believed, pervasive low mood in times of austerity may have increased the likelihood of psychosomatic illnesses and their report to NHS doctors.

Conclusion

The 1940s and 1950s witnessed two parallel phenomena relating to the stomach. First, Britain was hit by an epidemic of duodenal ulcer confirmed by post-mortem studies, which to this day has not been explained by gastroenterologists. Hypotheses have ranged from a high salt diet, increased levels of smoking through to the natural evolution of a disease process. Complementing this, and in cultural terms inextricably intertwined, was an epidemic of indigestion and abdominal pain. In most cases this did not reflect an underlying disease, evoking speculation as to its cause. Increasingly dyspepsia was interpreted as a stress-related disorder associated with the pressure of modern living, in particular industrial and commercial routines in large cities.

According to Ian Hacking particular concepts of illness 'will take only if there is a larger social setting that will receive it'.[109] Illness representations spread throughout a population if they offer a form of understanding that accords with popular beliefs and anxieties.[110] The British people, soldiers and civilians alike, had endured six years of war that had not only threatened their lives but also their lifestyle and the integrity of their nation. They had suffered austerity, uncertainty and, once the peace had been restored, were presented with constant reminders of their trauma: bombed towns, rationing and National Service. The idea that worry and anxiety could have physiological effects and undermine well-being had personal meaning for a significant section of the adult population in the late 1940s and early 1950s.

The scale and enormity of the Second World War underlined the impact that events could have on peoples' health. Heredity and infection were established causes of illness to which was now added stress. Psychologically-minded doctors, such as Taylor, emphasized the need to consider the environment, not only in terms of the workplace, but also in terms of the design of new settlements to replace housing destroyed by air-raids. Diet and lifestyle became increasingly important as common illnesses, such as asthma, hypertension, peptic ulcer, rheumatism and skin rashes, were linked to underlying psycho-biological processes. At a time when psychiatric diagnoses attracted stigma, it was not surprising that patients tended to emphasize physical symptoms and seek explanations that located causality with external agencies. Stress had the advantage that it could affect anyone who found themselves exposed to the new battlefield of industry and commerce. A nation recovering from the effects of total warfare readily took its aches and pains to the new NHS and thereby established a pattern of illness presentation that was to endure beyond the 1950s.

Acknowledgements

This research was supported by a grant from the Wellcome Trust, Grant No. 086071/Z/08/Z.

9 FOOD ALLERGY, MENTAL ILLNESS AND STRESS SINCE 1945

Matthew Smith

In 1976, British psychiatrist Richard Mackarness (1916–96) claimed that many of the mysterious, chronic and intractable ailments suffered by patients, including mental health problems, were caused by reactions to food, especially processed foods and synthetic additives.[1] He began with the case of one of his patients at Park Prewett Hospital in Basingstoke. 'Joanna', twenty-eight-years-old, had suffered from attacks of irritable, depressive, tense and violent behaviour ever since the birth of her third child in 1967. During the following six years, she had been admitted to Park Prewett thirteen times, often because of the danger she posed to her children, whom she had neglected and subjected to physical abuse. She was also a threat to herself, slashing her forearms with any nearby sharp object during 'her most disturbed phases ... as a way of relieving, if only temporarily, the unbearable tension and irritability mounting inside of her'.[2] Although her upbringing had not been ideal – Joanna's mother had beaten her as a child and they had slept in the same bed until she was eighteen years old – psychotherapy had not proven to be efficacious. Joanna's history was presented for a final time at a case conference, consisting of psychiatrists, psychiatric social workers, medical students, the consultant psychiatrist and Mackarness himself, and her prognosis for recovery was thought by all to be grim. Since Joanna had already been treated with 'every known combination of psychotropic drugs as well as several courses of ECT [electroconvulsive therapy]', most felt that psycho-surgery was the only solution, meaning that her three children would be most certainly taken into care.[3] Then Mackarness spoke up, speculating that Joanna might be suffering from 'a particularly severe case of food allergy'. Although the group generally felt that such an approach was 'bound to fail', the consultant was not eager to send Joanna to the neurosurgeons and, as a last resort, left her in Mackarness's care.[4]

Mackarness's first step was to place Joanna in Park Prewett's intensive care unit, where she fasted for five days. After the fast, during which time her behaviour had improved considerably, she was fed specific foods, one by one. Following the introduction of each food, Joanna and two independent observers assessed her reactions and Mackarness soon identified a number of foods that were likely triggers for Joanna's reactions, specifically coffee, egg, porridge, veal and bacon. Following a series of double-blind tests, Mackarness determined that these foods, as well as chocolate and cheese, were responsible for her symptoms and removed them from Joanna's diet. Before long, Joanna was discharged, taken off all medication and, within months, her general practitioner enthused that:

> Joanna has made a remarkable improvement. She is happy, gay, euphoric, sometimes almost hypomanic in her hearty enjoyment of life. She goes out to work, cares for the children without harming them, looks after her house and generally seems to be almost back to her old self before this illness first attacked her.[5]

Mackarness added that she continued to experience good mental health, apart from 'three short readmissions when she became ill through breaking her diet', lapses which were due to the 'addictive element in food and chemical allergy'.[6]

Joanna's story is emblematic of a prominent and controversial, yet enduring, trend in the history of allergic diseases, that is a tendency to blame food allergy for mental illness. Although the relationship between foods and mental illness arguably gained the greatest notoriety during the 1970s, when San Francisco allergist Ben Feingold (1899–1982) claimed that certain food chemicals could trigger hyperactivity in children, many other allergists had long believed that food allergy was a significant source of otherwise unexplained mental disorder.[7] The title of Mackarness's book, *Not All in the Mind*, was therefore a reminder to clinicians that the roots of psychiatric problems were not always to be found in disordered minds; allergic reactions to food could also be the explanation.

It is possible, however, that Mackarness's title carried other implications. While Mackarness and many food allergists claimed that symptoms of mental illness could be caused by food, critics argued the reverse: patients were mentally unbalanced and their complaints were psychosomatic, having nothing to do with food; in other words, their 'allergic' symptoms *were* all in the mind. As Mark Jackson and Carla Keirns have demonstrated, psychosomatic theories of allergic disease were common during the middle part of the twentieth century, particularly in cases of asthma.[8] While Jackson argues that psychosomatic theories of asthma not only played on stereotypes of the 'good mother', but also 'legitimated nascent radical, holistic, and ecological critiques of biomedical reductionism' that emerged during the post-war period, psychosomatic theories of food allergy were regarded by most allergists as being less radical and more credible than the suggestion that food allergy could cause mental illness.[9] Such assessments were partly due to the dominance of psychoanalysis in post-war Western culture and medicine, but also due to fundamental problems that many orthodox allergists had with respect to how food allergists defined, treated and understood allergy.[10] The issue of whether the symptoms experienced by food allergy sufferers were legitimately caused by food or were instead manifestations of psychosomatic illness would serve as a schism between food allergists and their more orthodox colleagues. While food allergists believed that allergic reactions to a wide range of foods and food chemicals could trigger a plethora of symptoms, orthodox allergists downplayed the prevalence of allergy, arguing that such reactions were psychosomatic. At the heart of these divisions were differences in how each group defined allergy. Orthodox allergists defined allergy narrowly, restricting it to only cases in which immune system involvement could be proven (chiefly through the use of skin tests). In contrast, food allergists employed a broad definition of allergy, encompassing both cases in which immune system involvement could be demonstrated and those in which such proof was elusive, resulting in fundamental differences in how food allergies, and allergic disease more generally, were understood. A patient entering an allergist's office during the 1950s, therefore, might leave with a prescription for an elimination diet or a referral to a psychiatrist.

This chapter explores how allergists came to conceptualize the relationship between food allergy and mental health during the post-war period, highlighting three themes that help to characterize and explain the irreconcilable split between food allergists and more psychosomatically-oriented allergists. First, allergists' disagreements about the legitimacy of food allergy reflected broader divisions about the nature of medical knowledge. While food allergists privileged inductive knowledge gained through repeated clinical encounters, advocates of psychosomatic allergy valued deductive knowledge that was rooted in psychoanalytical theory. Second, due to diagnostic challenges, food allergists were far more reliant on patient testimony in order to diagnose and treat food allergy. Such reliance meant that food allergists were more likely to trust their patients' accounts of their symptoms, unlike either conventional allergists, who relied on skin-prick tests for diagnosis and on desensitization as a treatment, or psychosomatically-oriented clinicians, who interpreted patient symptoms through the lens of Freudian theory. Finally, food allergists and their critics differed markedly in terms of how they interpreted stress as a contributor to allergic disease. Whereas psychosomatically-oriented allergists believed that stress was largely a psychological force that originated in traumatic life events, food allergists saw stress as an ecological phenomenon, a manifestation of the disjunction between human beings and their increasingly chemicalized environment.

Epistemological Differences

Many post-war debates about food allergy were rooted in epistemological issues, specifically whether deductive or inductive reasoning generated better knowledge about allergies. Within medicine, deduction was increasingly employed after the Second World War in the form of randomly-controlled trials (RCTs), the 'gold standard' of medical research, in order to test the effectiveness of treatments and to identify whether improvement might be due to the placebo effect. As sociologists Harry Collins and Trevor Pinch have suggested, the placebo effect was 'a massive embarrassment to the *science* of medicine', showing that 'at best, medical science has only partial control over its subject matter'.[11] Whereas deduction was increasingly associated with medical research, induction (or constructing generalizations from accumulated experiences) was closely associated with clinical practice. Clinicians developed hypotheses about clinical phenomena after observing, questioning and treating patients over a period of time. Some historians have argued that the split between clinical practice and laboratory research, one that parallels the dichotomy between inductive and deductive reasoning, has been overemphasized.[12] Indeed, allergists such as including John Freeman (1876–1962) cautioned against 'basing clinical decision merely on an accumulation of cases', and believed instead that a 'symbiotic' relationship should exist between the clinic and the laboratory.[13] But, in the case of food allergy, epistemological debates of this nature were prominent, especially with respect to the relationship between food allergy and mental illness.

A good example of how induction shaped food allergists' understanding of the relationship between food allergy and behavioural problems in children can be found in a 1950 survey of American and Canadian allergists by New York allergist T. Wood Clarke. Although most food allergists refrained from discussing the precise mechanism of such allergies, Clarke argued that so-called 'cerebral allergy' or 'neuro-allergy' was caused by cerebral oedema or impaired vascular function in the brain, which could cause not only migraine but also epilepsy, dizziness and abnormal behaviour.[14] Mental illness, therefore, was rooted in neurological dysfunction.[15] Such thinking contrasted fundamentally with psychoanalytically-oriented allergists who believed that allergic symptoms were primarily psychosomatic and that mental illness originated in traumatic early childhood experiences and interpersonal conflict, rather than brain pathology.[16] By surveying his fellow allergists, Clarke hoped to undermine psychosomatic notions and provide evidence that food allergy could cause a wide range of behavioural problems in children, a claim that allergists had been making for decades.[17]

Clarke reported that 95 of his 171 respondents acknowledged the relationship between food allergy and behavioural problems in children and included testimonies from dozens of allergists, all of whom supported a link between allergy and behavioural problems. According to the Boston physician Abraham Colmes, there 'is no doubt in the mind of any physician who is practicing allergy that food sensitivities do bring about definite changes in children's behavior'. Oklahoma paediatric allergist Fannie Lou Leney (1902–94) explained how 'every day since I have been practicing allergy, mothers come in with the statement that "Johnny is so irritable", or "his disposition is so much better since he is on his diet", or that " he is as mean as the devil when he eats a certain food"'.[18] Clarke's respondents also provided case studies that contributed to the accumulation of evidence about the wide range of behaviours linked to allergy:

> irritable, fretful, quarrelsome children, who could not get along with others, often had to be taken out of school as they upset the classes and were considered incorrigible, who after the nature of their allergy was discovered and proper steps taken to correct it, became friendly and happy and took active and joyous part in the occupations of their mates.[19]

Michigan allergist Gerald C. Grout recounted the case of a ten-year-old boy who was found to be sensitive to 'several of the more common foods, principally corn, wheat, chocolate and orange' and whose irritability and personality changes had gradually improved following avoidance of the offending allergens. The boy's mother stated that:

> it was difficult for her to believe, but she had finally been convinced that the complete reversal in the child's attitude and loss of irritability had accompanied improvement in the allergic symptoms. She further stated that prior to allergic management the child had never smiled and that now he is a very happy child.[20]

Most of the children described in these cases did not seek the assistance of an allergist because of 'character problems', but rather because of somatic symptoms, such as asthma, eczema or gastrointestinal complaints. After culpable foods were eliminated, however, allergists were informed by the child's parents that many additional behavioural problems had also abated. Since the allergic explanation suggested a simple, non-invasive and inexpensive solution, unlike many psychiatric theories, allergists such as Clarke emphasized that it was worth exploring further, suggesting that every child sent to a state hospital be given an allergic assessment. Not only was testing for allergies likely to be 'far more effective than either beatings or other forms of punishment', but through allergic treatment, 'psychic seeds may be rooted out and future psychoses forestalled'.[21]

Unlike many more dogmatic food allergists, Clarke advocated that allergists and child psychiatrists should 'co-operate in the study of the "problem child" from both the allergic and psychic angles'.[22] He acknowledged that the 'discomfort' caused by recurring respiratory, dermatological and gastrointestinal allergic symptoms could 'so affect the child's stability that his mental equilibrium is broken down and his character changed' due to the 'tension on his nervous system'.[23] He also conceded that the 'over-solicitous' parenting of an allergic child could result in further character problems.[24] Other researchers similarly commented that the 'stress' of dealing with allergies could result in secondary behavioural problems, including anxiety, anger and depression.[25] But Clarke's insistence that 'allergists ... pay more attention to the psyche of their child patients' and that 'child psychiatrists ... appreciate that psychosomatic medicine can travel in reverse gear, that physical allergy of the brain can cause emotional changes' indicates that many of his colleagues were unwilling to recognize a relationship between allergy and mental illness in such pluralistic terms.[26]

Leading allergist Leslie N. Gay (1891–1978), for example, argued that food allergists exaggerated their claims about food allergy and that other explanations were preferable. In a review of a textbook by prominent California allergist, Albert H. Rowe (1889–1970), Gay contended that: 'It is unfortunate that allergists rarely consider the psychosomatic side of human behavior ... permanent relief is obtained when a thorough study of his home environment and of his many mental problems is made, and when these all-important factors are adjusted'.[27] Gay's focus on the psychosomatic aspects of allergy was not unusual during the post-war period. Inspired by the writing of psychosomatic theorist Helen Flanders Dunbar (1902–59) and Freudian psychoanalysis, many allergists believed that allergy was essentially psychogenic.[28] Some individuals, according to Erich Wittkower (1899–1983), president of the American Psychosomatic Society, simply had 'an allergic personality'.[29] Listed among the possible treatments advocated for psychosomatic allergy were not only psychoanalysis and hypnosis, but also 'parentectomy' or the practice of removing children from asthma- or allergy-producing homes.[30] In one case, a ten-year-old girl with severe asthma was sent to a school where allergens to which she reacted were present. Abatement of her symptoms was explained in terms of her removal from psychodynamic triggers. According to the study's author:

> The allergist must begin now to consciously utilize all of these basic data of psychodynamics so that he may incorporate within his practice not only the information obtained from the basic sciences from physics and chemistry but also from the basic science of psychodynamics.[31]

Although clinical encounters certainly influenced how psychosomatically-oriented allergists – and many psychiatrists – came to understand the relationship between mental health and allergy,[32] analysis of the relevant medical literature suggests that, in comparison to food allergists, many physicians were chiefly driven by deductive reasoning rooted in psychoanalytical theory. In other words, the diagnosis and explanation of allergic complaints for psychosomatically-oriented physicians centred on the appropriate application of psychosomatic and psychoanalytical theory, rather than the incremental development of an explanation based on a series of clinical encounters, as was the case for food allergists. Such deduction was prevalent in a 1946 issue of *The Nervous Child* focusing on 'Psychosomatic Problems of Childhood', in which four out of the seven articles addressed allergic complaints, including itching, asthma and eczema.

One study focused on the relationship between mothers and their children. In one case, a girl with no family history of allergy developed asthma as she approached graduation from grammar school and found that her symptoms worsened whenever her relationship with her mother was threatened by physical separation or new relationships. According to the author, 'the longing to regress, to return to mother, apparently created sufficient tension to cause the attacks of asthma'.[33] In another case, a girl's eczema was blamed on the fact that her mother 'neglected her', returning to work soon after giving birth and leaving the infant in her grandmother's care. Whenever the girl visited her grandmother in later childhood, her eczema would disappear, only to break out even worse when she returned to her parents' home.[34]

Another article discussed the role that psychological factors played in dermatological problems, or 'cutaneous psychiatry', a topic boasting a body of literature 'so extensive that the selection of quotations would merely lead one astray'.[35] Although the authors acknowledged that dermatological reactions were atopic, meaning that a hereditary predisposition to allergy was involved, psychological factors were considered to be even more important:

> Now let us suppose that an infant endowed with these biological heredities has his first skin manifestations ... The child experiences stimulation in an organ system which has all the properties to be used for an adequate discharge of libidinal energies ... The child may then turn from curiosity to voyeurism; from pride and childish boasting to exhibitionism; from hostility, rage, and guilt feelings to sadomasochism; from love to self-love. All these can be acted out on the skin.[36]

If 'psychosomatic interplay' such as scratching an itch was prohibited by the child's parents, this would not only increase the pleasure derived from it, but also mean that scratching would serve as an outlet for any other conflicts between parent and child.[37] In the case of a fourteen-year-old girl with chronic atopic dermatitis, the mother prevented her daughter from sucking her thumb by putting her arms in braces and sprinkling pepper over her thumb. The treatment lasted until the girl was eight-years-old and because of it 'she hated her mother fiercely. Her hatred found the best outlet in scratching'.[38]

In these articles and others, psychotherapy was suggested as the primary means of treatment, although the details of such therapy are scant. One study described how the outcome of psychotherapy was 'somewhat impressive', but then intimated that such success might have been due to the fact that narcissistic patients enjoyed the attention that testing and psychoanalysis provided, stating that 'they tried to please and reward us with the improvement of their skin conditions'.[39] Sometimes avoidance of allergies and desensitization were attempted, but to no avail; what did work was either changing the behaviour of parents or resolving the underlying conflict.[40]

Discussions of psychotherapy were, however, largely overshadowed by descriptions of the patients' backgrounds, relationships, symptoms and the application of psychoanalytical theory. When therapy was mentioned, it was almost an afterthought, a dénouement after the climactic elucidation of what was truly at the heart of a patient's allergy. It is possible that, as with psychotherapy more generally, such a focus on explaining problems, rather than treating them, contributed to the eventual decline in psychosomatic explanations for allergy.[41] But it also represented a profoundly different way in which to construct knowledge about allergy. Unlike food allergists, who emphasized the incremental development of their insights, the knowledge generated by psychosomatically-oriented allergists was chiefly driven by pre-existing theoretical maxims which were rooted in psychoanalysis, and could be applied to allergy. Although some food allergists could also develop a similarly unilateral approach to their interpretation of the symptoms of allergy – by repeatedly insisting that food allergens were to blame – their predisposition to suspecting food was constantly moderated by another factor: a pronounced dependence on the recollections and insights of their patients.

Diagnosing Food Allergy

In 1953, former president of the American Academy of Allergy Will C. Spain articulated the difficulties inherent in diagnosing and treating food allergy in his review of *Food Allergy*, written by Theron Randolph (1906–95), Herbert Rinkel (1896–1963) and Michael Zeller (1900–77).[42] Unlike allergists dealing with inhalant allergies, food allergists could not rely on skin tests for effective diagnosis. Not only were skin tests potentially dangerous in cases of severe food allergy, but they were also inaccurate, producing many false negatives and positives. The capacity of food allergy to mimic the symptoms produced by other conditions also posed problems. Because of this, food allergists had to rely on their patients' testimony which, according to Spain, could be subject to 'whims, fancies, and aversions'.[43]

Although Spain's review of *Food Allergy* was cautiously positive, his description of patients' 'whims, fancies, and aversions' suggests that he was sceptical of patients' accounts of their symptoms. To a degree, Spain's approach to patient testimony was indicative of the allergist-patient relationship in conventional allergy. Patients were passive participants in the diagnostic and therapeutic approaches employed by allergists. Dust, pollen and pet allergies, for example, were detected through the use of skin tests. Allergists would inject the skin of a patient with suspected allergens and then see if the surrounding skin erupted in a wheal. Once an allergy was diagnosed, allergists would treat it through the use of desensitization therapy, injecting minuscule amounts of an allergen into the patient, gradually increasing the amount over time in the hope that the patient would develop resistance. In both diagnosis and treatment, therefore, allergists were the dominant party in the relationships that they had with patients.

A similar pattern existed in the relationship between the psychosomatically-oriented physician and their patient. While patient accounts of their life history and relationships were important, it was the physician's interpretation of these experiences, marinated in psychoanalytical theory, that was paramount in determining which psychodynamic factors were triggering allergies and which therapy was most appropriate. The opinions, beliefs and reasoning of patients, if anything, interfered with the diagnostic and therapeutic process. Perhaps more importantly, in both the conventional and the psychosomatic conceptualization of allergy, it was the patient, in body or mind, who was damaged or dysfunctional and who needed correction.

The relationship between food allergists and their patients differed significantly. Unable to rely on the same diagnostic tools as conventional allergists and wary of psychosomatic explanations, food allergists depended on the testimony of their patients to determine which foods were causing their allergies, largely through the use of elimination diets. Although the allergist would prescribe a specific diet, it was dependent on the patient to adhere to it and to observe their own responses to the introduction of particular foods by keeping a diet diary. Patients had an even more active role with respect to treatment, in that it was their responsibility to avoid the foods that caused their symptoms. In this way, food allergists and their patients developed a cooperative, almost symbiotic, relationship. As Rowe described, 'the absolute determination of all the allergenic causes of many allergic manifestations requires the intelligent and understanding cooperation and analysis of the patient'.[44] Rowe's reliance on the 'intelligent' patient for effective diagnosis and treatment was not unusual amongst physicians who suspected that food could cause otherwise unexplained symptoms. Unlike conventional or psychosomatically-oriented allergists, whose patients were essentially the passive recipient of medical expertise, the patients of food allergists were active agents, intimately involved in their own diagnosis and treatment.[45] Equally, if it was the patient's body or mind that needed to change in conventional or psychosomatic allergy, then for food allergists it was the patient's environment and diet that had to change. As food allergists, notably Theron Randolph, became more concerned about the allergenic nature of processed foods, additives and environmental pollutants, this mind-set intensified. It was not the patient who was dysfunctional, but their environment.[46]

The cooperative, sympathetic relationship food allergists enjoyed with their patients was enhanced by the fact that many individuals came to food allergists as a last resort. This was especially the case for patients who were suffering from psychiatric symptoms, as Joanna's story indicates. Unsurprisingly, food allergists often relished their ability to help such desperate people, as expressed in a 1950 letter to Theron Randolph: 'It is a grand life to be in allergy and get enthusiastic about curing the psychoneurotic, and the impossible'.[47] Part of this pleasure derived from demonstrating that patients should not be blamed for the behavioural symptoms that they exhibited. In a discussion of how food allergies could cause fatigue and irritability in children, for example, Randolph described how, before effective allergic management, 'a common reaction is to assume that the child is a "naughty brat" and to inflict various types of punishment to induce the child to "snap out of it"'.[48] In other cases, more intensive medical intervention would be attempted. Randolph described an eight-year-old boy who, in addition to nasal obstruction and hearing difficulties, presented a range of behavioural problems, including 'progressive fatigue, listlessness, irritability, crankiness ... restlessness, jitteriness, inattentiveness, and apparent difficulty in concentration', which hampered his scholastic achievement.[49] In order to treat the somatic symptoms, the boy underwent a tonsillectomy and two adenoidectomies to no avail. Once Randolph had determined that the boy was allergic to a range of foods, however, all symptoms disappeared.

Those sceptical of food allergy were quick to provide alternative explanations for such recoveries. The relationship between food allergists and their patients, changes in domestic routine caused by elimination diets, the hopes instilled in patients and parents by food allergists and the empowerment of patients, argued some, could act as a placebo.[50] Although many food allergists acknowledged these possibilities, they argued that it was not the decisive factor. Instead, the reduction of symptoms following the elimination of an allergenic food could ease household tensions more generally, contributing to better relationships, particularly between parents and their children.[51] Such a scenario was described by Connecticut physiologist and physician William Kaufman (1910–2000) in the case of Charles, a twelve-year-old who suffered from fatigue, headache and nausea. Although Charles's parents, especially his mother, simply dismissed him as a 'lazy dope', Kaufman determined that he was allergic to eggs. After eggs were eliminated from Charles's diet, 'his whole life changed', permitting 'him to attain his proper status in his family and at school'. Moreover, the 'change in attitude of other people toward him ... further helped him emotionally'.[52] Although Kaufman recognized that some reactions to food were psychogenic, due to 'life stresses', he emphasized that for many children 'the moment one can remove the etiologic agent, the child is restored'.[53]

In Charles's case, as in others, the blame for symptoms shifted from resting solely with the patient (and their faulty immune system or mental state) to outside agents, specifically, food. By seeing their patients as not inherently damaged and by perceiving them as intelligent, active partners in the diagnostic and therapeutic enterprise, food allergists not only attracted many sufferers who had failed to find help elsewhere, but also engendered a fierce loyalty in them. According to many patients, food allergists, unlike their psychosomatically-oriented counterparts, were on the side of their patients, both empathizing with and empowering them.[54] Relieved that their symptoms were 'not all in the mind', patients and parents played a key role in forming groups such as the Society for Clinical Ecology, founded by Theron Randolph in 1965 (renamed the American Academy of Environmental Medicine in 1984), and the Feingold Association of the United States, which stressed the link between food additives and hyperactivity in children. For these groups, clinicians such as Randolph and Feingold were granted near-hagiographic status; those who downplayed the role of food and additives were seen as villains. Such divisions were crystallized by the distinct ways in which food allergists and psychosomatically-oriented allergists defined stress.

Stress and Allergy

It is not surprising that Hans Selye's concept of stress was interpreted variously, given that his term was often stretched and modified to meet particular needs, not least by Selye himself.[55] In this way, use of the term stress mirrored that of allergy, which was also manipulated to suit the epistemological frameworks of allergists. For advocates of psychosomatic allergy, it was 'emotional stress' that was central in allergic diseases, as writers in the first volume of *Psychosomatic Medicine* attested in 1939.[56] Explaining the theory in *Introduction to Clinical Allergy*, Feingold described how 'under stress many physiological changes occur. If these protective physiological aberrations, used originally as emergency measures, become habitual ways of coping with continuous daily stresses, then permanent tissue damage may result, with concomitant clinical patterns of asthma, rhinitis, hay fever, hypertension, and so forth'.[57] Citing a study undertaken by New York neurologist Harold Wolff (1898–1962), Feingold noted how exposure to stress or even discussion of 'repugnant material' could be even more of an aggravating factor than the allergen itself.[58] Others observed that, in cases of asthma, physicians tended to 'over-emphasize physical-allergic factors in the precipitation of an asthma attack'.[59] In one study of psychosomatic allergy in a pair of identical twins, for instance, skin tests revealed that both brothers were equally sensitive to house dust and certain foods, but 'were strikingly different in their allergic manifestations', with brother 'A' having many more asthma attacks than brother 'B'.[60] The researchers determined that the explanation for this stemmed from the fact that 'A' was the favoured son and felt:

> a great need to succeed in order to please other people. His whole life is directed toward achieving success so that he will be acclaimed by his family and friends … when he is faced with a situation in which he must prove his ability to others … the tension is so great that it precipitates an attack of asthma.[61]

Such conclusions were echoed in a later study, in which women with various allergy symptoms were tested. Women who did not react strongly to skin tests were found to be more 'generally distressed and feeling unable to defend themselves against the onslaughts of everyday life', presenting symptoms of depression, withdrawal and anxiety.[62] These findings, according to the researchers, provided 'strong evidence that the allergy population is far from homogeneous either physiologically or psychologically'.[63]

For some physicians, such as Wolff, stress played such a prominent role in allergic diseases, such as asthma, urticaria, rhinitis and migraine (one of Wolff's specialities), that they could be described as 'stress diseases', along with hypertension and ulcers.[64] In 1952, Wolff and his co-investigators described how a checklist of 852 'prognostic factors', including 'life experiences' and how patients dealt with 'life problems', could be used with the help of an IBM sorting machine to determine which factors were most important for particular patients.[65] In another study, Wolff and his colleagues measured how 'life situations', including 'threats and assaults of widely varying character directed against bodily integrity', could exacerbate symptoms of hay fever.[66] One of their case studies involved a '57-year-old Negro housewife', who traced her 'ill-health' back to her marriage, at the age of eighteen, to a 'stern, demanding, unaffectionate husband', who 'took such advantage of her that she had four babies (one of whom died), one criminal abortion, and a pelvic operation within the period of six years'.[67] The woman had been suffering from hay fever for five years, since her three daughters had left home and her husband had become diabetic, with the result that he was even 'more demanding and less sympathetic to her many problems'.[68] She 'felt depressed and was often tearful' and began to exhibit the symptoms of hay fever, which were not eased by the prescription of 'rigid elimination diets' or desensitization therapy.[69] What did seem to abate her symptoms, however, was visiting the clinic, speaking about her domestic problems and receiving support from medical staff.

In order to test the relationship between the patient's 'life situation' and her hay fever, the clinicians subjected her to three experiments. The first measured her symptoms when exposed to pollen during an interview which required her to revisit some painful memories. As the patient discussed the more distressing details, she 'became anxious and restless' and began presenting 'a marked increase in the degree of nasal hyperfunction'.[70] Once 'she was given strong reassurance, support, and understanding by the examiner', not only did she regain 'her feelings of well being and tranquillity', but her nasal 'hyperfunction' also subsided, despite the fact that she was still being exposed to pollen.[71] While another experiment replicated the intense reaction when the patient was asked about her sexual experiences in a room with similar pollen levels, exposure to the same amount of pollen without the probing, personal interview only resulted in mild symptoms. For Wolff and his colleagues, such experiments demonstrated how pollen was not always 'the sole etiologic factor involved in the production of the hay fever syndrome'. Instead, 'a life situation engendering conflict and anxiety' could be required in many cases.[72]

In many of these studies, physicians expressed a subtly judgemental attitude towards their patients, hinting that, at some level, they were responsible for their allergies. Patients might have endured dysfunctional childhoods or marriages, but it was also their inability to cope with such situations that triggered or caused their symptoms.[73] As Jackson has observed, there were political ramifications to such thinking with respect to stress: physicians and politicians preferred 'to blame and treat individuals rather than attempt to overhaul the system: a demonstrable failure to thrive under the pressures created by advanced capitalist societies was more willingly accepted as a sign of personal weakness than as a symptom of the imminent collapse of social and moral order'.[74] This approach was anathema to food allergists who interpreted stress as an external, ecological phenomenon. Seeing stress as 'the struggle to adapt to a noxious agent', they argued, was more in line with Selye's theory of general adaptation.[75] Although some individuals might be more sensitive to such agents than others, it was those responsible for unleashing such agents who were responsible, not the patient.

For his part, Randolph claimed that his conception of 'specific adaptation syndrome', the adaptive process by which susceptible people succumbed to the 'long term inurement of environmental excitants', was a 'clinical counterpart of Selye's general adaptation syndrome'.[76] It was the failure of conventional allergists to reconcile their conceptualizations of allergy with Selye's notion of adaptation that spurred Randolph to theorize about the specific adaptation syndrome and contributed to his conversion from conventional allergy to clinical ecology by the mid-1950s.[77] Debates about whether reactive substances were 'allergens, irritants, or toxins', he argued, detracted from 'the fundamental facts that specific susceptibility and adaptation are the common denominators in the process':[78]

> The breadth of these observations ... is incompatible with the current immunologically restricted use of the word, allergy. Consequently, the broader term, *human ecology*, encompassing man's mutual relationship with his surroundings and other persons, seemed preferable. Clinical ecology ... is concerned with the demonstrated exogenous factors and health and behavior.[79]

Randolph believed that, by limiting the definition of allergy to specific biological processes, orthodox allergists were no longer in a position to deal with many of the reactions presented by patients in the clinic. They were:

> handicapped by self-imposed limitations of their field. Despite allergy having been originally defined as altered reactivity, the allergic concept of disease has since lost much of its usefulness ... A more clinically oriented and useful view is needed as a basis for understanding the long-term effects of a person's surroundings on his health and behavior.[80]

Psychiatric symptoms, in particular, were indicative that a patient had been suffering 'less advanced manifestations' of their allergies for quite some time.[81] The longer a sensitive individual was exposed to food chemicals and foods commonly used in food processing, such as corn and beet, the more likely they were to develop depression, paranoia, hostility, withdrawal and even hallucinations, amnesia and suicidal tendencies, symptomatic of the latter stages of the adaptation process.[82] Randolph estimated that patients suffering from such symptoms constituted at least one third of his Illinois practice, suggesting that clinical ecology would be 'competitive with psychiatry' in treating such patients.[83] As a 1950 letter to Randolph asserted: 'Psychosomatic medicine is going to be hard to fight. It is like Christian Science in that the onus is entirely on the patient to get himself better. Too bad someone cannot keep such stuff out of the *Annals* [*of Allergy*]'.[84] Widened by differing definitions of stress and allergy, by contrasting perceptions of patients and their role in the diagnostic and therapeutic process, and by dissimilar routes to attaining medical knowledge, the schism that existed between food allergists and their psychosomatically-oriented rivals would not be easily overcome.

Conclusion

As this chapter has suggested, the clinical and philosophical meanings of food allergy, mental illness and stress varied considerably during the decades following the Second World War. Orthodox allergists believed that patients who came to their clinic complaining of food allergy were most likely suffering from an underlying mental illness caused by emotional distress. Even in patients where there was immunological evidence of allergic disease, it was the stress of failed relationships, unresolved conflicts or other traumas that was most responsible for triggering or exacerbating the symptoms of hay fever, asthma or dermatitis. In contrast, food allergists and clinical ecologists asserted that food allergy was a manifestation of a completely different kind of stress. Processed foods and food chemicals represented physical stressors that could cause mental illness in susceptible humans. Underlying these conflicting ways of perceiving stress, both of which fitted into how Selye's term would come to be conceptualized, were fundamental differences about whether the most profound risks to human health came from the external environment or from within. Was the world becoming inherently more dangerous, requiring major ecological change? Or did people lack the fortitude of their ancestors and simply need either immunological or psychiatric adjustment? Behind the arguments about food allergy, mental illness and stress were basic questions such as these, which could also be applied to many other post-war debates about other chronic diseases, such as cancer, heart disease, diabetes and obesity. In order to further understand how ideas about stress, allergy and other medical concepts developed during the post-war period, it is important to acknowledge these underlying political and philosophical currents.

In 1966, however, an immunological discovery would deflate such debates within the allergy community. This was the identification of immunoglobulin E (IgE), 'the key antibody in the allergic response', by Japanese-American researchers Kimishige and Teruka Ishizaka.[85] Orthodox allergists now had a marker with which to distinguish 'true' food allergy, in which IgE was present, from food intolerance, in which it was absent. The emergence of IgE privileged certain allergic reactions, such as the sudden, severe and self-evident anaphylactic reactions to peanuts, over the chronic reactions early food allergists emphasized and often blamed for psychiatric problems.[86] Although many sufferers of unexplained health problems still turned to clinical ecologists – and even psychoanalysts[87] – in the decades that followed, anaphylaxis would come to symbolize the typical food allergy reaction, and the innocent, vulnerable child with a peanut allergy would become the archetypal allergy sufferer.

Since anaphylactic, IgE-mediated allergies could be fatal, a different kind of stress became associated with food allergy, namely, the stress of dealing with a life-threatening allergy.[88] Although seeing stress as a consequence, rather than a cause, of allergy was not new, having been acknowledged by Clarke as early as 1950, it nevertheless distracted from attempts to understand the subtler ways in which stress could impact on the functioning of the immune system. Often lost amongst the debates about food allergy and mental illness was the idea, long familiar to many allergists, that stress, however defined, played a secondary, rather than a primary, role in both normal and pathological immune response.[89] In other words, stress intensified, rather than caused, immune dysfunction.[90] While seeing stress in this way may have undermined the theories of the more ideological food allergists and psychosomatically-oriented allergists, it did not lessen the clinical significance of stress. Not only could stress inhibit one's ability to fight off viruses and bacteria, but it could also aggravate an individual's reaction to a food allergen, transforming it from an annoying symptom to a potentially life-threatening condition.

By understanding stress and its relation to food allergy in a more nuanced, and less dogmatic, way, it became possible to at least partially reconcile the views of food allergists and their psychosomatically-oriented rivals. In order to see how this might be the case, it is helpful to return to Joanna. Although Mackarness stressed that the root cause of Joanna's behavioural problems was her allergies to food, he did admit that her psychological state was also influential. Not only was Joanna abused by her mother, a possible explanation for her violent behaviour towards her own children, but Mackarness also observed that she had 'an attention streak in her personality', which spurred her to 'use her knowledge of the bad effects of certain foods upon herself to gain unconsciously desired ends, particularly when frustrated or angry with others in the ordinary course of living'.[91] The best way to deal with this, Mackarness suggested, was psychotherapy. For Joanna, mental illness might not have been *all* in the mind, but the mind still had its role to play.

Acknowledgements

The research on which this chapter is based was generously supported by a Wellcome Trust post-doctoral fellowship, Grant No. WT045705.

10 LABOURING STRESS: SCIENTIFIC RESEARCH, TRADE UNIONS AND PERCEPTIONS OF WORKPLACE STRESS IN MID-TWENTIETH-CENTURY BRITAIN

Joseph Melling

Recent records tell us that workplace stress is a formidable problem in modern society. Britain's Health and Safety Executive (HSE) estimated that in 2006–7 a total of 13.8 million working days were lost to work-related stress, depression and anxiety, and occupational stress was thought to be responsible for one third of all new incidents of ill-health.[1] The sharply rising incidence of stress in the workplace and wider society appears to be a relatively recent phenomenon, though the reasons for the global 'pandemic' of occupational illness remain obscure. Many researchers have argued that the origins of a modern epidemic of stress lies in our collective and distant past, documenting the intellectual lineage of the disorder from late-nineteenth-century psychology and physiology through to the work of Walter Cannon and others during the mid-twentieth century.[2] This chapter questions the familiar narrative of modern stress and suggests that workplace stress, in particular, was not recognized by a significant section of the professional scientific and medical world until the 1940s. It is argued that ideas about stress and the evidence of the phenomena of stress have had a complex and somewhat difficult relationship. The dissemination of the idea of occupational stress was largely an invention of the post-1945 era and more particularly of the late twentieth century. Stress linked to working life in ways that denoted a range of physiological, psychological and emotional effects, arising specifically from the work environment, was a product only of the last three or four decades of the century.

The claim that workplace stress is largely a creation of our own era appears eccentric; psychological unease linked to working life had been noted since at least the early nineteenth century. The genealogy of what has become known as workplace stress has been the subject of considerable discussion, led by social scientists such as Cary Cooper, who have emphasized the seminal influence of physiologists such as Walter Cannon, Hans Selye and Richard Lazarus.[3] Allan Young completed an influential study of the emergence of post-traumatic stress in the United States, using sociological and anthropological methods to situate scientific ideas about stress within an ideological, cultural and political nexus of modern capitalism.[4] Jackson's recent accounts of scientific and secular ideas of stress in the modern age similarly pay close attention to the physiological and biological models developed by Cannon, Selye and other north American researchers to explain the lack of bodily and social stability in the twentieth century, while also underlining the contributions of psychologists, psychiatrists and neurologists to understanding the degenerative impact of Western society on individual personalities.[5] Kitanaka has highlighted the role, and the limitations, of European psychological and psychiatric models of illness in providing modern Japan with ways of explaining personal distress related to employment.[6] All of these accounts note ambiguities in the usage of terms such as occupational stress and the attention called by key texts to varied personality characteristics, as well as the distinct ergonomic environment in which individuals were employed.

Many authors, including those contributing to the present collection, have outlined arguments about the sources of personal distress and the adaptation of individuals to identifiable stressors in their environment. The intention of this chapter is rather to consider the spreading influence of specific ideas about poor mental health in relation to work, and to critically assess the explanations of mental 'stress' by authorities in industrial research and professional medical communities. This technical vocabulary of stress may be compared with the understanding and adoption of the terminology of stress among the wider population during the middle years of the century. The well-known imprecision and elasticity in the terminology of stress should not discourage careful differentiation between models of fatigue and exhaustion and later notions of stress. The argument made here is that there was no consistent or critical application of models of work-related stress by professionals or by lay observers for most of the twentieth century, and the evidence indicates a marked and continued contrast between scientific commentators and other groups, within civil society, in the understanding of mental illness and emotional unhappiness, in regard to occupation.

This chapter shows that the critical transition in the making of a new era of stress was not in the application of a special model of organic stress (or even bodily strain) to expressions of anxiety and discomfort in the workplace. Rather the success of the vocabulary of stress depended on a particular conjunction of circumstances in the transformation of the global economy and in Western perceptions of mental disquiet. This combination of material, political and cultural expectations for individual effort served to legitimate an area or domain of discussion about the management of the self. While global corporations sought to change bargains agreed in full employment and to motivate or compel employees to accept tighter management of work, fostering a positive language of job quality control and fulfilment in customer satisfaction, labour organizations drew on discussions of personal responsibility to emphasize the hazards to health and safety in excessive workloads.[7] They utilized the articulation of personal anxiety, even of incapacity to meet job requirements, as evidence of a dilemma that led to an experience of worsening or chronic poor health.

The recording of occupational stress as a widespread phenomenon belongs to this period of transition, as the ending of the post-war boom and the beginnings of a major dislocation of the global economy and corporatist bargaining contracts, during the 1970s and early 1980s, accompanied a shift from extractive and manufacturing to service employment in many Westernized economies. This period saw a growing identification of stress amid a transformation of relations between employers, governments and citizen-workers, in which older certainties of post-War Fordist technologies and a broad consensus about secure employment gave way to chronic unemployment, increasing feminization and casualization of job markets and workplaces, bringing stronger management control and individual responsibility for work performance.

The terminology of stress acquired an accepted quasi-scientific status and mode of speaking through which people could engage in discussions about a sense of unease at work, articulating a space for anxiety about change and possibly offering respite by proposing symptoms, if elusive, of a recognized occupational disease. Early in the post-war period, incidents of psychological disturbance at work became apparent, including florid symptoms of strain that appeared to have roots in the industrial past. Britain's Trades Union Congress (TUC) noted, in the early 1970s, that there had been a significant rise in working days lost between the mid-1950s and later 1960s due to 'psychoneurosis and psychosis', as well as 'nervousness, debility and headaches'. The TUC itself registered received opinion that 'mental stress' involved a complex mix of domestic, social and workplace factors.[8] It was noticeable that these descriptions of workplace unease were framed in terms of serious mental illness, derived from clinical diagnoses rather than a fresh medical or lay terminology of workplace stress. The ailments, syndromes and experiential distresses that were specifically identified as 'stress' related to occupation appear to belong to a fresh domain of public and political (rather than specialized and scientific) debate about the nature of stress, which arose in the 1970s. To assume a biological continuity between recent depictions of stress and much older and different disorders, such as workplace fatigue, raises fundamental difficulties for a history which seeks to understand the particular cultural milieu in which diseases are recognized and named. Perceptions and pathologies attached to a disease may alter radically over time, more particularly where personal mentalities and emotional sensibilities are involved. Even physical injuries claim their own peculiar narrative histories and depend on ontological assemblages that were the product of distinctive periods and arguably of specific 'regimes' of industrial hazard.[9]

The analysis outlined thus far suggests social relationships, more particularly the exercise of social power, provided a basic context for the outbreak of what has been termed a 'stress pandemic' at the end of the last century. The language of stress connoted not merely a way of talking about bodily resources, equilibrium and health, but also expectations defined and framed by social and workplace relationships. Those who are said to experience or suffer from stress have become the subject of discussions of personal capacity for 'coping' with the demands of an environment which is shared with others who do not suffer similar levels of anxiety. The language of anxiety was expressed in different ways according to the social and cultural resources, or within the peculiar cultural horizons, of particular classes and communities. One important and surprising omission in our understanding of the evolution of workplace stress, now addressed directly by many chapters in this volume, has been a clear historical account of employees' perceptions of working life and the origins of disquiet.

Echoes of stress and distress can be more accurately heard within an analysis of the changing architecture of contemporary capitalism and the material realignment in the organization of production, affecting the role of employment in securing personal status and social identity, in Western societies during the late twentieth century. It can be argued that as workplace transactions became more personalized, involving less collective and more individual responsibility, so also the gendering of work was changed and diminished by employment trends. The language of workplace stress was developed and adapted to meet the needs of those facing contemporary capitalism whose spaces and boundaries were shifting. In this deep transition, the vocabulary of stress gained currency to become a global means of exchange between actors who possessed distinct and conflicting concerns about work and who gave the term 'stress' different inflexions to suit their needs and purposes. While workers and their representatives sought a space for the articulation of dissatisfactions, contributing to an emerging language of 'unhealthy' work environments, industrial researchers and medical scientists revised and relaxed the terms in which mental disquiet might be understood.

In addition to the reframing of workers' concerns about their personal experience of demanding employment conditions, fresh transactions were undertaken in the diagnosis and treatment of mental illness, which elaborated the ways in which psychiatric disorder was described, and reduced the stigma associated with such illnesses. This chapter does not examine the medical treatment of workers and their families for mental illness, which was another theatre for the development of the language of 'mental stress' in a specific intellectual and societal space during the middle decades of the twentieth century.[10] To understand the influence of ideas about stress in explaining illness in employment, and the remarkable spread in the currency of the term 'stress' within an expanding global economy, we need to consider how the domain of work was understood and the values attached to paid employment. Values were deeply embedded within scientific enquiry as well as lay transactions. The following section examines the relationships between industrial policy-makers and scientific experts, beginning with a narrative of discovery and discussion in the early 1970s.

Finding the Stress Problem in British Industry

In Autumn 1974 the Chief Psychologist at the Department of Employment (DE), Gilbert Jessup, contacted the Medical Research Council about the Labour Government's decision to commission research into two related subjects: 'mental stress in industry' and 'physiological and behavioural correlates of psychological well-being at work'. Jessup was based at the DE's new Work Research Unit and responding to current political demands for a fresh policy for labour relations, rather than developing a considered strategy for scientific investigation.[11] Surprisingly, the Medical Research Council (MRC) appeared equally unprepared for this emerging research agenda: they turned to a retired professor, Hywel Murrell (formerly of the University of Wales Institute of Science and Technology) to undertake a basic literature survey of the subject.[12] Given the long-standing responsibility of the MRC for the work of the Industrial Health Research Board since the 1930s, the ignorance and reticence of Britain's leading medical scientists is odd. Jessup visited the Applied Psychology Research Unit (APRU) at Cambridge in late 1974 to extend his network of contacts, since the APRU enjoyed an international reputation for research on cognition and skill performance, dating back to the Cambridge Psychology Laboratory under Frederic Bartlett, Kenneth Craik and Donald Broadbent.[13] Having moved to Oxford and collaborating with Dennis Gath, Broadbent was to seek funding from the MRC's Environmental Health Committee in early 1975 to investigate the mental health of paced assembly-line workers.[14]

The MRC's initial cautious response to government approaches may reflect their sensitivity to studies designed for a department directly involved in labour relations, rather than public health or medical research. The DE was clearly responding to industrial concerns in creating a working party with the Confederation of British Industry (CBI) and the TUC to discuss the impact of assembly-line work.[15] Union interest had been sparked by demands from Ford Motor workers in 1973 for an enquiry into 'mental breakdowns' among shift workers and those employed on high speed assembly lines.[16] In correspondence with the Employment Medical Advisory Service (EMAS), the TUC prepared a paper on 'mental stress' during early 1974, evaluating working days lost from the mid-1950s due to 'psychoneurosis and psychosis' and 'nervousness, debility and headaches', while noting the paucity of research into 'factors leading to stress'.[17] In summer 1974, the newly-formed Health and Safety Commission (HSE) joined the TUC, CBI and DE officials to discuss research into production-line work. Scientists employed by the civil service expressed the varied aspirations of the new Labour government; Jessup emphasizing the need to extend investigation beyond a 'clinical' definition of stress while Jacques insisted that the good health of workers rather than their productive capacity should guide research into 'symptoms of stress'.[18]

Tensions between political imperative and scientific interest were evident when Broadbent and other researchers met representatives of the DE, Health and Safety Commission (HSC), and TUC at the MRC offices in early 1975. Government officials explained official interest in assembly line work, since this was 'thought to be an area of high stress'. While the scientists agreed that society 'recognizes the problem of mental stress caused by work which ought to be studied' and accepted that 'stress' should be conceived 'in broad terms, spanning both the medical and psychological parts of the spectrum', they questioned whether 'the term "stress" could be omitted altogether and the proposal formulated as the study of the behavioural concomitants and problems of particular work environments', as a more 'practical formulation'.[19] Broadbent later asked the TUC for further guidance on factors behind workplace stress.[20] Congress had insisted that stress be tackled as a matter of human welfare rather than a means of raising productivity, suspicious of the EMAS proposal to investigate 'accident susceptibility' among workers.[21]

The MRC's uncertain response to fresh research funding cannot be explained solely in terms of scientists' aversion to political controversy, for labour unions were also critical of official approaches to injury and illness at work, as well as sceptical about business involvement. The MRC scientists displayed a lack of confidence in understanding 'stress' as well as an inability to relate the subject to the decades of applied research which had been undertaken on industrial output, fatigue and performance since the early twentieth century. These faltering discussions indicated that intellectual and commonsense understanding of 'stress' was not merely a question of recognizing another occupational disease or syndrome, but rather that knowledge of stress formed a distinct ontology of personal well-being. To understand the development of this ontology we need to take a longer perspective on the character of scientific research in British industry during the middle decades of the twentieth century.

Drawing the Stressed Worker: Knowledge and Regulation, 1930–70

One reason for the reticence of the MRC's scientists in responding to the stress research initiative was limited recent experience in dealing with government departments responsible for industrial relations.[22] The regulation of health and safety at work had been the responsibility of the Home Office before the Second World War, passing to the Ministry of Labour and thence to the Department of Employment. Early government research into occupational illness, conducted by Medical Factory Inspectors at the Home Office and by the IHRB, pioneered investigations of industrial disease before significant numbers of research scientists were employed after 1945. Psychologists such as Gilbert Jessup were late arrivals, which may explain the preference of MRC researchers to define the question of 'mental stress in industry', in terms of the physiological and behavioural dimensions of well-being.[23]

Cambridge remained a dominant influence in applied psychology research; the Cambridge Psychology Laboratory growing from the early work by Henry Head, Charles Myers and Rivers before 1914 and consolidated by Frederic Bartlett in the inter-war years.[24] The relationship that developed between the Cambridge psychologists, Myers at the National Institute of Industrial Psychology (NIIP), the IHRB and the Ministry of Labour in the 1930s largely defined the orientation of scientific research into workplace performance, though the IHRB remained formally accountable to the Ministry of Health. David Munro, as Secretary of the IHRB, fostered the work of the Committee on Industrial Psychology (CIP), chaired by Cyril Burt of London, particularly in regard to vocational guidance and accident-prone workers and incentives in industry. Munro sought Ministry of Labour support in 1934 for an ambitious scheme of vocational guidance using tests developed by IHRB industrial psychology researchers to monitor not only the intellectual capacity of children and young workers, but critically the 'temperamental and social qualities [which] play a large, if not a larger, part in contentment and efficiency'.[25] Frustrated by opposition from Charles Myers at NIIP and rival Scottish researchers, Munro still succeeded in attaching his 'Vocational Guidance Section' (VGS) and his protégé Eric Farmer to Bartlett's Psychology Department at Cambridge.[26]

Farmer developed aptitude and 'personality' tests to explore the relationship 'between social and industrial mal-adjustment and accident proneness', while Wyatt and Langdon's 1937 study of *Fatigue and Boredom in Repetitive Work* broke new ground in interviewing some 355 (generally younger) unmarried women in four different workplaces, considering physical fatigue and personal attitudes to self and status.[27] They found that educated and able workers were more likely to suffer boredom while less intelligent labourers worked harder and experienced 'a greater degree of strain'.[28] Their subsequent study, *The Machine and the Worker*, identified 'the strains and stresses' experienced by machine operators as a result of intense physical effort and increased pace, though unchanging speeds of work were also 'conducive to strain'.[29] Individual variations in attitudes and personality among workers were registered in responses to earnings and competitive effort.[30] At this point strain and stress were consistent with engineering models of fatigue due to physical demands on the human frame as distinct from the boredom of the intelligent mind. 'Depression' could afflict less able workers failing to complete intellectually demanding tasks, rather than from physical or mental effort.

The approach of war was to magnify strategic interest in this research, as Farmer's work on selection of personnel, aptitude testing and accidents attracted the attention of the Ministry of Labour and the armed services, as well as having (in Munro's view) considerable popular interest.[31] Farmer distinguished 'general mental ability' from specific mechanical aptitudes in tests that allowed rapid grading of recruits to the services and, with Alice Heim at Cambridge, he developed similar tests for civilian war work, arguing that the military had creamed off higher quality labour, and as people of lower intelligence and ability entered industry their inability to complete tasks would result in widespread 'depression'. Aptitude testing would reduce 'strain' and boredom, along with accidents, absenteeism and illness, as workers were directed to appropriate jobs within their abilities. Farmer's analysis of strain, elaborated in a study of female industrial conscripts, again found that women with a strong disinclination to factory work and tasks for which they were not mentally fitted could also lead to strain, accompanied by 'a good deal of weeping, minor sickness and absenteeism'.[32] Such conclusions appeared clearly gendered in assigning emotional disturbance to females who were unsuited to industrial employment, though Farmer emphasized the meritocratic features of testing where individuals with ability or special aptitudes would gain opportunities. His aptitude and selection tests were never adopted by wartime government for recruitment to essential industries. Heim's earlier research on aptitude tests for occupational fitness had been criticized by officials as lacking practical utility, though it is clear that the concerns of the Ministry of Labour lay in the fear of serious trade union opposition.[33] Farmer conceded that educated persons performed better in his general ability tests but complained bitterly that his proposals were effectively ditched on 'the ground that it is regimenting people to give them tests', even though his scheme would remove gross inefficiencies in wartime labour dilution and help post-war reconstruction planning.[34] Farmer had some success in advising individual firms on labour selection but attracted little interest from business organizations.[35]

Farmer's efforts to apply his aptitude tests to the wartime civilian workforce also aroused the suspicions of Bartlett, who noted in a report on research conducted at Cambridge in 1940–1 that Farmer's studies had 'gradually converted the Army from scepticism on the matter of psychological selection tests', and had potential value for post-war reconstruction, though in private correspondence to the MRC he insisted on his authority over the ambitious Farmer.[36] The manoeuvres prompted by these research efforts reveal divergent approaches to scientific method and rival ambitions to claim recognition for the public value of scientific research beyond the confines of laboratory experimentation. Bartlett strove to defend Heim's education research against official criticism in 1937, acknowledging to Munro that her work offered limited insight into 'social factors outside the school', but insisting that his team's work had wide medical, as well as intellectual, implications. Emphasizing the competitive challenge from American as well as German scientists, Bartlett argued that 'research about temperament, personality, vocational diagnosis and prognosis, or whatever you like to call it, is just as much a contribution to public health as investigations into physical disease, or mental defect'. Exasperated by the lack of official vision, Bartlett insisted that many psychologists wanted to undertake practical researching and engage the listening public, vividly illustrating the point from his own best-selling texts on noise:

> As regards noise, I think the next step ought to be out of the laboratory ... Collecting opinions and following them up, watching results, not in terms of measureable fatigue, but in the increase of irritability, and the growth of attitudes akin to neuroses. Noise wants treating not as an individual problem, but as a public affair ... I mean we want to know whether the amount of social discord that is produced this way is worth taking a lot of public notice of, or whether it is just the infrequent crank who sits up and howls about it. I've had a lot of letters ... nearly all from people who say that certain specific and inescapable noises are driving them to distraction.[37]

Bartlett's aspirations to engage with public concerns by undertaking some form of mass observation of 'attitudes akin to neuroses' were never realized, and his claim to a broad vision for social research was to be tested in the post-War years when, as a member of the MRC's Psychology Committee, he considered unorthodox applications from social scientists at the Tavistock Institute and elsewhere.[38]

Research into industrial 'strain' conducted at Cambridge and elsewhere during these years hardly departed from the specialized concern with highly-controlled studies of manual and mental dexterity, rarely integrating social health concerns with those of efficient output.[39] Cambridge and IRHB psychologists did make increasing use of fieldwork questionnaires to elicit workers' opinions, including Wyatt's study to investigate 'morale' at two car plants in 1946. His fellow researchers identified eight aspects of the industrial environment that influenced workplace attitudes at Vauxhall's Luton plant, though little attention was offered to variations in personality and very few references made to 'strain' or 'stress' as payment systems again figured as a dominant factor in workers' evaluations of employment.[40] High levels of job satisfaction were recorded alongside complaints about monotonous track line work.[41] Limited attention was given to individual attitudes and little effort made to describe the nature of labour relations or the implications of management models of leadership. The authority-centred and gendered orientation of studies in the interwar years was moderated by the empowerment of labour during the 1940s. However, there was a notable shift in concerns after the war with management leadership and workplace supervision becoming key determinants of workplace relations, reflecting contemporary American and European management literature.[42] Extricating themselves from state regulation and determined to reassert management control, major automobile firms declined to cooperate in scientific studies, though Ford's Personnel manager, Marsden-Jones, assured the Cambridge researchers that employers had 'now seen the writing on the wall as regards human relations'.[43]

The writing that management was reading, and itself writing, on the wall of the industrial workplace was influenced by particular narratives of post-war business. In the age of Fordist production and consumer affluence that extended into the 1970s, Ford and other employers relied on high wages and rising demand to secure consensus while developing a strategic vision for management that accommodated union bargaining without conceding control over work. Narratives shared between management strategists and academic researchers, including those composing 'industrial stress' literature surveyed by Murrell, included portraits of industrial supervisors squeezed by the growth of specialist managers and union bargainers, leading to (it was claimed) a frustrating loss of authority and human contacts on the assembly lines.[44] Psychological studies of workplace relations in the 1950s included Norah Davies' study of incentive wages, funded by the MRC, which again focused on wage incentives but also revealed the ways in which workers absorbed and adapted scientific knowledge and contemporary language regarding workers' health and mental well-being, mediated by collective culture and occupational tradition.[45]

At this period there appeared some divergence between empirical studies of workplace production and industrial bargaining over effort, on the one hand, and the controlled laboratory studies of perception, learning and skill adaptation undertaken by leading psychologists, such as the notable Cambridge stress researcher Donald Broadbent, on the other.[46] Murrell's survey of research into industrial stress noted that the impetus for detailed empirical research into industrial psychology had been lost before 1970. Substantive investigations into workers' attitudes had been largely undertaken by management researchers and industrial administration specialists rather than scientists and psychologists. The orientation of scientific interest away from the investigations of occupational health registered, in part, a broader 'environmental turn' of social medicine in the 1950s and 1960s.

The weakness of research noted by Murrell may also reflect a distancing of elite medical science from the radical commitment of occupational and epidemiological researchers in the earlier era of Philip D'Arcy Hart, Richard Schilling and Archibald Cochrane. These institutional and professional barriers were overcome not by scientific discourse or novel forms of medical practice, but primarily through cultural responses to a changing material world, as the consensus which underpinned the Fordist economic settlement and state welfare provisions began to fracture. 'Stress' became an effective means of describing and explaining the world anew, connecting the personal and the existential with the turbulent environment of capitalism in crisis and renewal, most vividly in the life of the workplace. The world of maddening industrial and social noise remained remote from the secluded Cambridge laboratory, even as Bartlett sought a popular resonance for his research. As the political landscape altered and governments again sought, as they had in the 1940s, to articulate a language in which to comprehend production relationships, elite scientists struggled to find their own voice in response. This reading of institutional science in the post-war years provides a way of understanding the scientific conversations and confused discussions of the early 1970s, when 'industrial stress' was raised as a matter of political concern.

Recovering 'Industrial Stress': Psychologists and the Return of Industrial Research

Those who still recalled the post-war years may have noticed the irony that Ford Motor Company, which had denied entry to industrial researchers such as Wyatt, provided the arena in the early 1970s for fresh trade union demands for an investigation of mental disturbance among assembly-line workers.[47] Those demands were not yet framed in the language of 'stress' and it is evident that this language was to be embraced, if not initially coined, in the evolving relationships between experts, sponsors and subjects. An MRC Environmental Health Committee agreed, in April 1975, on the scope for research into machine-paced work, as well as a broader study of an industrial population and a literature survey.[48] In conducting his survey, H. Murrell warned his sponsors at the outset that 'the meaning of the word "stress" was unclear and depended upon the context in which it was used', since stress might be considered to result from 'anything causing disruption or dissent'.[49] Avoiding the 'semantic morass' in regard to stress (or more precisely 'mental strain'), Murrell was sharply critical of biologists and physiologists, including Hans Selye, for confusing 'stress' and 'strain', while Lazarus had allegedly shifted attention from human physiology to the interplay of psychology and environment – raising, but not resolving, complex problems of motivation.[50] Murrell preferred to talk about 'short-term and long-term behavioural and physical effects' of work, concluding that the usage of terminology such as 'stress/strain in industry' offered little value, 'rather it is a positive embarrassment'.[51]

Murrell's overview confirmed the opinions of MRC scientists that little guidance could be gained from earlier research, while civil servants, research directors and academic researchers failed to agree on 'the best mechanical analogy for the human phenomenon' in examining the causes of personal stress. They pragmatically concluded that this omission might not obstruct new research, though the specific character of such research remained vague.[52] The Department of Employment's Research Committee agreed that it should commission 'strategic research', rather than funding work 'aimed at short-term problems originating in DE or from political pressures'.[53] Yet they insisted that stress should be defined 'sufficiently broadly' to be of interest to their political masters, and the MRC accepted that the Department would formulate the 'specific research questions' to be addressed, as well as monitoring research undertaken at groups such as the MRC's Social and Applied Psychology Unit (SAPU) in Sheffield.[54]

Murrell emphasized the difficulties in distinguishing pressures that were not linked to the mechanical pacing of work and those that were. Such fieldwork hazards persuaded some researchers to retreat to laboratory testing of physiological and psychological correlations rather than rely solely on industrial observation.[55] Among the diverse range of projects developed by MRC researchers, only Cox and Mackay drew directly on the research of Selye, Lennart Levi and Lazarus in discussing cognitive appraisal and coping mechanisms. Even so, their philosophical and scientific axioms remained general: 'We are still essentially Man the hunter physically, but not so psychosocially'. As Cox studied the psychosocial effects of short-cycle repetition work, methodological difficulties persisted.[56] Broadbent's specific study of assembly-line workers, replicating Arthur Kornhauser's (1965) Detroit research, utilized the idea of anxiety rather than stress, and proposed to combine industrial study and an examination of medical symptoms among employees, though the latter goal was never realized.[57]

Researchers had always depended on business cooperation to gain entry to private establishments, even in wartime. The ability of scientists to observe and interrogate workers as subjects had required less consent. This facility altered in the 1940s with the growing influence of labour unions, as Farmer discovered. By the 1970s, trade unions were again demanding research scientists take workplace health seriously and to take the views of workers seriously. Following a meeting of MRC researchers with the TUC in 1975, Broadbent asked an insider at the organization to help him secure basic information about 'the sort of job which worries people, and hearing any grumbles they might have, rather than getting into the sort of interrogation we were discussing at the meeting!'[58] At the same period the EMAS, now part of the HSE, strove to assure suspicious trade unions that a study of the 'accident susceptibility' of industrial workers, utilizing the Goldberg questionnaire, would not weaken the factory inspectorate's commitment to highest standards of workplace safety.[59] By early 1976, the EMAS was itself moving to study mental health of occupations, including psychiatric staff.[60] In practice, the research agenda of 'stress', sponsored by the Labour Government at this period, was now steadily distinguished from mental health as prominent sectors of manufacturing and construction were considered for study.[61]

This flowering of political and scientific interest in workplace stress was to be brief. Research undertaken by the MRC groups at Sheffield and elsewhere faced sharp criticism from scientists, particularly in the neurological field, within the MRC as frictions between the Council and the DE over research development and supervision continued into 1978.[62]From the outset, senior figures in the MRC doubted the intellectual dividends of scientific exchange, with Joan Faulkner commenting on 'the general poverty' of many research gatherings.[63] None of the initial research projects delivered a clear model or method by which 'mental stress' in industry could be defined, measured and controlled.[64] Amidst the turbulent industrial relations of 1978–9 in Britain, the policy agenda of workplace stress shifted: concerns about industrial strife extended to employment and moves were made to close the DE's Work Research Unit and remove Gilbert Jessup. The election of a Conservative Government in 1979 marked the effective end of the early experiment in government-scientific cooperation concerning stress, though the HSE employed increasing numbers of psychologists in the years that followed.

The thin intellectual and political fruits of industrial stress research might have been richer had participants followed their own declared intention of embracing a historical perspective on the origins and growth of the phenomena that came to be identified as 'stress'. Research undertaken on workplace output and attitudes conducted in the middle decades of the century had similarly sought to address questions of motivation and to investigate the selection of individuals for different tasks at a time when governments were concerned with industrial and military efficiency. The institutional basis for cooperation and dissemination of expertise between policy-makers, scientists and management remained tentative and uncertain, while shop floor workers continued to be considered in terms of authoritarian and gendered assumptions by senior researchers. The anti-state ethos of business and scientific elites during the 1950s and 1960s provided poor ground for empirical scientific research, as ideas about stress developed in specialist military and laboratory studies of perceptual and cognitive performance in conditions of duress. Little interest was shown in more popularized approaches to the subject until Western capitalism began to enter a new period of crisis and transformation, with profound implications for a post-war global settlement founded on Fordist production and the expansion of a welfare-medical system arranged around large institutional funding.[65] The epoch of stress was about to arrive.

Conclusion

At the beginning of the twenty-first century, five million Britons were reported to have experienced 'stress' as a result of their work, and an estimated half a million people reported stress-related illnesses, costing the economy £3.7 billion pounds per year.[66] Nor was stress confined to mature European societies facing relative decline, as the matrix of global capitalism was dramatically recast and the balance of economic strength tipped eastwards; for stress has become a guiding global narrative in which multiple physical, mental and emotional disorders have been fused to capture and explain the unease of late modernity. To be 'stressed' became a way of identifying and knowing the self as well as the body, an affirmation of existence within a demanding environment. Recognition of such vulnerability became an issue of contention in the workplace as well as civil society and the acknowledgement of a condition of stress formed part of the sensibility of contemporary life: social citizenship had extended to the realm of stress. Injury by stress expressed a civic and political as much as a physical condition.

There is little doubt that we can, without straining credibility, link the characteristics of personal stress to the symptoms of neurasthenia and other mental disorders described by Charles Beard and others in the late nineteenth century. This chapter has not sought to challenge the diverse scientific lineages of organic stress, but has argued that these ideas had relatively little impact on popular and political opinion in Britain (and other countries) before the 1970s. We have argued elsewhere that scientific models of stress devised by physiologists and psychologists from the late nineteenth century had little impact even in the larger scientific and medical community before the 1940s, even though the idea of 'mental stress' was well established in the early twentieth century.[67] Stress remained, in theory and experience, a relatively marginal phenomenon until a particular conjuncture of societal and cultural shifts in the expectations of populations in affluent countries from the 1960s. Stress did not become a significant social fact for Britain and other Westernized countries until the rediscovery of what Marx had termed alienation and what sociologists later identified as anomie, notions that were rearticulated and refined in the peculiar and particular historical conditions of the late twentieth century.

The dawn of the era of workplace stress signified not a steady dissemination of scientific knowledge, but rather the creation of particular kinds of regimes in regard to knowledge and ways in which knowledge about the world might be validated. In Britain we can trace the emergence of a language of workplace and occupational 'stress' to a specific historic setting where an established structure of knowledge and the existing interest groups in society shifted as employees' own expectations altered. These changing aspirations registered a broader transformation in the industrial division of labour across the world, as innovations in the globalized economy eroded earlier hierarchies of male seniority. The spread of occupational maladies has been historically associated with the expansion of the global economy, leading to recognizable structures of exploitation and regulation that formed distinct regimes of industrial hazard in the modern world.[68] The re-articulation of male and female health needs within the established manufacturing sectors and production lines, as we have seen, gave rise to a significant extension in the understanding of labour protection from physical and mental damage to personal anxiety.

While registering the importance of a vernacular language of duress and anxiety in this period, the relationship between the acknowledged holders of expertise – recognized authors of empirical practice as well as scientific elites advising states – and the subjects of their observation remains an important question for historians of stress. It was the discussion of harm inflicted in production itself that gave stress discourses one of their most vivid forms of contestation in the period surveyed here. The evidence presented in this chapter indicates that the groundwork and methodologies, developed by British scientists and social scientists, to examine workplace attitudes between the late 1930s and the early 1950s first led researchers towards, and then away from, models of human behaviour that were later to be linked to occupational stress. From the outset, research into effort at work was guided by an over-riding concern with efficiency and economy. Projects conducted by industrial psychologists into the education, abilities and selection of labour were primarily concerned with aptitude and incentives. The Second World War appeared to provide an impetus to psychological work with an anthropological and sociological turn, including a more holistic approach to workplace relationships. Bartlett espoused a broader social approach, although he watched this orientation diminish rather than increase among research psychologists in the 1950s, with a parallel decline of interest in industrial psychology at the MRC. The divergence of scientific biology and medical psychology from the sociological understanding of work was reinforced by organizational and leadership models of industrial behaviour, which remained largely detached from medical investigation of mental disorder and dysfunction.

Public and political conversations about 'workplace stress' began in earnest in Britain during the 1970s. The evidence discussed here indicates that a lay language of 'stress' was sustained and elaborated by contemporary concerns about industrial life and the impact of technology on the human subject. These concerns did not originate in contemporary scientific enquiry or arise directly from medical discussions of psychological illness, though each contributed to wider understanding of mental well-being. The emergence of workplace stress as an urgent concern in the 1970s reflected a growing recognition of the impact of different industrial environments on the well-being of the wider community and a growing consciousness of the place of employment in mental health and the rights of citizens to freedom from unease. Existential expressions of unease took different forms and were identified in regard to different areas of social life, although 'stress' assumed the character of a distinctly individual and personal response to external pressures.

As the end of the long post-war boom led to crises in Fordist models of bargaining and welfare security for working populations, the appropriation of the ideas and vocabulary of stress to the changing global economy of the late twentieth century emerged as a product of the shifting structures and patterns of the division and mobilization of labour across the developed world. Stress can be traced to the anxieties generated as older work hierarchies were transformed and non-manual white collar employment expanded, fostering self-evaluation of personal careers based on individual performance. While the changing fortunes of ageing industrialized countries within the global economy provided a shared material context for the discussion of workplace stress in the late twentieth century, to search for a direct causal relationship between such conditions and contemporary 'stress' at work is only to recreate the conundrum faced by MRC researchers in the 1970s.

11 CREATING 'THE SOCIAL': STRESS, DOMESTICITY AND ATTEMPTED SUICIDE

Chris Millard

'The social' is everywhere. It is difficult to imagine any action or interaction that is outside this pervasive category of modern thought. However, just as the body and the emotions have been found to be historically contingent,[1] 'the social' also has a history. This chapter uncovers a specific production of 'the social' and its consequences, which must be evaluated rather than simply presumed to be inevitable. Despite the sweeping claims made in its name, 'the social' is not monolithic, but is made and remade through various overlapping instances of practical and intellectual labour.

One iteration of this fluid organizing idea is rooted in the encounter between British psychiatry and two world wars, and reinforced by the socialized medicine of the National Health Service (NHS). It gains further prominence through shifts in mental healthcare towards 'care in the community', the emergence of psychiatric epidemiology and the rise of social work, particularly psychiatric social workers (PSWs). These post-1945 arrangements presume and construct a psychosocial realm, an environment connected to mental pathology and well-being through the concepts of 'stress' and 'distress'. These concepts relate diverse social situations to various mental disorders. The aim of this chapter is to historicize this space, variously known as the 'psychosocial', 'social constellation' or 'psychosocial matrix'. It is part of an historically contingent way of seeing the world that informs and underwrites sociology, social work, social psychiatry, psychiatric epidemiology, social history and the social sciences.

This psychosocial space is explored through the emergence of an 'epidemic of attempted suicide as a cry for help' in the 1950s and 1960s in Britain. This involves young people – increasingly female – arriving at Accident and Emergency (A&E) departments having taken an amount of medication deemed excessive, but insufficient to kill them. This action becomes securely cast by psychiatrists and PSWs not as a genuine suicide attempt, but as a communication with an environment: a spouse, lover, friends or family. This environment is accessed and brought to prominence by PSW practices of spouse interviews, home visits and follow-up. Self-poisoning becomes a female pathology, corresponding to a feminine domestic environment.

Rates charting this phenomenon – termed 'attempted suicide', 'self-poisoning' or 'parasuicide' – fall away after the late 1970s. In one sense, this phenomenon captures the psychosocial at its purest: psychopathology as social action. An act securely associated with mental pathology is performed as a communication with a social circle. Ideas of communication and the social environment are not simply mutually reinforcing, they emerge as part of the same idea: the social environment cannot exist without meaningful information passing between humans, just as communication requires more than one self-contained individual. Communicative action, and the increasing stability of the 'cry for help' as a category, feeds into the self-evidence of a psychologically significant, interpersonal, psychosocial space.

Concepts of 'stress' and 'distress', which are interrelated but not interchangeable terms, are crucial here. Today, 'distress' is more often used in a way that implies a raw emotional state, on which human definitions or interpretations work, shaping it into a form of pathology or disorder through diagnosis. Ian Hacking's work on multiple personality disorder uses distress in this basic sense, arguing that this category 'provided a new way to be an unhappy person ... it has become, to use one popular phrasing, a culturally sanctioned way of expressing distress'.[2] In *The Myth of the Chemical Cure*, Joanna Moncrieff similarly decries the lack of consideration given to the impact that psychoactive drugs have 'on someone experiencing emotional distress'.[3] Emotional distress is here an attempt to step back from using more loaded categories such as 'mental illness'.[4]

By contrast, stress is more often used to express a connection between an environment and a mental or physical state; that is a response to environmental stimuli. In the mid-twentieth century, influential stress theorist Hans Selye redefined the word stress as '"the nonspecific response of the body to any demand upon it" [which] was so persuasive that it persisted and remains widely used today'.[5] Thus stress is neither normal nor pathological. However, as with many conceptual innovations, these categories are used rather loosely. Richard Lazarus, author of the influential *Psychological Stress and the Coping Process* (1966), and Susan Folkman quote a prescient passage from 1964 which argues that 'when the word stress came into vogue, each investigator, who had been working with a concept he felt was closely related, substituted the word stress ... and continued in his same line of investigation'.[6] However, in broad terms, stress signifies the effect of environmental stimuli on an organism, whilst distress attempts to capture an unstructured mental state or emotional raw material.

Stress has been variably cast as an endocrine reaction, disturbed physiological balance[7] or the source of mental problems in exogenous depression (caused by the stress of life events), and has been incorporated into psychological rating scales.[8] This is sometimes claimed to derive from 'the chrysalis of psychobiology generated by Adolf Meyer [1866–1950] through his invention and use of the "life chart"'.[9] Jackson cites the influential works of Harold Wolff, Daniel Funkenstein, Roy Grinker and John Spiegel as evidence that it was this psychosocial approach 'rather than Selye's experimental physiology that came to dominate clinical and epidemiological accounts of stress'.[10] The most influential twentieth-century articulation of stress is found in post-traumatic stress disorder (PTSD), the genesis of which Allan Young has meticulously charted through Veterans' Administration hospitals in the aftermath of the American war in Vietnam.[11]

Because stress and distress are neither normal nor pathological, they enable the boundary between mental health and illness to become porous. Every human experience in a psychosocial realm has the potential to provoke pathology. This chapter asks four interrelated questions. First, what relationships exist between the psychosocial, stress and attempted suicide as a cry for help? Second, how do stress and distress help to produce the psychosocial as a realm for intervention, surveillance and management? Third, what are some of the specific qualities of this psychosocial environment, in terms of gender-specificity and a particular vision of pathological domesticity? Finally, what roles do 'the social' and 'social stress' play in the diagnostic expansionism of psychiatry, through the mobile boundary between mental health and pathology that they enable?

Psychiatric Epidemiology and 'The Social'

Over thirty years ago, David Armstrong theorized a shift from what he called 'panoptic' to 'dispensary' medicine in the early twentieth century:

> the dispensary radiated out into the community. Illness was sought, identified and monitored by various techniques and agencies in the community ... The new gaze, however, identified disease in the spaces between people, in the interstices of relationships, in the social body itself.[12]

The concern of this new gaze with the social body and the relationships between people is charted through a number of medical registers, including psychiatry, paediatrics, geriatrics and general practice. He argues that at 'the beginning of the twentieth century the "social" was born as an autonomous realm',[13] referencing Jacques Donzelot's French-focused *The Policing of Families* (1979).[14]

It is important not to overstate the novelty of this 'social' in the twentieth century. In Armstrong's analysis, moves towards community care in psychiatry are reduced to expressions of power relations. He claims that from 1948, comprehensive healthcare in Britain and 'the contemporary invention and importance placed on community care are simply manifestations of a new diagram of power', arguing that the 'community was the term deployed to describe that truly social space that had emerged in the calculated gap between bodies'.[15] Consequently the 'social gaze' appears almost totally novel, the result of a radical rupture. However, it has been argued that this social gaze is not new at all. Charles Webster has suggested that the seventeenth-century 'dominance of Baconian natural history' undercuts the claim for the 'Dispensary as an invention of a later age'.[16] Diverse connections can be made and many genealogies traced. Trevor Pearce follows ideas of organism-environment interaction back to the nineteenth-century philosopher Herbert Spencer,[17] and Mary Poovey traces notions of the social body to reformers such as Edwin Chadwick.[18] The extent to which the novelty of the psychosocial is undermined by apparent precursors remains open to question.

However, it can be stated confidently that *something* is new about the links between mental disorder and environment after 1945. The encounter of British psychiatry (especially workers at the Tavistock Institute) with the practicalities and casualties of the Second World War generates many interpersonally-focused psychotherapeutic practices, including Maxwell Jones's work on therapeutic communities,[19] the Northfield experiments of Wilfred Bion, John Rickman, S. H. Foulkes, Tom Main and others,[20] and Adam Curle and Eric Trist's notion of transitional communities resettling prisoners of war.[21] All of these focus upon interpersonal relationships and the importance of communities to mental health and disorder.

These endeavours presume or imply a relationship between environmental conditions and mental states, generating unsettling conceptual gaps. In this way, they can be said to be significantly novel. This is well-illustrated by the rise of psychiatric epidemiology, a set of techniques designed to survey mental disorder in the community and playing a central role in the construction of the psychosocial. The essence of epidemiology is the ability to relate 'findings in the "cases" ... to the defined population in which those cases arose'.[22] Thus, there must exist a credible conceptual apparatus for this relationship between cases and population (for example, the germ theory of disease). The novelty of *psychiatric* epidemiology is clear in light of 'traditional' epidemiological concerns. Up until the Second World War, this approach makes most sense in the quest to control and prevent infectious diseases such as typhoid, cholera and influenza. However, Joseph Goldberger's 'impeccable studies of pellagra', at the turn of the twentieth century in the American South, show that the diseases do not have to be infectious; pellagra is found to be associated with dietary deficiencies.[23]

After 1945, epidemiological methods are increasingly applied in psychiatry, advancing in step with the shift towards community care. Mark Parascandola argues that 'by the 1950s epidemiologic methods and thinking had expanded beyond the mere study of epidemics'.[24] The concept of the 'epidemiology of mental disorders' begins to make sense as a way to describe the distribution and incidence of mental problems within a defined area. However, without an agreed or stable model for the relationship between environment and mental disorder, this proves to be 'a difficult transition that still troubles epidemiology'.[25] This is exemplified by the reaction of a professor of bacteriology in 1952, who is furious at:

> an undoubted debauchery of a precise and essential word, 'epidemiology' which is being inflated by writers on social medicine and similar subjects to include the study of the frequency or incidence of diseases whether epidemic or not ... to speak of the epidemiology of coronary thrombosis, or of hare lip, or diabetes, or of any non-epidemic disease, is a debasement of the currency of thought. It is of no use saying that the word is being used in its wider sense. It has no wider sense.[26]

Social medicine is singled out for criticism, highlighting the presence of 'the social' at the core of this new epidemiology. Michael Shepherd – the first ever Professor of Epidemiological Psychiatry[27] – quotes and contests the above passage, citing J. C. F. Hecker's *The Epidemics of the Middle Ages* (1859), which deals with an epidemic of 'disordered behaviour, the Dancing Mania [and] makes no distinction between epidemics of infectious disease and those of morbid behaviour'.[28] Richard de Alarcón recycles Jerry Morris's 1957 observation that there are 'many interesting analogies between the dynamics of infectious disease and that of mental illness: from the dancing mania of the Middle Ages to epidemic benzedrine addiction'.[29] However, G. M. Carstairs, head of a research unit on the 'Epidemiology of Mental Disorders', is uneasy about the meaning of the word in 1959, noting that 'I find that this term "Epidemiology" is in the process of acquiring a new, specialized meaning which is at a variance with its generally accepted one: the study of epidemics. As a result I find that even with medical men the term "epidemiology of mental disorders" usually requires some explanation'.[30] Morris's mention of 'interesting analogies' sidesteps conceptual issues, specifically the lack of a single agreed model to relate mental disorder to groups of human beings, rather than individuals. This field is new and contentious and people are cautious and uncertain about what it might mean and how much conceptual sense it makes. Concepts of the psychosocial have not always been self-evident.

Psychiatric epidemiology emerges with the shift towards community care in mental health, both implying and relying on a concept of 'the psychosocial'. Mental disorder is embedded in populations by stress, via social relationships. George Rosen concludes in 1959 that from 'the 18th century to the present there has existed the concept that social stress is in some way related to the causation of mental illness'.[31] However, Rhodri Hayward argues that while such easy associations between personal adversity and physical distress seem long lasting, the component parts of these connections have repeatedly been reconstituted around different goals, using different investigative techniques.[32] The relationship between investigative techniques and models of distress is crucial. Jackson notes 'the capacity for the language of stress to clearly articulate the relationship between organisms and their environment ... in debates about the social and cultural determinants of mental illness'.[33]

Thus stress and distress are centrally implicated in the psychosocial. Psychiatric epidemiology and social psychiatry begin to make sense in the twentieth century through these broad terms which are neither inherently normal nor pathological. They are instead the fabric of social psychiatry, enabling a porous boundary between mental health and illness. Stress performs significant conceptual, sense-making work for psychiatric epidemiology, the bedrock investigative technique of social psychiatry, associating mental disorder with the environment. Thus by the early 1950s, 'the psychiatrist ... is incessantly forced to consider the social relations of his patient'.[34] This is the shift with which Armstrong is concerned, describing 'a body constituted by its social relationships and relative mental functioning'.[35] The link between stress and this idea of 'the social' is made clear: within psychiatry, 'sociology has provided a rich and diverse contribution to the extension of the medical gaze ... theoretically it, together with psychology, has helped to define basic concepts, such as stress and coping ... sociology has reinforced the shift of the psychiatric gaze'.[36] Hayward argues that 'the sheer number of concepts deployed ... and the broad variety of narratives that these make possible have attracted widespread critical comment'.[37] This broad variety is precisely the point, enabling stress to bear the conceptual load of bridging environment and mental disorder.

Like 'the social', attempted suicide as a cry for help is often presumed to have existed throughout history.[38] However, an epidemic in Britain between the 1950s and the 1970s has its roots in inter-war mental observation wards, attached to general hospitals.[39] It is publicized by Erwin Stengel, during the 1950s in London, and then by Neil Kessel, in Edinburgh during the 1960s, where it is renamed 'self-poisoning' in order to emphasize that it is not *suicide* that is being attempted, but *communication*. Norman Kreitman arrives at Edinburgh in the mid-1960s, and in 1969 proposes the neologism 'parasuicide'.

The relevance of this epidemic of attempted suicide to the psychosocial is made clear by Stengel and Nancy Cook's foundational monograph, *Attempted Suicide: Its Social Significance and Effects* (1958). Not only does the subtitle bring *social* significance explicitly to the fore, but the text's most-quoted passage leaves no doubt about its centrality:

> There is a *social* element in the pattern of most suicidal attempts. Once we look out for the element we find it without difficulty in most cases ... If we think in terms of a social field we may say that those who attempt suicide show a tendency to remain within this field. In most attempted suicides we can discover an appeal to other human beings.[40]

Stress and distress are crucial in Kessel's work. He is not the first to use these terms around this phenomenon, but he is the first to unify it under such a concept.[41] Distress is what makes his self-poisoners a cohesive group. He asks whether there is 'a unifying basis to self-poisoning acts? Is there some feature that informs them all?' He answers that it is distress that 'drives people to self-poisoning acts: distress and despair, unhappiness and desperation'.[42] He also links this unifying concept to 'the social', arguing that distress, 'whether it stems from depression or from intolerable social circumstances, is always present at the time of the act', a usage that casts 'distress' as more like 'stress', as emanating from circumstances.[43] Irving Kreeger claims in 1966 that 'suicide is not a circumscribed entity but a method of reacting to stress which cuts across most of the formal diagnostic categories'.[44] He argues that in every patient 'an attempt should be made to identify the nature of the appeal, whether this is for amelioration of environmental stress or for protection against overwhelming internal conflict'.[45] Two of Kessel's former colleagues declare in 1972 that they 'firmly endorse Kessel's statement that "*distress drives people to self-poisoning acts.*"'[46] Stress, as cause and connection, and distress, as both connection and basic category, are explicitly emphasized at the core of the behaviour.

This unifying distress enables the porous boundary of psychopathology that emerges in community mental health, because it straddles both normal and pathological reactions to environments. Indeed, Kessel's rooting of self-poisoning in distress is explicitly part of this complicated relationship between abnormal action and psychiatric pathology: 'It has often been argued that to poison oneself is such an abnormal act that everyone who does so must be psychiatrically ill. We have not fallen into that tautological trap'. The troublesome borderline is made possible by a concept that passes through it. The position of distress as negotiating the uncertain boundary of psychopathology is clear: it is distress that 'drives people to self-poisoning acts, and distress is not the exclusive province of the mentally ill'.[47]

A focus on communication is also a basic part of 'the social'. A distress-based, psychosocial approach casts certain 'self-inflicted injuries' as communications with that social environment. In Jurgen Ruesch and Gregory Bateson's *Communication: The Social Matrix of Psychiatry* (1951), Ruesch notes that psychiatrists 'have moved out of the enclosing walls of mental institutions and have found a new field of activity in the general hospitals of the community and in private practice'. This leads to the argument that 'it is necessary to see the individual in the context of his social situation'.[48] He further claims that it is 'the task of psychiatry to help those who have failed to experience successful communication' and that psychopathology is 'defined in terms of disturbances of communication'.[49] Ruesch admits that such a formulation might be a little surprising, but that the sceptical reader need only open a textbook of psychiatry to find that terms such as 'illusions', 'delusions', 'dissociation' or 'withdrawal' in fact 'refer specifically to disturbances of communication'.[50]

Conceptualizing psychiatric disorders as essentially communicative shows how ideas of stress and coping feed into communicative action. Not only does social stress prompt the communication, but the social environment is also where help is sought through communication. Stress is what enables mental illness and environment to be mutually reconstituted and for that environment to take on psychological importance as 'the psychosocial'. In 1992, Raymond Jack surveys the models that have been used to explain self-poisoning. He acknowledges that stress has been seen as key and emphasizes how closely stress comes to stand for the social environment: 'stress is external to individuals and emanates from the social conditions which govern their everyday lives'.[51]

Knowing and Managing 'The Social'

Having shown that stress and distress are foundational to 'the social', which is co-constituted with understandings of attempted suicide as a cry for help, we turn now to the practical ways in which this realm is envisaged and actively constructed by psychiatric and social work professionals, a process principally achieved through home visiting and spouse and family interviews. Social work is vital to self-poisoning because, according to Kessel, it offers therapeutic possibilities across the unstable psychopathological boundary. For him, it 'does not follow that the patient can benefit from treatment only if he has a psychiatric illness. Nearly half of those without such illness were judged to be helpable by further care, a term which embraces social work as well as psychiatric therapy'.[52] Furthermore, Kessel puts psychiatric social workers (PSWs) right at the heart of this phenomenon.

The roots of psychiatric social work lie in mental after-care and the child guidance movement. Vicky Long notes that, in the late nineteenth and early twentieth centuries, 'the Mental After Care Association deployed lady volunteers to visit its charity cases in their homes or places of work to check on their progress and resolve any difficulties'.[53] John Stewart shifts focus, arguing that PSWs emerge 'after 1918 in an organic relationship with child guidance'.[54] Noël K. Hunnybun, Senior PSW in the Children's Department at the Tavistock Institute, agrees, plotting psychiatric social work's development through 'the medium of child guidance',[55] and tracing the profession back through concerns expressed in Cyril Burt's *The Young Delinquent* (1925), which emphasizes 'the importance of studying the child in relation to his family and social background'.[56] These concerns with 'families' and 'social background' are absolutely crucial, both to PSWs and attempted suicide.

In 1929 the London School of Economics establishes the first PSW training course for social science graduates. The Universities of Edinburgh (1944), Manchester (1946) and Liverpool (1954) follow suit,[57] and the government is also concerned to increase the number of social workers. Eileen Younghusband notes in 1951 that the Cope and the Mackintosh Committees are, at that point, considering 'the supply and demand, recruitment and training of almoners, and of psychiatric social workers and other social workers in the mental health service'.[58] She also sees wider acknowledgement during the 1950s of 'the profound influence which the family and social environment had on the well-being and social functioning of mentally disordered people'.[59] Political intervention is also noted by Richard Titmuss in 1961, when he claims that numerous 'Royal Commissions and committees of enquiry have discovered in recent years the virtues of the normal social environment – or as near "normal" as possible'.[60]

Of critical importance to British child guidance and to psychiatric social work are the explanatory schemes of John Bowlby.[61] His work reconfigures the psychological crux of the parent-child relationship away from the intricate fantasies, envies and anxieties of orthodox psychoanalysis, focusing on what Anthony Storr revealingly labels 'real life'. According to Storr, while 'most psychoanalysts assume that neurotic symptoms originate from the patient's inner world of fantasy, Bowlby remained firmly convinced that traumatic events in real life were more significant – not only actual separation and loss, but also parental threats of abandonment and other cruelties'.[62] This constitutes a crucial emphasis on the social origins of psychopathology, where 'the social' is elided with 'real life'.

PSWs are an obvious expression of this psychologized turn towards 'the social' as well as key instruments in the development of such perspectives. In 1951 Aubrey Lewis claims that 'until comparatively recently explicit concern about these matters was rare ... Times have changed. The psychiatric social worker is an essential member of the mental hospital or clinic staff'.[63] Younghusband notes the need for a new kind of social work in mental health which calls for 'a social frame of reference, a fuller recognition of the complexity of human motivation and behaviour, and particularly of family and social interaction'.[64] The broad shift, after 1959, towards 'community care' brings social work to renewed prominence. In the foreword to Alistair Munro and Wallace McCulloch's *Psychiatry for Social Workers* (1968), it is claimed that psychiatry 'is showing a healthy tendency to emerge from hospital into the community and in doing so it leans much more heavily than before on the assistance of every type of social worker'.[65]

It is this 'social frame of reference' that becomes increasingly dominant, part of a broad political project. Influential studies from Aubrey Lewis's Social Psychiatry Research Unit focus upon the role of the family in the recovery from conditions such as schizophrenia.[66] Felix Post – who conducts studies around the same time and on the same ward as Stengel[67] – also becomes involved with the role of the family in mental illness, citing H. B. Richardson's *Patients Have Families* (1945) as a 'pioneer work'.[68] Nikolas Rose describes this post-war project in terms of 'minimizing social troubles and maximizing social efficiency',[69] and notes that psychiatric social case work, through ideas about familial relations, is able to access and intervene upon 'the internal world of the home ... in a new way'.[70] Mathew Thomson argues that social workers are seen during the 1950s and 1960s as 'shock troops' of a movement to spread psychological and psychiatric understandings of self and surroundings, with 'an ability to reach into the home'.[71] Eghigian, Killen and Leuenberger describe a 'new wave of state interventionism ... directed at women, children, and families' in the decades after the Second World War.[72] The goal of this intervention, counselling and casework is to produce what Rose calls the 'responsible autonomous family', a nuclear, private, productive unit comprising well-adjusted, physically and psychologically healthy citizens.[73]

PSWs occupy an increasingly prominent place in Kessel's studies of self-poisoning, which dominate his four years in Edinburgh (1961–5). Edinburgh is the first place outside London to offer PSW training courses. Here, the Meyerian influence of D. K. Henderson, Professor of Psychiatry at Edinburgh (1932–54), makes it a conducive place for PSWs to work. They flourish, for whilst lip service was 'paid to Adolf Meyer's more global picture ... only a minority of psychiatrists seemed to take this seriously in practice. These were the best friends of the PSWs, and valued their support in demonstrating the ... tensions and conflicts in the family and social situation'.[74] PSWs are intimately concerned with access to the 'social situation'. It is through home visiting and the taking of social histories that 'the centrality of the home to child guidance and the part therein of the psychiatric social worker' is established.[75] Indeed, sometimes social workers 'sought to visit the home even before a clinic visit'.[76] The social history is the most basic building block for reliable access to 'the social setting', and Stewart notes that psychiatrists 'appreciated such "social history"'.[77] This is central to PSW practice and takes up considerable time.

Kessel works most closely in collaboration with PSWs Elizabeth Lee and J. Wallace McCulloch. It is noted that 'in Edinburgh the Medical Officer of Health was an enthusiastic exponent of home treatment for the mentally ill and had been training his Health Visitors to act as P. S. W.s'.[78] When mental healthcare becomes increasingly organized around outpatient departments, especially after 1959, the PSW staples of home visiting and social history-taking have even more potential to fabricate a credible social space around any given case of mental disorder.[79] There is thus significant 'socially-focused' expertise upon which Kessel can draw, but it is still not enough. He complains in 1962 that a shortage of 'psychiatric social workers makes it difficult to obtain additional information; when their services are available it is more often to provide after-care than to augment the history'.[80] However, a footnote acknowledges that this paper 'was submitted for publication in 1961. Since then there has been an increase in the allocation of psychiatric and social work time. This now permits a fuller investigation of each case'.[81]

Kessel is explicit about PSW prominence in investigations into self-poisoning. In 1963, he argues that 'we need as much of the P. S. W.'s time as of the psychiatrist's' which 'reflects the importance we place upon social work both in elucidating the circumstances leading to the overdosage and in dealing with the complicated social nexuses and tangled personal relationships that beset so many of these patients'.[82] In addition, arrangements are made for the PSW to interview key informants such as a spouse or relative.[83] Then 'a clinical conference is held at which the patient is seen by the whole team; social and clinical details are put together and the disposal of the patient is arranged'.[84] These are the practices upon which an interpersonal social nexus is built. In Edinburgh, a routine clinical conference with PSWs has emerged by February 1963, when Kessel writes to *The Lancet* advising that in all cases of attempted suicide a friend or family member of the patient should be interviewed, and that multiple times 'we found that we erred before we made this a rule'.[85] PSWs broaden investigations through follow-up home visits, enhancing the credibility of the resulting social spaces. These projections bring out an explicitly normative social setting which is built into the foundations of attempted suicide:

> There is no simple explanation of the high rate of self-poisoning among young women in their early twenties ... These women, although fully engaged in their normal social setting, mothering and running a home, are emotionally isolated ... they have not yet had time to adjust to the confines of domesticity ... Unhappiness mounts, and then suddenly explodes, at a moment of special crisis.[86]

This 'social' is explicitly normal, domestic and potentially psychopathogenic.

Kessel's 'distress' is also informed (through PSWs again) by the marriage guidance movement. This reinforces another crucial practice for constructing 'the social': spouse interviews. Post-1945, psychiatric social work transcends its child guidance heritage, moving closer to marriage guidance, a movement founded in the 1920s with historic connections to PSWs.[87] The Family Discussion Bureau is founded in 1948 by the Family Welfare Association and becomes attached to the Tavistock Institute of Human Relations in 1956.[88] Elizabeth Irvine reveals of PSW training schemes that the 'psychology of family relations was introduced in the late 1950s, largely taught by members of the Family Discussion bureau (later the Institute of Marital Studies), who sometimes narrowed the subject to marital relations alone'.[89]

The increasingly marital focus of PSWs is evident at Edinburgh: 'marital conflict is the chief aetiological factor in many cases; generally the attempt follows swiftly upon an acute domestic quarrel in a chronically disturbed matrimonial situation'. Kessel and Lee 'stress the importance of the breaking home' rather than a Bowlbian 'broken home' caused by parental divorce or absence.[90] In 1964 Noel Timms registers temporal changes in the 'social history': it is 'possible that the purpose and method of taking the social history have changed, since psychiatric social workers now think they are called on not so much for a detailed expression of family history but for an assessment of the present situation'.[91] The environment imagined around 'attempted suicide' shifts from Bowlbian parent-child relations, becoming more recognizably 'social'. Social work practice implies a *present* social space, a web of relationships, of which attempted suicide is a symptom.

Present marital conflict is only a short step from broader communicative, interpersonal concerns, founded upon distress. Kessel argues that admission to the ward, 'having poisoned oneself, can be for instance a powerful weapon in bringing back errant boy friends. The girls who resort to it are, all the same, very much distressed; in their despair they do something stupid and senseless, and it works'.[92] Self-poisoning is imagined as a powerful weapon by being situated in a social, communicative field founded upon distress. The social constellation allows pathology to be projected onto (or articulated through) somebody who has not even been poisoned. McCulloch and Philip put this most clearly in 1972:

> the Edinburgh studies have shown that among married women pathological jealousy in the husband was found in almost a quarter of the cases. Indeed, the persistent suspicions of the 'jealous husband' were frequently found to be a precipitating factor for the attempt. In all but a tiny proportion of such cases, the husbands themselves reported that their jealousy had been completely unfounded.[93]

This idea of illness emerges at the point where marriage guidance and psychiatry intersect. J. H. Wallis's influential marriage guidance text includes a chapter on 'The Jealous Husband', where a flexible and potentially expansive sense of psychopathology emerges when considering whether to refer such a husband to a psychiatrist: there 'cannot be a categorical answer to this question since the dividing line between sickness and health is not precise. One has to consider the whole situation'.[94] The social constellation, allied to marriage guidance-inspired spouse interviews, is credible enough to support the redistribution of pathology away from the presenting action (self-poisoning) onto a social relationship. Again, the boundary of psychopathology is radically mobile, buttressed by specific ideas and practices.

Spouse interviews are central to Kessel's social setting, as he 'noted one phenomenon over and over again. An insensitive spouse, generally the husband, although he cared for his wife had failed to notice either her need for emotional support and encouragement or the growing sense of isolation within the home that stemmed from their lack'.[95] Here, domestic stress is gendered through a feminine lack of resilience, or a masculine lack of support.

The social space, painstakingly constructed through interviews, visits and assumptions, fundamentally informs Kessel's way of framing and answering questions: 'Confirmation was thus provided of the clinical impression derived from dealing with the patients, especially the women in the ward, that marital conflict is the chief aetiological factor in many cases'.[96] PSW practices bring in credible information, accessed through an interview with somebody who is *not a patient*, opening up a space where Kessel's clinical impression gains empirical validation or confirmation. This enables him to speak about a social, domestic space through what he observes in a hospital ward. Once this clinical impression is confirmed, it can predominate, even to the point of overriding PSW input that helps to enable it: the psychiatric social worker, Kessel argues 'who had seen both partners, graded only half the marriages as poor or bad ... Perhaps, however, one has to be inside a marriage really to assess its satisfactions and its failures'.[97]

These practices build a 'social' around marriages, spouses and homes. The clinical conferences and Kessel's clinical impression articulate a socially situated self-poisoning through PSWs, even though their input is sometimes overridden. Visions of the home are created in these analyses, co-constituted with the aetiology of self-poisoning through distress. This is a significant part of the wider project inscribing mental health and mental disorder onto the social, interpersonal fabric of everyday life. This pathological domesticity is crucial in stabilizing the attempted suicide during the 1960s.

Kessel differentiates this feminized, domesticated 'psychosocial' from more traditional readings. He asks whether self-poisoning is 'perhaps the female counterpart of delinquency in young men? Such a hypothesis would suggest that women turn their aggression against themselves, while men act against society'.[98] He rejects this, arguing instead that clinical study leads him to explain self-poisoning through the abovementioned 'emotional isolation' and failure to adapt to the 'confines of domesticity'. Through rehearsal and rebuttal of this hypothesis, Kessel moves away from conventionally masculine, sociological concerns such as crime and delinquency. His analysis recalls Elliot Slater and Moya Woodside's observations gathered during home-interviews of the wives of selected soldiers in the late 1940s, where Woodside reports witnessing 'struggles and ambitions eventually adapting themselves to the limitations of a restrictive environment'.[99] This is not new; marriage, domesticity and psychopathology are historically well-connected.[100] This connection is enabled anew and reiterated by the PSW-founded interrogation of domesticity, which has a fundamental effect on the kind of 'social' that is imagined.

This domesticated social space becomes increasingly gendered throughout the 1960s, interacting with other concerns. The self-conscious nature of Kessel's self-poisoning (compared to Stengel's more unconscious-focused framework) feeds into stereotypes of feminine manipulation, exemplified by Kessel's above-quoted comment about bringing back errant boy friends. Self-poisoning – rather than slashing one's own throat, for example – is also seen as a passive (read: feminine) method which interacts with a gendered imbalance in the prescription of barbiturates. As Ali Haggett states, '[s]ince the 1970s, feminist historians have suggested that the lack of opportunities afforded to women and the banality inherent in the domestic role caused symptoms of anxiety and depression in post-war housewives. Correspondingly, they have argued that the primary motive for prescribing psychotropic drugs was to ensure that women "adapted" to their domestic role'.[101] Finally, distress has resonances with supposed feminine emotionality and hysteria, but is also explicitly articulated as part of this feminized domestic role.

Psychiatry, the social setting and women are closely connected during the 1960s. The classic *Psychiatric Illness in General Practice* (1966) goes so far as to say that 'it would be a justifiable exaggeration to say that in the eyes of the general practitioners, psychiatry in general practice consists largely of the social problems of women'.[102] A gender imbalance in attempted suicide as a cry for help does not seem exceptional in the wider context of reading mental illness into interpersonal, domestic relationships. The idea that women are physically, emotionally, psychologically or evolutionarily more suited to domestic, home or family spaces is a durable plank in circular sexist arguments that feminize domesticity *a priori*.

This is not all. PSWs have their own gendered freight to contribute to the domesticated, psychopathological 'social'. John Stewart notes that during the interwar period, 'social work was ... a predominantly female occupation',[103] an assessment echoed by Noel Timms in the post-war period.[104] Of course, the presence of those gendered women in any given profession *does not* mean that the work produced will necessarily be gendered in any particular way. The problem arises from the gendered assumptions that are articulated through the imagery and associations of a supposedly female profession. The child guidance roots of PSWs carry significant gendered associations, and Timms is well aware of the belittling of PSWs by psychiatrists. He recalls an article in the *British Medical Journal* in 1950 on 'The Role of the Psychiatric Social Worker' where:

> Dr J. B. S. Lewis appeared to give full recognition to the psychiatric social worker. 'She should', a report of the meeting states, 'of course, work in close conjunction with a psychiatrist; but it must be remembered that she had a skill of her own, and he could learn from her as she from him. Her duties were multifarious. She had to explain to the patient, his relatives, employers, etc. what the hospital or clinic was doing; to take a social history; to follow-up and help discharged patients; to co-operate with other social services; to help in administration and therapeutic work and in research; and, in fact, to carry out many *other chores*'.[105]

This earnest and patronizing picture is assessed with Timms's sardonic comment that the 'fairly high status accorded to the psychiatric social worker is somewhat diminished by the ambivalent comment in (my) italics'.[106] Scrutiny of domesticity is elided into domestic work (chores). The sexism upon which pathological domesticity is founded is the same sexism that saturates the profession of psychiatric social work.

Through the routine deployment of practical social work arrangements, the establishment of this particular domestic, gendered 'social' around attempted suicide is highly successful. Stress and psychiatric social work are, respectively, the conceptual and practical means through which circumstances and pathological behaviour become connected. Hence, statements that 'marital disharmony causes self-poisoning' are possible when the latter is encountered on a hospital ward. Once this process begins to recur predictably, when social spaces and pathogenic relationships become presumed and thus self-reinforcing, this particular 'social' can be considered established. To quote Hacking, 'new possibilities for action' can become 'a culturally sanctioned way of expressing distress'.[107] However, as has been argued here, this concept of distress is linked to socially directed or communicative behaviour in such a comprehensive way that there is not much value in using one to explain the other in the case of attempted suicide. Indeed, explaining a psychological epidemic of *anything* during the twentieth century using the language of distress begs more questions than it answers given the way that stress and distress are constituted at the heart of – and are conceptual guarantors for – the new project of psychiatric epidemiology and its psychogenic social space.

Conclusion

Attempted suicide drives and expresses the broad and eclectic turn to 'the social' in mental health; this 'social' still undergirds the controversial justifications for community care. In addition, the psychosocial environment provides the terrain that makes possible the 'psychologisation' or 'psychiatrisation' of society. It seems obvious today that everybody exists in a social environment and is subject to various stresses in some degree. Through stress, everything is potentially psychopathological, every (social) relationship and (social) situation is on a continuum and carries a mental health risk.

Acknowledging the central role of stress and the psychosocial in the relentless diagnostic expansion of psychiatry allows a more precise position to be taken on the ethics and desirability of this expansion. Stress is a vital conceptual plank in various mental health-care arrangements that create an ever-widening psychosocial field of action. This sounds superficially like the 1960s anti-psychiatry that protests that mental illness is a social, rather than biological, phenomenon. The anti-psychiatric position criticizes the psychiatric profession for conflating the two and participating in 'social control'. Thomas Szasz characterizes 'psychiatry as social action' and the psychiatrist as a 'social manipulator of human material [who] punishes, coerces or otherwise influences people'.[108] These arguments are fully embedded in 'the social'. His work also finds a link between distress, characteristically mobilized as a basic category, and 'the social': 'in so far as physicians try to help persons who are in distress – rather than *only* repair bodies that are deranged – they must have some familiarity with man as a social being'.[109] Whilst Szasz uses distress to step back from labelling phenomena as illness, this usage comes with assumptions of its own; Szasz is merely the logical end point for rolling back the unstable boundary of pathology built into this 'social'. 'The social' becomes a self-evident battleground, the prerequisite for these arguments. Thus it is also largely invisible, undergirding both sides, self-evident and beyond comment. Lives are psychologized (some more than others due to their gender identity) by the seemingly banal fact that the social and the psychopathological are intimately connected in the 'psychosocial', a connection enabled by the concept of stress.

In the twenty-first century, stress is increasingly understood neurochemically, but not to the exclusion of 'social stress'; that concept still functions to bridge the gap between mental state and environment.[110] It still underwrites 'the social' – with its overlapping assumptions, aetiologies and concepts – which remains one of the most basic categories for understanding human action. The aim of critical history is to uncover the premises for our understandings of the world, to defamiliarize that which seems most natural, to make visible that which is most difficult to see. It roots these premises in time, in space, in context; they are therefore up for debate, subject to review, able to be changed. The ethical consequences (involving diagnostic expansionism, surveillance, enduring sexism and individual rights) of understanding and governing the world through this idea of 'the social' take on new pertinence when placed in context. The idea that we should simply manage or contest, 'roll back' or 'advance', the unstable boundary of pathology is no longer the only thinkable binary. This critique brings into view how the boundary becomes constituted as unstable in the first place.

Acknowledgements

This research was made possible by a Wellcome Trust Studentship 089708/Z/09/Z. I would like to acknowledge the rigorous and critical comments of Mark Jackson and Rhodri Hayward at various stages of this research.

NOTES

Jackson, 'Stress in Post-War Britain: An Introduction'

1. T. Benedek, *Insight and Personality Adjustment: A Study of the Psychological Effects of War* (New York: Ronald Press, 1946), p. 89. Born in Hungary, Benedek emigrated in 1936 to America, where she worked in the Chicago Institute of Psychoanalysis until 1970.
2. Sir J. Marchant (ed.), *Rebuilding Family Life in the Post-War World: An Enquiry with Recommendations* (London: Odhams Press, 1945).
3. Sir A. MacNalty, 'Influence of War on Family Life', in *Rebuilding Family Life*, pp. 128–36, on p. 135.
4. For a vision of the centrality of physical and mental well-being to state planning, see E. F. M. Durbin, *The Politics of Democratic Socialism: An Essay in Social Policy* (London: George Routledge and Sons, 1945). I am grateful to Rhodri Hayward for this reference – see R. Hayward, 'The Pursuit of Serenity: Psychological Knowledge and the Making of the British Welfare State', in S. Alexander and B. Taylor (eds), *History and Psyche: Culture, Psychoanalysis, and the Past* (Basingstoke: Palgrave Macmillan, 2012), pp. 283–304. Parallel strategies to link urban planning and social reconstruction to psychological health in North America are the focus of on-going research by Ed Ramsden, Queen Mary University of London.
5. Close attention to family structure, patterns of work, and health is evident in a number of contemporary surveys of family life: R. Fletcher, *Britain in the Sixties: Family and Marriage* (London: Penguin, 1962); M. Young and P. Willmott, *The Symmetrical Family* (London: Routledge and Kegan Paul, 1973). The formulation of the notion of work-life balance in the context of growing concerns about the impact of working on women's mental health is the focus of on-going work by Fred Cooper at the University of Exeter.
6. D. Goodhart, *The British Dream: Successes and Failures of Post-War Immigration* (London: Atlantic Books, 2013).
7. For contemporary discussion of the housing, education and health and welfare aspects of immigration, see *Race Relations in Britain: Central Office of Information Reference Pamphlet 108* (London: HMSO, 1972).
8. During the 1970s and 1980s, a number of studies explored the social, political and personal benefits and costs of immigration: C. Holmes (ed.), *Immigrants and Minorities in British Society* (London: George Allen and Unwin, 1978); R. C. Nann (ed.), *Uprooting and Surviving: Adaptation and Resettlement of Migrant Families and Children* (Dordrecht: D. Reidel, 1982); K. Lunn, *Race and Labour in Twentieth-Century Britain* (London: Frank Cass, 1985); C. Holmes, *John Bull's Island: Immigration and British*

Society, 1871–1971 (Basingstoke: Macmillan, 1988).

9. L. Abrams, 'Liberating the Female Self: Epiphanies, Conflict and Coherence in the Life Stories of Post-War British Women', *Social History*, 39 (2014), pp. 14–35.
10. Abrams, 'Liberating the Female Self', pp. 14–35.
11. For detailed accounts of various aspects of life in post-war Britain, see: D. Kynaston, *Modernity Britain, Book One: Opening the Box, 1957–59* (London: Bloomsbury, 2013); and D. Kynaston, *Modernity Britain, Book Two: A Shake of the Dice, 1959–62* (London: Bloomsbury, 2014).
12. Historical debates about best how to interpret the 1960s in particular can be found in: D. Farber (ed.), *The Sixties: From Memory to History* (North Carolina, NC: University of North Carolina, 1994); A. Marwick, *The Sixties* (Oxford: Oxford University Press, 1998); S. Robotham, *Promise of a Dream: Remembering the Sixties* (New York: Verso, 2001); D. Sandbrook, *White Heat: A History of Britain in the Swinging Sixties* (London: Abacus, 2007); M. Collins (ed.), *The Permissive Society and its Enemies: Sixties British Culture* (London, Rivers Oram, 2007); J. Diski, *The Sixties* (London: Profile, 2009).
13. Abrams, 'Liberating the Female Self', p. 35.
14. Abrams, 'Liberating the Female Self', p. 19.
15. C. Steedman, *Landscape for a Good Woman* (London: Virago, 1986), pp. 5–6, 143–4.
16. For examples of recent literature on the history of stress, see: A. Young, 'The Discourse on Stress and the Reproduction of Conventional Knowledge', *Social Science and Medicine*, 14 (1980), pp. 133–46; K. Pollock, 'On the Nature of Social Stress: Production of a Modern Mythology', *Social Science and Medicine*, 26 (1988), pp. 381–92; R. Kugelmann, *Stress: The Nature and History of Engineered Grief* (Westport, CT: Praeger, 1992); R. Viner, 'Putting Stress in Life: Hans Selye and the Making of Stress Theory', *Social Studies of Science*, 29 (1999), pp. 391–410; A. Young, *The Harmony of Illusions: Inventing Post-Traumatic Stress Disorder* (New Jersey, NJ: Princeton University Press, 1995); S. Doublet, *The Stress Myth* (Sydney: Ipsilon Publishing, 2000); B. Shephard, *A War of Nerves: Soldiers and Psychiatrists 1914–94* (London: Pimlico, 2002); C. R. Brewin, *Post-Traumatic Stress Disorder: Malady or Myth?* (New Haven: Yale University Press, 2003); C. L. Cooper and P. Dewe, *Stress: A Brief History* (Malden, MA, and Oxford: Blackwell, 2004); E. Jones and S. Wessely, *Shell Shock to PTSD: Military Psychiatry from 1900 to the Gulf War* (Hove and New York: Psychology Press, 2005); A. Patmore, *The Truth About Stress* (London: Atlantic Books, 2006); M. Jackson, *The Age of Stress: Science and the Search for Stability* (Oxford: Oxford University Press, 2013); and D. Cantor and E. Ramsden (eds), *Stress, Shock and Adaptation in the Twentieth Century* (Rochester: University of Rochester Press, 2014).
17. For further discussion of these late-nineteenth and early-twentieth-century accounts, see Jackson, *The Age of Stress*, pp. 21–55.
18. For a summary of this argument, see the discussion in Jackson, *The Age of Stress*, pp. 265–70.
19. P. J. Bracken, 'Post-Modernity and Post-Traumatic Stress Disorder', *Social Science and Medicine*, 53 (2001), pp. 733–43; A. Harrington, *The Cure Within: A History of Mind-Body Medicine* (New York: W. W. Norton, 2008), p. 139.
20. See Chapter 7 'Men and Women Under Stress', by Jackson, in this volume.
21. See, in particular, E. S. Watkins, 'Stress and the American Vernacular: Popular Perceptions of Disease Causality', in Cantor and Ramsden (eds), *Stress, Shock and Adaptation*, pp. 49–70.
22. For further discussion, see Jackson, *The Age of Stress*, pp. 1–20. On the stress epidemic,

see P. Blythe, *Stress Disease: The Growing Plague* (London: Arthur Barker, 1973). For a discussion of the 'unwanted tempo' of life causing stress and disorientation, see A. Toffler, *Future Shock* (London: Bodley Head, 1970).

23. The research was funded by a Wellcome Trust programme grant, No. 082834/Z07/Z.
24. Some historical work has focused on migrants and health, largely in the context of labour migration, but scope exists for further research on the experiences of, and reactions to, stress amongst immigrant and host communities. For a useful discussion of issues relating to the history of health and migration, see L. Marks and M. Worboys (eds), *Migrants, Minorities and Health: Historical and Contemporary Studies* (London: Routledge, 1997).
25. A. Toffler, *Future Shock* (London: Bodley Head, 1970), pp. 330–1. On Selye's insistence on distraction or deviation as a coping strategy, see M. Jackson, *The Age of Stress: Science and the Search for Stability* (Oxford: Oxford University Press, 2013).
26. For contemporary discussions of the stresses under which families were placed, see: Sir J. Marchant (ed.), *Rebuilding Family Life in the Post-War World: An Enquiry with Recommendations* (London: Odhams Press, 1945); and R. Hill, *Families Under Stress* (New York: Harper and Brothers, 1949).
27. For a discussion of smoking as relief from stress, see Mass Observation, *Man and His Cigarette*, File Report 3192 (Mass Observation, December 1949), pp. 184–5.
28. This pattern of behaviour has persisted. A number of social scientists have highlighted the impact of masculine norms (or what has been termed 'hegemonic masculinity') on illness behaviour: W. H. Courtenay, 'Constructions of Masculinity and Their Influence on Men's Well-Being: A Theory of Gender and Health', *Social Science and Medicine*, 50 (2000), pp. 1385–401; C. Lee and R. G. Owens, 'Issues for a Psychology of Men's Health', *Journal of Health Psychology*, 7 (2002), pp. 209–17; R. O'Brien, K. Hunt and G. Hart, '"It's Caveman Stuff, But That is to a Certain Extent how Guys Still Operate": Men's Accounts of Masculinity and Help Seeking', *Social Science and Medicine*, 61 (2005), pp. 503–16; P. Crawshaw, 'Governing the Healthy Male Citizen: Men, Masculinity and Popular Health in *Men's Health* Magazine', *Social Science and Medicine*, 65 (2007), pp. 1606–18.
29. On the socio-economic and cultural determinants of this process of individualizing stress, see Jackson, *The Age of Stress*, pp. 198–210. For a contemporary discussion of the challenges of adapting to novel occupational practices, see R. Dubos, 'Man adapting to working conditions', in L. Levi (ed.), *Society, Stress, and Disease: Volume 4: Working Life* (New York: Oxford University Press, 1981), pp. 3–7.
30. See D. Thomson, 'Civil Service Sick Leave 1967' (28 January 1970), National Archives, HX5/1, 1.16. For contemporary discussions of the pressures on women to balance work and family and of provisions for women's welfare, see for example: A. Myrdal and V. Klein, *Women's Two Roles: Home and Work* (London: Routledge and Kegan Paul, 1956); and E. Wilson, *Women and the Welfare State* (London: Tavistock Publications, 1977).
31. For examples of some of the early literature in this area, see: R. and R. Rappaport, 'Work and Family in Modern Society', *American Sociological Review*, 30 (1965), pp. 381–94; and M. Young and P. Willmott, *The Symmetrical Family* (London: Routledge and Kegan Paul, 1973), pp. 165–8, 251–5.
32. For a discussion of debates about the aetiology of 'busman's stomach' in the inter-war years, see R. Hayward, 'The Pursuit of Serenity: Psychological Knowledge and the Making of the British Welfare State', in S. Alexander and B. Taylor (eds), *History and*

Psyche: Culture, Psychoanalysis, and the Past (Basingstoke: Palgrave Macmillan, 2012). See M. Jackson, *The Age of Stress: Science and the Search for Stability* (Oxford: Oxford University Press, 2013), pp. 88–98, for an account of constitutional and psychosomatic medicine and stress-related disorders in the same period.

33. This notion was elaborated in the 1960s by two American psychiatrists, Thomas H. Holmes and Richard H. Rahe, to explain the impact of adverse circumstances, such as bereavement, unemployment and divorce, on physical and mental health. The relative effects of these events were measured in the Social Readjustment Rating Scale. For further discussion, see Jackson, *The Age of Stress*, pp. 191–8.
34. See the various contributions to R. Hayward (ed.), 'Special Issue: Inventing the Psycho-social: Stress and Social Psychiatry', *History of the Human Sciences*, 25 (2012).
35. H. Selye (ed.), *Selye's Guide to Stress Research* (New York: Van Nostrand, 1980), vol. 1, p. vii.
36. J. Heller, *Something Happened* (London: Jonathan Cape, 1974). Heller's novel depicts the gradual collapse of an executive, Bob Slocum, and his family in the face of social demands, occupational pressures and personal expectations.

1 Richardson, 'From War to Peace: Families Adapting to Change'

1. H. Selye, *The Story of the Adaptation Syndrome* (Montreal: Acta, 1952).
2. R. Lazarus and S. Folkman, *Stress, Appraisal and Coping* (New York: Springer, 1984).
3. R. Lazarus, *Stress and Emotion: A New Synthesis* (London: Free Association Books, 1999), Part IV and 'Foreword' by S. Folkman, p. xii.
4. http://senate.universityofcalifornia.edu/inmemoriam/richardlazarus.html, p. 2. [accessed April 2012].
5. R. R. Grinker and J. P. Spiegel, *Men Under Stress* (Philadelphia, PA: Blakiston, 1945), p. vii.
6. R. Hill, *Families Under Stress* (New York: Harper, 1949).
7. These case histories were recorded in the 1990s when Lizzie, Nancy and Rose, all in their sixties, and Robbie, in his seventies, took part. They all answered the same twenty questions based on their lives and reactions to events in the period 1939 to 1950. There were also oral discussions separately (and sometimes together for the girls) and family records of letters and photographs were accessible. Permission was given to use these primary sources, with name changes to protect identities.
8. There is evidence of these words in the case studies of the period – see A. Haggett, 'Housewives, Neuroses and the Domestic Environment in Britain, 1945–1970', in M. Jackson (ed.), *Health and the Modern Home* (London: Routledge, 2007), pp. 84–110.
9. Title quoted from Prime Minister, Neville Chamberlain, BBC radio broadcast, 3 September 1939.
10. S. Isaacs (ed.), with the co-operation of S. C. Brown and R. H. Thoules, *The Cambridge Evacuation Survey* (London: Methuen & Co., 1941).
11. S. Isaacs, *Childhood and After: Some Essays and Clinical Studies* (London: Routledge and Kegan Paul, 1948); S. Isaacs, *Troubles of Children and Parents* (London: Methuen, 1948); J. Bowlby, *Separation, Anxiety and Anger: Attachment and Loss*, 2 vols (London: Hogarth Press, 1973), vol. 2; J. Bowlby, *A Secure Base-Parent and Child Attachment and Healthy Home Development* (London: Routledge, 1988); D. Winnicott, *The Child and the Family* and *The Child and the Outside World* (London: Tavistock, 1957); and A. Freud, *The Writings of Anna Freud,* 8 vols (New York: Indiana University of Pennsylvania, 1966–80).

12. 'Nancy' was diagnosed with tuberculosis in her left hip when the family returned from Singapore in 1937. She was admitted to the Lord Mayor Treloar Hospital at Alton later that year to undergo long-term treatment consisting of fresh-air, a balanced diet, physiotherapy and light treatment.
13. The loss of personal power is a stressor explored by H. Selye in *The Stress of Life* (London: McGraw-Hill, 1956), p. 297.
14. 'Rose', Oral history, 1990.
15. Selye, *The Stress of Life*, p. 297.
16. For discussion of smoking as an antidote to stress see M. Jackson, *The Age of Stress. Science and the Search for Stability* (Oxford: Oxford University Press, 2013), pp. 245–7. Also Mass Observation, *Man and His Cigarette,* File Report 3192 (Mass Observation, December 1949).
17. The hospital closed to visitors in December, January and February, except for extreme cases and opened one day a month from March to November.
18. The care of long-term child patients, at this hospital, in the thirties, was based on strict discipline for nurses and patients – see the Hampshire Record Office Archive 47M94.
19. 'Nancy', Oral history, 1990.
20. S. Hayes, 'The Medicalisation of Maladjustment: The Conceptualisation and Management of Child Behavioural Problems in Britain *c.*1890–1955' (PhD thesis, University of Exeter, 2008), p. 316.
21. This view of a maladjusted child is supported by F. Dodd: one 'who is unable to cope with the circumstance with which it is faced', and by A. S. Neill: 'simply angry 'cos of [perceived] lack of love mostly'. J. Bowlby also wrote of 'feelings of jealousy' between siblings as a reason for aberrant behaviour. See these quotes in S. Hayes, 'Rabbits and Rebels: The Medicalisation of Maladjusted Children', in M. Jackson (ed.), *Health and the Modern Home* (London: Routledge, 2007), pp. 139, 147.
22. 'Rose', Oral history, 1990.
23. A. Haggett 'Housewives, Neuroses and the Domestic Environment in Britain 1945–1970', in Jackson (ed.), *Health and the Modern Home*, p. 92.
24. 'Rose', Oral history, 1990. Being the youngest and last to leave home, it seems that her mother confided in her.
25. M. North, *The Secular Priests* (London: George Allen and Unwin, 1972), pp. 17–28.
26. Ali Haggett comments on the value of joining something outside the home and of having a Christian faith in difficult times, which she found in her study of women of the post-war period: Haggett, 'Housewives, Neuroses and the Domestic Environment in Britain', p. 92.
27. Selye discusses the damaging effect of stress-produced hormones on the immune system in *The Stress of Life*, p. 115.
28. Letter dated 3 November 1940.
29. He was recalled by the Navy in 1939 and posted to Alexandria.
30. 'Robbie', Oral history, 1992.
31. His wartime letters to his parents remain in the family archive.
32. Selye, *The Stress of Life*, pp. 178–82. See also: I. Miller, 'The Mind and Stomach at War: Stress and Abdominal Illness in Britain, *c.*1939–1945', *Medical History*, 54 (2010), pp. 95–110; and Chapter 8 'Stomach for the Peace' by E. Jones in this volume.
33. Information about 'Maria' has come from oral interviews with 'Robbie' and from the recollections of their children.
34. 'Robbie', Oral history, 1992. He said how difficult it was to discuss the situation with

his parents and spoke of his feeling of guilt and helplessness at having to go back to sea, trying to re-assure Maria, but knowing that he might not return.

35. Her daughter (Robbie's sister) disclosed that the subject was discussed with her and she was aware of her mother's distress. Oral history, 1990.
36. S. McKay, *The Secret Life of Bletchley Park* (London: Aurum Press: 2011), pp. 200–1, comments on this subject and the class distinctions revealed.
37. 'Robbie' wrote 'So Michael and I are in together! I must send him a line it's great'. Letter 31/10/1943. On his own situation, he wrote, 'there are many in the same boat and I have been more fortunate than most' – letter 18/1/1944.
38. 'Robbie's' letters to his parents refer to the bright and cheerful letters he received from 'Maria', Correspondence 1944–5.
39. Selye, *The Stress of Life*, p. 268.
40. Title quoted from Winston Churchill, BBC broadcast London and the House of Commons, 8 May 1945.
41. R. R. Grinker and J. P. Spiegel, *Men Under Stress* (Philadelphia, PA: Blakiston, 1945), p. vii.
42. J. Groen, 'Foreword, Association for Research in Nervous and Mental Diseases', *Life Stress and Bodily Disease* (Baltimore, MD: Williams and Wilkins, 1950), p. xviii.
43. R. Hill, *Families Under Stress* (New York: Harper and Brothers, 1949).
44. The girls recalled the general feeling of excitement, tidying their bedrooms, choosing their prettiest frocks and favourite things to show Daddy and cleaning their shoes with special care to impress him. 'Lizzie', 'Nancy' and 'Rose', Oral history, 1992.
45. J. Summers, *Stranger in the House: Women's Stories of Men Returning from the Second World War* (London: Simon and Schuster, 2008), p. 3.
46. G. Field, 'The Working Class in World War II: Perspectives on the Working Class Family in Wartime Britain, 1939–1945', *International Labor and Working Class History*, 38 (1990), published on-line 2008: www.researchgate.net/publications/231877518 [accessed June 2012].
47. Summers, *Stranger in the House*, p. 4.
48. 'Robbie', Oral history, 1992.
49. *Woman's Own*, January 1945, quoted by Summers, *Stranger in the House*, p. 15.
50. T. Benedek, *Insight and Personality Adjustment: A Study of the Psychological Effects of War* (New York: Ronald Press, 1946), p. 89. See also Summers, *Stranger in the House*, p. 4.
51. Thomas Forrest Main served in the Royal Army Medical Corps (RAMC) during the war and afterwards worked in the rehabilitation of psychiatrically disturbed servicemen.
52. B. Cartland, *The Years of Opportunity, 1939–1945* (London: Hutchinson, 1948), pp. 194–6.
53. *British Medical Journal*, correspondence, 1:809 (24 April 1948), p. 809.
54. Burt's work is discussed at length by S. Hayes, 'Rabbits and Rebels: The Medicalisation of Maladjusted Children', in M. Jackson (ed.), *Health and the Modern Home* (London: Routledge, 2007), pp. 135–9.
55. 'Rose', Oral history, 1990.
56. M. Jackson, *The Age of Stress: Science and the Search for Stability* (Oxford: Oxford University Press, 2013), p. 265.
57. www.ons.gov.uk/ons/dcp171778 _351693.pdf.3[accessed March 2015].
58. Letter from an Orthopaedic Surgeon, Royal Hants County Hospital, dated 28 July 1949.

59. Letter to the Officer Commanding, British Army of the Rhine (BAOR), 34, Krefeld, 25 January 1950, Family archive.
60. The local doctor had looked after May and the girls since 1940. Note his use of the word 'worry'.
61. 'Rose', Oral history 1992.
62. J. Finch and P. Summerfield, 'Marriage and Family in Sociological Writing', in L. Burgoyne and D. Clark (eds), *Marriage, Domestic Life and Social Change: Writings for Jacqueline Burgoyne 1944–1959* (London: Psychology Press, 1991), p. 7.
63. This was strongly evident in their written answers to questions, 1990.
64. Knowledge of Maria's character and behaviour comes from Robbie's oral history record.
65. A. Haggett, 'Housewives, Neuroses and the Domestic Environment in Britain 1945–1970', in Jackson (ed.), *Health and the Modern Home*, p. 104.
66. R. Cooperstock and H. L. Lennard, 'Some Social Meanings of Tranquilliser Use', *Sociology of Health and Illness*, 1 (1979), pp. 331–47.
67. H. Selye, *The Stress of Life* (London: McGraw-Hill, 1956), pp. 185–7, 304.
68. T. Benedek, *Insight and Personality Adjustment: A Study of the Psychological Effects of War* (New York: Ronald Press, 1946), p. 89.
69. H. Selye emphasized the capacity of stress to stimulate adaptation and resilience, describing the general adaptation syndrome as '*adaptive* because it [stress] stimulates defence and thereby helps the acquisition and maintenance of a state of inurement' – see Selye, *The Stress of Life* (London: McGraw-Hill, 1956), p. 32.
70. 'Robbie', Oral history 1992.
71. Current research indicates the therapeutic potential of music and movement for patients suffering from dementia: http://www.npr.org/2012/04/18/150891711/for-elders-with-dementia-music-sparks-great-awakenings?sc=emaf [accessed April 2012].
72. R. Lazarus, *Adjustment and Personality* (New York: McGraw-Hill, 1961); R. Lazarus, *Psychological Stress and the Coping Process* (New York: McGraw-Hill, 1966); R. Lazarus, *Personality*, 2nd edn (Eaglewood Cliffs: N. J., Prentice Hill, 1971); R. Lazarus, *Patterns of Adjustment*, 3rd edn (New York: McGraw-Hill, 1976); R. Lazarus, *Emotion and Adaptation* (New York: Oxford University Press, 1991).
73. A. D. Kanner, J. C. Coyne, C. Schafer and R. S. Lazarus, 'Comparison of Two Modes of Stress Measurement: Daily Hassles and Uplifts Versus Major Life Events', *Journal of Behavioural Medicine*, 4 (1981), at https://connects.catalyst.harvard.edu/Profile/display/1144172 [accessed August 2013]. The research suggested that it was 'these day to day events that have proximal significance for health outcomes and whose cumulative impact, therefore, should also be assessed', pp. 2–3.
74. www.combatstress.org.uk [accessed April 2012].

2 Baur, 'Families, Stress and Mental Illness in Devon, 1940s to 1970s'

1. Uncatalogued correspondence regarding OP, Devon Record Office (hereafter DRO). Confidential – access restricted. In order to protect patients and relatives' identities, only initials will be used in this chapter when referring to people.
2. M. Jackson, *The Age of Stress: Science and the Search for Stability* (Oxford: Oxford University Press, 2013), p. 22.
3. I. C. Huang, 'Family Stress and Coping', in S. J. Bahr (ed.), *Family Research: A Sixty-Year Review, 1930–1990* (New York: Lexington, 1991), pp. 289–334; R. A. Settersten and K. U. Mayer, 'The Measurement of Age, Age – Structuring and the Life Course',

Annual Review of Sociology, 23 (1997), pp. 233–61; and S. Cohen, 'After Effects of Stress on Human Performance and Social Behaviour: A Review of Research and Theory', *Psychological Bulletin*, 88 (1980), pp. 82–108.

4. E. W. Burgess, 'Mental Health in Modern Society', in A. M. Rose (ed.), *Mental Health and Mental Disorder: A Sociological Approach* (New York: W. W. Norton, 1955); M. R. Yarrow, J. R. Clausen and P. R. Robbins, 'The Social Meaning of Mental Illness', *Journal of Social Issues*, 11 (1955), pp. 33–48; M. R. Yarrow, C. G. Schwarz, H. S. Murphy and L. C. Deasy, 'The Psychological Meaning of Mental Illness in the Family', *Journal of Social Issues*, 11 (1955), pp. 12–24; C. E. Vincent, 'Mental Health and the Family', *Journal of Marriage and the Family*, 29 (1967), pp. 18–39; J. Grad and P. Sainsbury, 'Evaluating a Community Care Service', in H. Freeman and J. Farndale (eds), *Trends in the Mental Health Services* (New York: Macmillan Company, 1963), pp. 303–17; J. Grad and P. Sainsbury, 'Mental Illness and the Family', *Lancet*, 1 (1963), pp. 544–7; J. Hoenig and M. Hamilton, *The Desegregation of the Mentally Ill* (London: Routledge and Kegan Paul, 1969); J. Hoenig and M. Hamilton, 'The Schizophrenic Patient in the Community and His Effect on the Household', *International Journal of Social Psychiatry*, 12 (1966), pp. 165–76; A. Hatfield, 'Psychological Costs of Schizophrenia to the Family', *Social Work*, 23 (1978), pp. 355–9; and M. Herz, G. Endicott and R. Spitzer, 'Brief Versus Standard Hospitalization: The Families', *American Journal of Psychiatry*, 133 (1976), pp. 795–801.
5. H. I. McCubbin and M. A. McCubbin, 'Research Utilization in Social Work Practice of Family Treatment', in A. J. Grasso and I. Epstein (eds), *Research Utilization in the Social Sciences: Innovations for Practice and Administration* (New York: Haworth, 1992), pp. 149–92; J. Haley, 'The Family of the Schizophrenic: A Model System', *Journal of Nervous and Mental Disease*, 129 (1959), pp. 357–74; S. Cohen and T. Wills, 'Stress, Social Support, and the Buffering Hypothesis', *Psychological Bulletin*, 98 (1985), pp. 310–57; R. Lazarus and S. Folkman, *Stress, Appraisal, and Coping* (New York: Springer, 1984); and D. Marsh, *Families and Mental Illness: New Directions in Professional Practice* (New York: Praeger, 1992).
6. R. Hill, 'Generic Features of Families Under Stress', *Social Casework*, 49 (1958), pp. 139–50, on p. 143.
7. R. Hill, *Families Under Stress: Adjustments to the Crises of War Separation and Reunion* (Westport, CT: Greenwood Press, 1949); and Hill, 'Generic Features', pp. 139–50.
8. W. Burr, *Theory Construction and the Sociology of the Family* (New York: Wily and sons, 1973); H. I. McCubbin and J. M. Patterson, 'The Family Stress Process: The Double ABCX Model of Adjustment and Adaptation', in H. I. McCubbin, M. S. B. Sussman and J. M. Patterson (eds), *Social Stress and the Family: Advances and Developments in Family Stress Theory and Research* (New York: Haworth, 1983), pp. 7–37; T. H. Holmes and M. Masuda, 'Life Change and Illness Susceptibility', in B. P. Dohrenwend and B. S. Dohrenwend (eds), *Stressful Life Events: Their Nature and Effects* (New York: Wiley, 1974), pp. 45–72; and A. Meyer, 'The Life Chart and the Obligation of Specifying Positive Data in Psychopathological Diagnosis', in E. Winters (ed.), *The Collected Papers of Adolf Meyer: Vol. III. Medical Teaching* (Baltimore, MD: The Johns Hopkins Press, 1951), pp. 162–94.
9. H. Selye, *The Stress of Life* (New York: McGraw-Hill, 1956); and B. P. and B. S. Dohrenwend (eds), *Stressful Life Events*.
10. A. DeLongis, S. Folkman and R. Lazarus, 'The Impact of Daily Stress on Health and Mood: Psychological and Social Resources as Mediators', *Journal of Personality and*

Social Psychology, 54 (1988), pp. 486–95; M. S. Goldstein, 'The Sociology of Mental Health and Illness', *Annual Review of Sociology*, 5 (1979), pp. 381–409; B. P. and B. S. Dohrenwend, 'Life Stress and Illness: Formulation of the Issues', in Dohrenwend and Dohrenwend (eds), *Stressful Life Events and Their Contexts* (New York: Neale Watson Academic, 1981), pp. 1–27; and J. Rabkin and E. Struening, 'Life Events, Stress and Illness' *Science*, 194 (1976), pp. 1013–20.

11. Goldstein, 'The Sociology of Mental Health'; J. K. Myers, J. J. Lindenthal and M. P. Pepper, 'Life Events, Social Integration and Psychiatric Symptomatology', *Journal of Health and Social Behavior*, 16 (1975), pp. 421–7; Rabkin and Struening, 'Life Events'; A. Dean and N. Lin, 'The Stress-Buffering Role of Social Support', *Journal of Nervous and Mental Disease*, 165 (1977), pp. 403–17; and S. Gore, 'The Effect of Social Support in Moderating the Health Consequences of Unemployment', *Journal of Health and Social Behavior*, 19 (1978), pp. 157–65.
12. A. D. Kanner, J. C. Coyne, C. Schaefer and R. Lazarus, 'Comparision of Two Models of Stress Measurements: Daily Hassles and Uplifts Versus Major Life Events', *Journal of Behavioral Medicine*, 4 (1981), pp. 1–39; and J. Zubin and B. Spring, 'Vulnerability – A New View of Schizophrenia', *Journal of Abnormal Psychology*, 86 (1977), pp. 103–26.
13. R. Lazarus, *Emotion and Adaptation* (Oxford: Oxford University Press, 1991); and Goldstein, 'The Sociology of Mental Health', p. 394.
14. D. Meichenbaum, 'Disasters, Stress, and Cognition', in S. E. Hobfoll and M. W. de Vries (eds), *Extreme Stress and Communities: Impact and Intervention* (Dordrecht: Kluwer), pp. 33–61.
15. E. Paykel, 'Life Stress and Psychiatric Disorder: Applications of the Clinical Approach', in B. P. Dohrenwend and B S. Dohrenwend (eds), *Stressful Life Events: Their Nature and Effects* (New York: Wiley, 1974), pp. 135–49.
16. W. Stroebe and M. Stroebe, 'Bereavement and Health: Processes of Adjusting to the Loss of a Partner', in L. Montada, S. H. Filipp and M. J. Lerner (eds), *Life Crisis and Experience of Loss in Adulthood* (Hillsdale, NJ: Erlbaum, 1992), pp. 3–22; and P. J. Clayton, 'Bereavement', in E. Paykel (ed.), *Handbook of Affective Disorders* (New York: Guilford Press, 1982), pp. 403–15.
17. Uncatalogued correspondence regarding SD, Devon Record Office (hereafter DRO). Confidential – access restricted.
18. Uncatalogued correspondence regarding BS, DRO. Confidential – access restricted.
19. Uncatalogued correspondence regarding CT, DRO. Confidential – access restricted.
20. Uncatalogued correspondence regarding AM, DRO. Confidential – access restricted.
21. R. Hill, *Families Under Stress: Adjustments to the Crises of War Separation and Reunion* (Westport, CT: Greenwood Press, 1949); and T. Benedek, *Insight and Personality Adjustment: A Study of the Psychological Effects of the War* (New York: Ronald Press, 1946).
22. Uncatalogued correspondence regarding AM, DRO.
23. R. Day, J. A. Nielsen, et al., 'Stressful Life Events Preceding the Acute Onset of Schizophrenia: A Cross-National Study from the World Health Organization', *Culture, Medicine and Psychiatry*, 11 (1987), pp. 123–205, on p. 194.
24. R. Lazarus and S. Folkman, *Hassles and Uplifts Scales* (Palo Alto, CA: Consulting Psychologists Press, 1989).
25. See Chapters 1, 'From War to Peace', and 3, 'Gender, Stress and Alcohol Abuse', in this volume by Pamela Richardson and Ali Haggett.
26. Uncatalogued correspondence regarding AW, DRO. Confidential – access restricted.
27. Uncatalogued correspondence regarding RF, DRO. Confidential – access restricted.

28. A. Haggett, 'Housewives, Neuroses and the Domestic Environment in Britain, 1945–70', in M. Jackson (ed.), *Health and the Modern Home* (London: Routledge, 2007), pp. 84–110.
29. Uncatalogued correspondence regarding GB, DRO. Confidential – access restricted.
30. Uncatalogued correspondence regarding WD, DRO. Confidential – access restricted.
31. Uncatalogued correspondence regarding MD, DRO. Confidential – access restricted.
32. Uncatalogued correspondence regarding EB, DRO. Confidential – access restricted.
33. Uncatalogued correspondence regarding WC, Devon Record Office (hereafter DRO). Confidential – access restricted; and J. Northover, 'Rehabilitated Long-Stay Schizophrenics in the Community' *British Journal of Psychiatry*, 111 (1965), pp. 258–67.
34. E. Goffman, *Stigma: Notes on the Management of a Spoiled Identity* (Englewood Cliffs, NJ: Prentice Hall, 1963). For more recent studies, see A. Jorm, 'Mental Health Literacy', *British Journal of Psychiatry*, 177 (2000), pp. 396–401; W. Gaebel, A. Baumann, A. Witte and H. Zaske, 'Public Attitudes Towards People with Mental Illness in Six German Cities', *European Archives of Psychiatry and Clinical Neuroscience*, 252 (2002), pp. 278–87; and G. Schomerus, H. Matschinger and M. Angermeyer, 'Public Beliefs about the Causes of Mental Disorders Revisited', *Psychiatry Research*, 144 (2006), pp. 233–6.
35. Uncatalogued correspondence regarding WW, DRO. Confidential – access restricted.
36. Uncatalogued correspondence regarding RF, DRO. Confidential – access restricted.
37. Uncatalogued correspondence regarding WG, DRO. Confidential – access restricted.
38. Uncatalogued correspondence regarding TL, DRO. Confidential – access restricted.
39. Uncatalogued correspondence regarding FS, DRO. Confidential – access restricted.
40. Uncatalogued correspondence regarding MM, DRO. Confidential – access restricted.
41. A. Horwitz, 'Family, Kin, and Friendship Network in Psychiatric Help-Seeking', *Social Science and Medicine*, 12 (1978), pp. 297–304.
42. Uncatalogued correspondence regarding RW, DRO. Confidential – access restricted.
43. Uncatalogued correspondence regarding WG, DRO.
44. Uncatalogued correspondence regarding MH, DRO. Confidential – access restricted.
45. R. Sommer, 'Visitors to Mental Hospitals: A Fertile Field for Research', *Mental Hygiene*, 43 (1959), pp. 3–15.
46. M. R. Yarrow, J. R. Clausen and P. R. Robbins, 'The Social Meaning of Mental Illness', *Journal of Social Issues*, 11 (1955), pp. 33–48; K. Rawnsley, J. B. Loudon and H. L. Miles, 'Attitudes of Relatives to Patients in Mental Hospitals', *British Journal of Preventive and Social Medicine*, 16 (1962), pp. 1–15; and C. Rose, 'Relatives' Attitudes and Mental Hospitalization', *Mental Hygiene*, 43 (1959), pp. 194–203.
47. Uncatalogued correspondence regarding GP, DRO. Confidential – access restricted.
48. Uncatalogued correspondence regarding WH, DRO. Confidential – access restricted.
49. Uncatalogued correspondence regarding TP, DRO. Confidential – access restricted.
50. Uncatalogued correspondence regarding WB and WD, DRO. Confidential – access restricted.
51. Uncatalogued correspondence regarding WH, DRO.
52. Uncatalogued correspondence regarding RS, DRO. Confidential – access restricted.
53. Uncatalogued correspondence regarding MF and OT, DRO. Confidential – access restricted.
54. Uncatalogued correspondence regarding TP, DRO.
55. Uncatalogued correspondence regarding ST, DRO. Confidential – access restricted.
56. Uncatalogued correspondence regarding TN, DRO. Confidential – access restricted.

57. Uncatalogued correspondence regarding HW, DRO. Confidential – access restricted.
58. Uncatalogued correspondence regarding VS, DRO. Confidential – access restricted.
59. E. Mills, *Living with Mental Illness: A Study in East London* (London: Routledge and Kegan Paul, 1962); and J. Wing, E. Monck, G. Brown and G. M. Carstairs, 'Morbidity in the Community of Schizophrenic Patients Discharged from London Mental Hospitals in 1959', *British Journal of Psychiatry*, 110 (1964), pp. 10–21.
60. Uncatalogued correspondence regarding WP, DRO. Confidential – access restricted.
61. Uncatalogued correspondence regarding WD, DRO.
62. Uncatalogued correspondence regarding WG, DRO. Confidential – access restricted.
63. Uncatalogued correspondence regarding WB, DRO.
64. Uncatalogued correspondence regarding WF, DRO. Confidential – access restricted.
65. Uncatalogued correspondence regarding WB, DRO.
66. G. M. Carstairs, 'The Social Limits of Eccentricity: An English Study', in M. K. Opler (ed.), *Culture and Mental Health: Cross-Cultural Studies* (New York: Macmillan Company, 1959), pp. 373–89; and Wing, Monck, Brown and Carstairs, 'Morbidity in the Community'.
67. G. Brown, E. Monck, G. M. Carstairs and J. Wing, 'Influence of Family Life in the Course of Schizophrenic Illness', *British Journal of Preventive and Social Medicine*, 16 (1962), pp. 55–68.

3 Haggett, 'Gender, Stress and Alcohol Abuse in Post-War Britain'

1. See J. Greenaway, *Drink and British Politics Since 1830: A Study in Policy Making* (Basingstoke: Palgrave Macmillan, 2003); J. Nicholls, *The Politics of Alcohol: A History of the Drink Question in England* (Manchester: Manchester University Press, 2009); B. Thom, *Dealing with Drink: Alcohol and Social Policy, From Treatment to Management* (London: Free Association Books, 1999); and V. Berridge, R. Herring and B. Thom, 'Binge-Drinking: A Confused Concept and its Contemporary History', *Social History of Medicine*, 22 (2009), pp. 597–607.
2. See figures from Thom relating to alcohol treatment units prior to the 1970s in *Dealing with Drink*, p. 57; and recent research in D. Wilkins (ed.), *Untold Problems: A Review of the Essential Issues in the Mental Health of Men and Boys* (London: Men's Health Forum, 2010), p. 29; For figures on women and psychiatric disorder, see, for example, C. A. H. Watts, *Depressive Disorders in the Community* (Bristol: John Wright, 1966), pp. 34–5; and more recent analysis in D. Freeman and J. Freeman, *The Stressed Sex: Uncovering the Truth about Men, Women and Mental Health* (Oxford: Oxford University Press, 2013).
3. MIND, *Men and Mental Health: Get it off your Chest* (London: MIND, 2009), cited in Wilkins, *Untold Problems*, p. 30.
4. M. Jackson, *The Age of Stress: Science and the Search for Stability* (Oxford: Oxford University Press, 2013).
5. For a full account of these developments, see Jackson, *The Age of Stress.*
6. See Jackson, *The Age of Stress*, p. 177.
7. See Jackson, *The Age of Stress*, p. 216.
8. See, for example, B. Thom, *Dealing with Drink: Alcohol and Social Policy, From Treatment to Management*, (London: Free Association Books, 1999); and N. Heather and I. Robertson, *Problem Drinking* (Oxford: Oxford University Press, 2004).
9. Thom, *Dealing with Drink*, p. 15. Thom cautions that although there have been broad

shifts in explanatory models, differing perceptions have continued to co-exist. Current disease theories are still contested. See, for example, S. Peele, 'Addiction as a Disease: Policy, Epidemiology and Treatment Consequences of a Bad Idea', in J. Henningfield, W. Bickel and P. Santora (eds), *Addiction Treatment in the 21st Century: Science and Policy Issues* (Baltimore, MD: Johns Hopkins University Press, 2007), pp. 153–63.

10. E. M. Jellinek, 'Phases of Alcohol Addiction', *Quarterly Journal of Studies on Alcohol*, 13:4 (1952), pp. 673–84.
11. Heather and Robertson, *Problem Drinking*, p. 58.
12. G. Edwards and M. M. Gross, 'Alcohol Dependence: Provisional Description of a Clinical Syndrome', *British Medical Journal*, (1 May 1976), pp. 1058–61.
13. G. Watts, 'James Griffith Edwards', Obituary, *The Lancet*, 338 (6 October 2012), p. 1224.
14. Heather and Robertson, *Problem Drinking*, p. 31.
15. Heather and Robertson, *Problem Drinking*, p. 31.
16. Heather and Robertson, *Problem Drinking*, p. 31.
17. 'Conversation with Max Glatt', *British Journal of Addiction*, 78 (1983), pp. 231–43, on p. 233.
18. 'Conversation with Max Glatt', p. 236.
19. Thom, *Dealing with Drink*, p. 75.
20. Camberwell Council on Alcoholism (hereafter CCA), Miscellaneous Correspondence, SA/CAA/17, 'An Alcohol Information and Discussion Week', *Medical Officer* (31 December 1965), pp. 353–5, on p. 353, Wellcome Archives and Manuscripts. The Council first met in 1961. It consisted of members drawn from medicine and psychiatry, the clergy, the police, social services and the Chamber of Commerce. It worked to educate doctors and other interested parties and became nationally influential.
21. M. Bennett, 'Drinking as a Career', *Journal of Alcoholism*, 11 (1976), pp. 150–2, on p. 151.
22. Bennett, 'Drinking as a Career', p. 150.
23. Thom, *Dealing with Drink*, p. 20.
24. Thom, *Dealing with Drink*, pp. 22, 25, 34, 39.
25. Thom, *Dealing with Drink*, p. 46.
26. Correspondence, Rowntree Trust Steering Group on Alcohol 1957–64, PP/AWD/H6/2, Wellcome Archives and Manuscripts.
27. Correspondence, Rowntree Trust Steering Group, PP/AWD/H6/2.
28. SA/CCA/44, CCA, 'Seminars on Alcoholism', 1970, pp. 5–7.
29. SA/CCA/44, 'Seminars on Alcoholism', p. 12.
30. 'Conversation with Max Glatt', p. 234.
31. Thom, *Dealing with Drink*, pp. 41, 63.
32. 'Conversation with Max Glatt', p. 237.
33. Thom, *Dealing with Drink*, p. 65.
34. Thom, *Dealing with Drink*, pp. 57–8. The term 'skid row' originated from the USA during the 1930s. It is a derogatory term applied to disreputable parts of a town known for high levels of vagrancy and poor maintenance – often frequented by alcoholics.
35. SA/CCA/62, CCA 'Women Alcoholics: Seminars, Student Surveys, Agencies and Work-Group Meetings', 1973–5.
36. P. Borsay, 'Binge Drinking and Moral Panics, Historical Parallels?', *History and Policy* website at http://www.historyandpolicy.org/papers/policy-paper-62.html [accessed 28 January 2013]. This debate continues today, see V. Berridge, R. Herring and B. Thom,

'Binge-Drinking: A Confused Concept and its Contemporary History', *Social History of Medicine*, 22 (2009), pp. 597–607, where the authors argue that the government and media continue to focus on women drinkers while mortality rates from alcohol are twice as high in men than women.

37. SA/CCA/62, 'Women Alcoholics', minutes of meeting from the planning group.
38. SA/CCA/62, 'Women Alcoholics', minutes.
39. A. B. Sclare, 'The Female Alcoholic', *British Journal of Addiction*, 65 (1970), pp. 99–107.
40. SA/CCA/62, 'Women Alcoholics'.
41. SA/CCA/62, 'Women Alcoholics'.
42. SA/CCA/44, CCA '"Cured" by a Recovering Alcoholic', Seminars on Alcoholism, Paper Number 5, Autumn 1970.
43. SA/CCA/62, 'Women Alcoholics'.
44. D. Parr, 'Alcoholism in General Practice', C1957, Papers of Sir Allen William Daley PP/AWD/H6/3/2, Wellcome Archives and Manuscripts.
45. SA/CCA/32, Camberwell Council on Alcoholism (hereafter CCA), CCA 'Information Week', Transcripts of seminar proceedings, 1967, pp. 50–1.
46. Correspondence, Rowntree Trust Steering Group on Alcohol, 1957–64, PP/AWD/H6/2.
47. Interview with Dr Robin Edwards, Devon. Interviewed 5 October 2009.
48. G. Edwards, 'Patients with Drinking Problems', *British Medical Journal* (16 November 1968), pp. 435–7, on pp. 436–7.
49. A. Alibone, 'The Health of Doctors', in D. J. P. Gray (ed.), *The Medical Annual* (Bristol: Wright, 1983), pp. 141–50, on p. 142.
50. Fifteen retired GPs were interviewed as part of this research. All GPs had experience of practice during the late 1950s, 1960s or 1970s. They were recruited from a range of rural, provincial and urban practices across England. Pseudonyms have been used. The broad consensus among them was that men regularly used alcohol as a coping mechanism.
51. Papers of John Fry, Research Notes: Peptic Ulcers *c.*1950-*c.*1980, Royal College of General Practitioners' Archive.
52. See J. Fry and D. Finer, 'Peptic Ulcer in General Practice', *British Medical Journal* (16 July 1955), pp. 169–72.
53. L. I. Zander and J. Bennett, 'A Case of Peptic Ulcer', *British Medical Journal* (16 April 1977), pp. 1017–19.
54. Interview with Dr Richard Long, Devon, interviewed 6 October 2009.
55. C. A. H. Watts, *Depressive Disorders in the Community* (Bristol: John Wright, 1966), p. 35.
56. Watts, *Depressive Disorders*, p. 120.
57. D. L. Crombie, 'The Prevalence of Psychogenic Illness in General Practice', *Journal of the College of General Practitioners,* Research Newsletter, 4 (1957), pp. 218–27. For an overview of all studies, see A. Ryle, 'The Neuroses in a General Practice Population', *Journal of the College of General Practitioners*, 3 (1960), pp. 313–28.
58. Ryle, 'The Neuroses in a General Practice Population', p. 319.
59. W. P. D. Logan and E. M. Brooke, *The Survey of Sickness 1943–1952, Studies on Medical and Population Subjects* (London: HMSO, 1957), p. 54.
60. H. J. Walton, 'Effect of the Doctor's Personality on his Style of Practice', *Journal of the Royal College of General Practitioners,* 17:82 (1969), supplement 3, pp. 6–17, on p. 6.
61. Walton, 'Effect of the Doctor's Personality', p. 6.

62. Walton, 'Effect of the Doctor's Personality', p. 8.
63. Walton, 'Effect of the Doctor's Personality', p. 11.
64. Walton, 'Effect of the Doctor's Personality', p. 14.
65. Interview with Dr Richard Mitchell, Shrewsbury, interviewed on 4 January 2012.
66. Interview with Dr Richard Mitchell, January 2012.
67. Interview with Dr Richard Mitchell, January 2012.
68. M. Shepherd and A. Clare, *Psychiatric Illness in General Practice* (Oxford: Oxford University Press, 1981), p. 133.
69. Shepherd and Clare, *Psychiatric Illness*, p. 149.
70. Shepherd and Clare, *Psychiatric Illness*, p. 175.
71. Contribution From a General Practitioner, Transcript of Seminar Proceedings, SA/CCA/32, Camberwell Council on Alcoholism (hereafter CCA), 'Information Week', 1967, p. 14.
72. SA/CCA/32, 'Information Week', p. 21.
73. SA/CCA/23, CCA, 'Conferences and Meetings', Industrial symposium.
74. SA/CCA/23, 'Conferences and Meetings', Industrial symposium.
75. R. M. Murray, 'Alcoholism and Employment', *Journal of Alcoholism*, 10 (1975), pp. 23–6, on p. 25.
76. SA/CCA/32, 'Information Week', p. 9.
77. 'Menace of Monday Morning Blues', *Daily Express*, 19 January 1970.
78. 'Why 25000 Men Did Not Go to Work', *Daily Express*, 22 October 1968.
79. SA/CCA/32, 'Information Week', p. 4.
80. SA/CCA/32, 'Information Week', p. 15.
81. A debate discussed in R. S. F. Shilling, 'Assessing the Health of the Industrial Worker', *British Journal of Industrial Medicine*, 14 (1957), pp. 145–9. See also J. K. C. Jones, C. A. Brown and N. Nicholson, 'Absence from Work: Its Meaning, Measurement and Control', *International Review of Applied Psychology*, 22 (1973), pp. 137–53; and J. K. C. Jones, *Social Psychology of Absenteeism* (New York: Praeger, 1982). 'Absenteeism' was defined as short-term unconfirmed absence which may or may not be due to sickness, as distinguished from 'sickness absence' which was formally certified by a doctor or medical officer.
82. This problem is discussed in C. Gordon, A. R. Emerson and D. S. Pugh, 'Patterns of Sickness Absence in a Railway Population', *British Journal of Industrial Medicine*, 16 (1959), pp. 230–43.
83. For a study of neurosis in British workers, see R. Fraser, *The Incidence of Neurosis among Factory Workers* (Industrial Health Research Board, Report No. 90: HMSO, 1949); and P. J. Taylor, 'Personal Factors Associated with Sickness Absence', *British Journal of Industrial Medicine*, 25 (1968), pp. 106–18. For an international study correlating alcohol abuse with neurosis, see D. Furguson 'Some Characteristics of Repeated Sickness Absence', *British Journal of Industrial Medicine*, 29 (1972), pp. 420–43.
84. W. D. Ross, *Practical Psychiatry for Industrial Physicians* (Springfield, IL: Charles C. Thomas, 1956). For an Australian study, see Furguson, 'Some Characteristics'; and for debates in Sweden see S. Lokander, 'Sick Absence in a Swedish Company', *Acta Medica Scandinavica*, 171 (1962), Suppl. 377.
85. J. A. C. Brown, 'Review of Ross, *Practical Psychiatry for Industrial Physicians*', in *British Journal of Industrial Medicine*, 16 (1959), pp. 176–7.
86. T. M. Ling (ed.), *Mental Health and Human Relations in Industry* (London: H. K. Lewis, 1954).
87. J. Archer, 'Occupational Alcoholism: A Review of Issues and a Guide to the Literature',

in C. J. Schramm (ed.), *Alcoholism and its Treatment in Industry* (Baltimore, MD and London: John Hopkins University Press, 1978), pp. 2–28, on p. 2.

88. O. Jones, 'Kennecott's INSIGHT Program', in Schramm (ed.), *Alcoholism and its Treatment*, pp. 76–81, on p. 76.
89. D. Caldwell, review of Schramm (ed.), *Alcoholism and its Treatment in Industry*, in *British Journal of Industrial Medicine*, 36 (1979), pp. 244–5.
90. H. Berger, 'The Prevention of Alcoholism', *British Journal of Addiction to Alcohol and Other Drugs*, 2 (1963), pp. 47–54, on pp. 47–8.
91. H. Berger, 'The Prevention of Alcoholism', p. 51.
92. See Chadwick-Jones, *Social Psychology of Absenteeism*, pp. 120–1; Jones, Brown and Nicholson, 'Absence from Work', p. 144; Fraser, *The Incidence of Neurosis*, p. 37; for material on the British Civil Service see M. Jackson, *The Age of Stress: Science and the Search for Stability* (Oxford: Oxford University Press, 2013), pp. 202; and Chapter 6 'Cultural Change' by Debbie Palmer in this volume.
93. V. Isambert-Jamati, 'Absenteeism Among Women Workers in Industry', *International Labour Review*, 85 (1962), pp. 248–61, on p. 249.
94. Isambert-Jamati, 'Absenteeism Among Women', p. 255.
95. Fraser, *The Incidence of Neurosis*, pp. 13, 18.
96. J. F. Ager and P. A. B. Raffle, *Patterns in Sickness Absence: Experience of London Transport Staff over Two Decades* (London Transport Executive, 1973), p. 15; *Off Sick* (London: Office for Health Economics, 1971); and see also W. Gardner (ed.), *Proceedings of the Symposium on Absence from Work Attributed to Sickness* (Society of Occupational Medicine, 1968), p. 17.
97. Ager and Raffle, *Patterns in Sickness Absence*, p. 11.
98. C. L. Cooper and J. Marshall, 'Occupational Sources of Stress: A Review of the Literature Relating to Heart Disease and Mental Ill Health', *Journal of Occupational Psychology*, 49 (1976), pp. 11–28, on p. 12.
99. R. Jenkins, 'Minor Psychiatric Morbidity in Employed Young Men and Women and its Contribution to Sickness Absence', *British Journal of Industrial Medicine*, 42 (1985), pp. 147–54, on p. 150.
100. Jenkins, 'Minor Psychiatric Morbidity', p. 152. See also P. J. Taylor and J. Burridge, 'Trends in Death, Disablement and Sickness Absence in the British Post Office since 1891', *British Journal of Industrial Medicine*, 39 (1982), pp. 1–10.
101. A. Cherns, 'Perspectives on the Quality of Working Life', *Journal of Occupational Psychology*, 48 (1975), pp. 155–67.
102. Jackson, *The Age of Stress*, p. 208.
103. B. Thom, *Dealing with Drink: Alcohol and Social Policy, From Treatment to Management* (London: Free Association Books, 1999), pp. 157–8, 161.
104. Thom, *Dealing with Drink*, p. 130.
105. An advert for Black and White Scotch Whisky, *The Times*, 28 June 1939, for example, claimed that it was 'a most effective stimulant' which was 'especially helpful in these days of stress and strain'.
106. R. Lemle and M. E. Mishkind, 'Alcohol and Masculinity', *Journal of Substance Abuse Treatment*, 6 (1989), pp. 213–22.
107. Lemle and Mishkind, 'Alcohol and Masculinity', p. 214.
108. Mass Observation, *The Pub and the People* (1943; London: Faber and Faber, 2009), pp. 42, 46.
109. M. Micale, *Hysterical Men: the Hidden History of Male Nervous Illness* (Harvard, MA:

Harvard University Press, 2008), p. 280.
110. Micale, *Hysterical Men*, p. 284.
111. D. Wilkins and M. Kemple, *Delivering Male: Effective Practice in Male Mental Health* (Men's Health Forum, 2011), p. 65.
112. C. Wyllie et al., *Men, Suicide and Society: Why Disadvantaged Men in Midlife Die by Suicide* (Samaritans, 2012).

4 Kirby, 'Working too Hard: Experiences of Worry and Stress in Post-War Britain'

1. Interview with James Lyon, 13 October 2003, Lives in the Oil Industry, British Library, F14738-F14741. None of the oral history interviews referred to in this chapter have been anonymized. However, all the names in Miss Richmond's reports, except her own, have been anonymized at the request of the archivist.
2. 'Working Days Lost', Latest information from the Labour Force Survey for 2010/11, Office of National Statistics, accessed 15 October 2012.
3. R. Viner, 'Putting Stress in Life: Hans Selye and the Making of Stress Theory', *Social Studies of Science*, 29 (1999), pp. 391–410, on p. 399.
4. M. Spring-Rice, *Working-Class Wives: Their Health and Conditions*, 2nd edn (London: Virago, 1981), p. 69.
5. I. H. Pearse and L. H. Crocker, *The Peckham Experiment: A Study in the Living Structure of Society* (London: George Allen and Unwin Ltd, 1943), p. 254.
6. H. Jones, *Health and Society in Twentieth-Century Britain* (London: Longman, 1994), pp. 60–1.
7. Mass Observation Archive (hereafter MOA), Spring 1997 Directive, 'You and the NHS', G2134. Mass Observation was founded in 1937 as a social research organization based on a panel of correspondents, replying to themed questions (directives), but also collecting material from diarists and reports from observers recording the events around them. It was restarted in 1981 as the Mass Observation Project and correspondents continue to reply to three or four directives every year. It provides a rich source of personal experience, opinion and insight into the lives of British citizens.
8. Anon., *The Household Doctor* (London: English Universities Press, 1938), p. 5.
9. Jones, *Health and Society*, p. 76.
10. MOA, July 1939 Directive, 'Age Differences', 2325.
11. A. S. Jackson and E. O. Kennedy, *The Answer is ... Your Nerves* (Kingswood, Surrey: World's Work, 1947), p. 2.
12. M. Tebbutt, *Women's Talk? A Social History of 'Gossip' in Working-Class Neighbourhoods, 1880–1960* (Aldershot: Scolar Press, 1995), p. 84.
13. Jones, *Health and Society*, p. 117.
14. E. S. Watkins, 'Stress and the American Vernacular', in *Stress, Shock, and Adaptation in the Twentieth Century*, ed. D. Cantor and E. Ramsden (Rochester, NY: University of Rochester Press, 2014), pp. 53–66.
15. For further discussion of the language of stress see M. Jackson, *The Age of Stress: Science and the Search for Stability* (Oxford: Oxford University Press, 2013); R. Hayward, 'Stress', *The Lancet*, 365 (2005), p. 2001; A. Patmore, *The Truth About Stress* (London: Atlantic, 2006), pp. 38–46; and S. Doublet, *The Stress Myth* (Chesterfield, MO: Science & Humanities Press, 2000), pp. 65–78.

16. J. Kirby, 'Troubled by Life: The Experience of Stress in Twentieth-Century Britain' (Unpublished thesis, University of Sussex, 2014), pp. 29–77.
17. H. J. S. Guntrip, *You and Your Nerves: A Simple Account of the Nature, Causes and Treatment of Nervous Illness* (London: George Allen & Unwin, 1951); H. B. Harris, *How to Live With Your Nerves and Like It: A Family Doctor Book* (London: British Medical Association, 1956); and C. Weekes, *Peace from Nervous Suffering* (London: Angus and Robertson, 1972).
18. H. Gavron, *The Captive Wife: Conflicts of Housebound Mothers* (London: Routledge & Kegan Paul, 1966); and B. Friedan, *The Feminine Mystique* (Harmondsworth: Penguin, 1963).
19. R. McKibbin, *The Ideologies of Class: Social Relations in Britain, 1880–1950* (Oxford: Clarendon, 1994), p. 148; W. Ronco and L. Peattie, 'Making Work: a Perspective from Social Science', in *On Work: Historical, Comparative and Theoretical Approaches*, ed. R. E. Pahl (Oxford: Basil Blackwell, 1988), p. 710; and M. Roper, *Masculinity and the British Organisation Man since 1945* (Oxford: Oxford University Press, 1994), p. 21.
20. For example, J. L. Halliday, 'Psychoneurosis as a Cause of Incapacity Among Insured Persons', *British Medical Journal*, 1 Supplement 1584, 3870 (1935), pp. S85–S92; and P. Eisenberg and P. F. Lazarsfeld, 'The Psychological Effects of Unemployment', *Psychological Bulletin*, 35 (1938), pp. 358–90.
21. Eisenberg and Lazarsfeld, 'Psychological Effects', p. 378; M. Jahoda, 'Work, Employment and Unemployment: An Overview of Ideas and Research Results in the Social Science Literature', in *Science Policy Research Unit Occasional Papers* (University of Sussex, 1980), pp. 1–70, on pp. 11–12.
22. Mass Observation Archive (hereafter MOA), Summer 1983 Directive, 'Work', A005 and B787.
23. MOA, 'Work', A012.
24. M. Thomson, *Psychological Subjects: Identity, Culture, and Health in Twentieth-Century Britain* (Oxford: Oxford University Press, 2006), pp. 227–8 and 243.
25. MOA, 'Work', P440.
26. MOA, 'Work', A008.
27. E. Jones and S. Wessely, 'War Syndromes: The Impact of Culture on Medically Unexplained Symptoms', *Medical History*, 49:1 (2005), pp. 55-78, on pp. 69–71.
28. Mass Observation Archive (hereafter MOA), Personal Collections: Miss Richmond, 'Welfare Visitor's Report', 22 September 1949.
29. MOA, 'Welfare Visitor's Report', 22 September 1949.
30. See Chapter 6 'Cultural Change' by Debbie Palmer in this volume.
31. For further discussion of military views on inherent weakness and shell shock see M. Jackson, *The Age of Stress: Science and the Search for Stability* (Oxford: Oxford University Press, 2013), pp. 50–3; B. Shephard, *A War of Nerves: Soldiers and Psychiatrists in the Twentieth Century* (Cambridge, MA: Harvard University Press, 2001), pp. 165–8; and P. Barham, *Forgotten Lunatics of the Great War* (New Haven, CT and London: Yale University Press, 2004), pp. 235–6.
32. MOA, 'Welfare Visitor's Report', 24 May 1954.
33. MOA, 'Welfare Visitor's Report', 24 May 1954. Shaws was a subsidiary of Hunter and Sons.
34. MOA, 'Welfare Visitor's Report', 22 September 1949.
35. J. Kennedy, *Worry: Its Cause and Cure* (London: The Psychologist, 1950), p. 28; and F. Preston, 'Good Health is Your Birthright', in *Healthy Minds and Bodies*, ed. Dr T.

Traherne (London: Waverley Book Company Ltd, 1956), p. 11.
36. M. Culpin and M. Smith, *The Nervous Temperament: Medical Research Council Report 61* (London: Industrial Health Research Board, 1930), p. iii.
37. Culpin and Smith, *The Nervous Temperament*, p. iii.
38. Jackson, *Age of Stress*, pp. 91–2; A. Hull, 'Glasgow's "sick society"?: James Halliday, Psychosocial Medicine and Medical Holism in Britain *c.*1920–48', *History of Human Sciences*, 25 (2012), pp. 78–80; and R. Hayward, 'Enduring Emotions: James L. Halliday and the Invention of the Psychosocial', *Isis*, 100 (2009), pp. 834–5.
39. Roffey Park Rehabilitation Centre, 'Health and Human Relations in Industry: The Courses at Roffey Park' (Horsham, 1947), Wellcome Library.
40. Roffey Park Rehabilitation Centre Advisory Panel, 'Confidential Report of the Advisory Panel Appointed by the Governors of St Thomas' Hospital in Connection with Roffey Park Rehabilitation Centre' (London: St Thomas's Hospital, 1949), Point 10.
41. Roffey Park Rehabilitation Centre, 'Courses at Roffey Park'.
42. Interview with Don Thompson, 16 March 2006, Oral History of British Athletics, British Library, C790/38.
43. Interview with Jeff Mills, 9 December 1998, Millennium Memory Bank Collection, British Library, C900/05537 © BBC.
44. Interview with Jeff Mills, 9 December 1998.
45. Interview with Jeff Mills, 9 December 1998.
46. Interview with Jeff Mills, 9 December 1998.
47. Interview with Jeff Mills, 9 December 1998.
48. Interview with Jeff Mills, 9 December 1998.
49. 'The Seven Ages of Stress', *Daily Mirror*, 20 October 1972, p. 25; 'Man "Broken by Stress"', *The Guardian*, 13 June 1974, p. 6.
50. M. Roper, *Masculinity and the British Organisation Man since 1945* (Oxford: Oxford University Press, 1994), p. 40.
51. C. M. Callahan and G. E. Berrios, *Reinventing Depression: A History of the Treatment of Depression in Primary Care, 1940–2004* (Oxford: Oxford University Press, 2005), p. 107.
52. D. Healy, *Let Them Eat Prozac* (New York and London: New York University Press, 2004), p. 226; A. Haggett, *Desperate Housewives, Neuroses and the Domestic Environment, 1945–1970* (London: Pickering & Chatto, 2012), pp. 131–4. For further discussion of the role of pharmaceutical companies, see A. Tone, *The Age of Anxiety: A History of America's Turbulent Affair with Tranquilizers* (New York: Basic Books, 2009); and D. L. Herzberg, *Happy Pills in America: from Miltown to Prozac* (Baltimore, MD and London: Johns Hopkins University Press, 2009).
53. Interview with Peter Allen, 10 November 1998, Millennium Memory Bank Collection, British Library, C900/07016 © BBC.
54. Interview with Peter Allen, 10 November 1998.
55. Interview with Peter Allen, 10 November 1998.
56. Interview with Peter Allen, 10 November 1998.
57. Callahan and Berrios, *Reinventing Depression*, p. 111.
58. Interview with Peter Allen, 10 November 1998.
59. Interview with Peter Allen, 10 November 1998.
60. D. Wainwright and M. Calnan, *Work Stress: The Making of a Modern Epidemic* (Buckingham: Open University Press, 2002), p. 1.
61. Interview with Peter Allen, 10 November 1998.

62. F. Füredi, *Therapy Culture: Cultivating Vulnerability in an Uncertain Age* (London and New York: Routledge, 2004), p. 114.
63. H. Selye, *The Stress of Life* (New York: McGraw-Hill, 1956).
64. For further discussion of anti-anxiety medication, see A. Haggett, *Desperate Housewives, Neuroses and the Domestic Environment, 1945–1970* (London: Pickering & Chatto, 2012).
65. D. Wainwright and M. Calnan, *Work Stress: The Making of a Modern Epidemic* (Buckingham: Open University Press, 2002), p. 125.
66. C. M. Callahan and G. E. Berrios, *Reinventing Depression: A History of the Treatment of Depression in Primary Care, 1940–2004* (Oxford: Oxford University Press, 2005), pp. 35, 109–10.

5 Hayes, 'Industrial Automation and Stress, *c.*1945–79'

1. Sir W. Puckey, 'The Automatic Factory – Dream or Nightmare?', in *The Automatic Factory – What Does it Mean? Report of Conference of Institution of Production Engineers, Margate 16–19 June 1955* (London, 1955), p. 8.
2. R. C. Browne, 'Automation and Stress', *Journal of Psychosomatic Research*, 10 (1966), pp. 73–5, on p. 73.
3. For studies into the history of occupational health in factories, see A. J. McIvor, *A History of Work in Britain, 1880–1950* (Basingstoke: Palgrave, 2001); M. D. McFeely, *Lady Inspectors: The Campaign for a Better Work Place, 1893–1921* (Oxford: Basil Blackwell, 1991); and P. Weindling (ed.) *Social History of Occupational Health* (London: Croom Helm, 1985).
4. See J. Melling, 'Fordism and the Foreman: Labour Relations and Supervisory Trade Unionism in the American and British Automobile Industries, *c.*1939–1970', in J. Melling and A. Booth (eds), *Managing the Workplace: Productivity, Politics and Workplace Culture in Post-War Britain* (Aldershot: Ashgate, 2008), pp. 27–47; and S. Tolliday and J. Zeitlin (eds), *The Automobile Industry and its Workers: Between Fordism and Flexibility* (Cambridge: Cambridge University Press, 1986).
5. Department of Scientific and Industrial Research (hereafter DSIR), *Automation in Perspective* (London: HMSO, 1956), p. 2. For a discussion of Harder's definition, see: Sir W. Puckey, 'The Automatic Factory – Dream or Nightmare?', in *The Automatic Factory – What Does it Mean? Report of Conference of Institution of Production Engineers, Margate 16–19 June 1955* (London, 1955), p. 8.
6. This phrase featured repeatedly in government departmental sources relating to the Board of Trade and the Ministry of Labour in the immediate post-war period – for example, Ministry of Labour and National Service, *Chief Inspector of Factories Annual Report 1946* (London: HMSO, 1948), p. 1.
7. F. Allaun, *Automation – Blessing or Curse?* (Manchester: Co-operative Press, 1957); Puckey, 'The Automatic Factory – Dream or Nightmare?'.
8. W. Wingo, 'Automation's Impact', *The Science Newsletter*, 84:18 (2 November 1963), p. 278.
9. Puckey, 'The Automatic Factory – Dream or Nightmare?'.
10. A. Rabinbach, *The Human Motor: Energy, Fatigue and the Origins of Modernity* (Berkeley, CA: University of California Press, 1990), p. 11.
11. Sir L. Bagrit, *The Age of Automation: The BBC Reith Lectures 1964* (London: Weidenfield & Nicolson, 1965), p. 11.

12. DSIR, *Automation in Perspective*, p. 3.
13. World Health Organization (hereafter WHO), *Mental Health Problems of Automation: Technical Report Series No.183* (Geneva, 1959).
14. Bagrit, *The Age of Automation*, p. 11.
15. Ford Branch Communist Party, *Fords – Whose Hands on the Wheel? (A Look at the Present and Future)* (Dagenham, 1962).
16. WHO, *Mental Health Problems of Automation.*
17. This term had been widely used in the inter-war period following scientific studies instigated by Elton Mayo: E. Mayo, *The Human Problems of an Industrial Civilization* (Boston, MA: Macmillan, 1933).
18. P. Sadler, *Social Research on Automation: A Social Science Research Council Review of Current Research* (London: Heinemann, 1968), p. 2.
19. WHO, *Mental Health Problems of Automation*, p. 9.
20. WHO, *Mental Health Problems of Automation*, p. 8.
21. F. Garner, 'Automation – Some Problems for the Manager', in *The Automatic Factory – What Does it Mean?*, p. 41.
22. F. G. Woollard, 'Machines in the Service of Man', in *The Automatic Factory – What Does it Mean? Report of Conference of Institution of Production Engineers, Margate 16–19 June 1955* (London, 1955), pp. 198–206.
23. Bagrit, *The Age of Automation.*
24. Many historical studies have focused on this issue. For the origins of this social construct, see L. Davidoff and C. Hall, *Family Fortunes: Men and Women of the English Middle Class, 1780–1850* (Routledge: London, 1987).
25. M. Glucksman, *Women Workers and the New Industries in Inter-War Britain* (London: Routledge, 1990), p. 3.
26. E. Hagen and J. Jenson, 'Paradoxes and Promises: Work and Politics in the Post-War Years', in J. Jenson, E. Hagen and C. Reddy (eds), *Feminization of the Labour Force: Paradoxes and Promises* (Cambridge: Polity Press, 1988), p. 4.
27. See Debbie Palmer's chapter, 'Cultural Change', in this volume.
28. A. Mydral and V. Klein, *Women's Two Roles: Home and Work* (London: Routledge and Kegan Paul, 1956).
29. Interviews conducted by S. Hayes with workers at J. & C. Clarks' Mayflower factory, Plymouth, 26 June, 2013.
30. WHO, *Mental Health Problems of Automation,* p. 9.
31. WHO, *Mental Health Problems of Automation,* p. 9.
32. This definition of automation appears in, for example, F. Allaun, *Automation – Blessing or Curse?* (Manchester: Co-operative Press, 1957), p. 4.
33. R. C. Browne, 'Automation and Stress', *Journal of Psychosomatic Research*, 10 (1966), pp. 73–5; and J. D. Sutherland, 'Industry and Stress Disorder', *Journal of Psychosomatic Research*, 10 (1966), pp. 71–2. For a seminal analysis of the emergence of medical models of stress in the post-war period see M. Jackson, *The Age of Stress* (Oxford: Oxford University Press, 2013).
34. World Health Organization (hereafter WHO), *Mental Health Problems of Automation: Technical Report Series No.183* (Geneva, 1959), p. 9.
35. WHO, *Mental Health Problems of Automation,* p. 9.
36. WHO, *Mental Health Problems of Automation,* p. 9.
37. WHO, *Mental Health Problems of Automation,* p. 9.
38. Allaun, *Automation*, p. 4.

39. WHO, *Mental Health Problems of Automation,* p. 12.
40. Allaun, *Automation*, p. 5.
41. Modern Records Centre – Transport & General Workers' Union Archives: MSS 126/TG/RES/GW/72-1 'Tobacco Trade – Report of Industrial Disputes Tribunal: Award 914' (3 October 1956).
42. MRC: MSS 126/TG/RES/GW/72-1 – 'Tobacco Trade'.
43. Joint Ford Shop Stewards Committee, *What's Wrong at Ford* (1962), p. 5.
44. WHO, *Mental Health Problems of Automation,* p. 12.
45. H. Beynon, *Working for Ford* (Harmondsworth: Penguin, 1973).
46. WHO, *Mental Health Problems of Automation,* p. 12.
47. WHO, *Mental Health Problems of Automation*, p. 13.
48. E. R. F. W. Crossman, *Automation and Skill: Problems of Progress in Industry No. 9* (London: Department of Scientific and Industrial Research, 1960), p. 50.
49. H. G. Woolf, *Stress and Disease* (Springfield, IL: Charles C. Thomas, 1953), p. 15.
50. H. G. Woolf, *Stress and Psychiatric Disorder* (Oxford: Blackwell, 1960).
51. Sutherland, 'Industry and Stress Disorder', p. 71.
52. R. Passmore and C. N. Swanston, *Industrial Health: An Introduction for Students* (Edinburgh: E & S Livingstone Ltd, 1950).
53. Department of Scientific and Industrial Research, *Automation in Perspective* (London: HMSO, 1956), p. iii.
54. A. Reid, 'Employers' Strategies and Craft Production: The British Shipbuilding Industry, 1870–1950', in S. Tolliday and J. Zeitlan (eds), *The Power to Manage? Employers and Industrial Relations in Comparative-Historical Perspective* (London: Routledge, 1991), p 35.
55. Crossman, *Automation and Skill.*
56. Browne, 'Automation and Stress', p. 73.
57. [Anon.], 'Automation and Industrial Health', *British Medical Journal*, 1:5026 (4 May 1957), p. 1059.
58. V. Long, *The Rise and Fall of the Healthy Factory: The Politics of Industrial Health in Britain, 1914–60* (Basingstoke: Palgrave Macmillan, 2010), pp. 65–8.
59. WHO, *Mental Health Problems of Automation,* p. 12.
60. [Anon.], 'Automation and Industrial Health', p. 1059.
61. R. Cavendish, *Women on the Line* (London: Routledge & Kegan Paul, 1957), p. 40.
62. MRC: MSS 126/TG/RES/GW/72-1 – 'Tobacco Trade'.
63. H. J. Graves, 'The Automatic Mechanical Project Factory: A Sight of Things to Come', in *The Automatic Factory – What Does it Mean? Report of Conference of Institution of Production Engineers, Margate 16–19 June 1955* (1955).
64. Browne, 'Automation and Stress', p. 75.
65. Ministry of Labour and National Service, *HM Chief Inspector of Factories: Annual Report 1946* (London: HMSO, 1948), p. 20.
66. S. Tolliday and J. Zeitlan (eds), *The Power to Manage? Employers and Industrial Relations in Comparative-Historical Perspective* (London: Routledge, 1991).
67. F. W. Taylor, *The Principles of Scientific Management* (New York: Harper & Brothers, 1911).
68. R. Kanigel, *The One Best Way: Frederick Winslow Taylor and the Enigma of Efficiency* (London: Little Brown & Company, 1997).
69. F. B. Gilbreth, *Motion Study* (New York: D. Van Nostrand Co., 1911).
70. M. J. Nadworny, 'Frederick Taylor and Frank Gilbreth: Competition in Scientific Man-

agement', *Business History Review*, 31 (1957), pp. 23–34.

71. Remark made by Emile Pouget, French trade union leader, in 1913, quoted in A. Rabinbach, *The Human Motor: Energy, Fatigue and the Origins of Modernity*, (Berkley, CA: University of California Press, 1990), p. 241.
72. Emile Pouget, quoted in Rabinbach, *The Human Motor*, p. 239.
73. Melling has argued that this is too simplistic a view of Fordism, which should be seen as as an ensemble of techniques, policies and practices – J. Melling, 'Fordism and the Foreman: Labour Relations and Supervisory Trade Unionism in the American and British Automobile Industries, *c.*1939–1970', in J. Melling and A. Booth (eds), *Managing the Workplace: Productivity, Politics and Workplace Culture in Post-War Britain* (Aldershot: Ashgate, 2008), p. 30. For further analysis of international interpretations of Fordism, see H. Shiomi and K. Wada (eds), *Fordism Transformed: The Development of Production Methods in the Automobile Industry* (Oxford: Oxford University Press, 1995).
74. R. Cavendish, *Women on the Line* (London: Routledge & Kegan Paul, 1957), p. 19.
75. Joint Ford Shop Stewards Committee, *What's Wrong at Ford* (1962), p. 5
76. Article, 'The Other Person's Job: Work Study', *Clarks Courier*, 16 (24 January 1958), p. 7.
77. H. Ford, *My Life and Work* (New York, 1922).
78. Cavendish, *Women on the Line*, p. 40.
79. *HM Chief Inspector of Factories Annual Report* (1963), pp. 55–6.
80. *HM Chief Inspector of Factories Annual Report* (1963), p. 56.
81. Joint Ford Shop Stewards Committee, *What's Wrong at Ford*, p. 5
82. Modern Records Centre: MSS 292/571/3 'Work Study 1934–52': National Production Advisory Council (General Council Side), *Motion and Time Study* (24 February 1949).
83. H. Beynon, *Working for Ford* (London: Allen Lane, 1973), p. 86.
84. Beynon, *Working for Ford*, p. 86.
85. Beynon himself highlights these reactions in the preface to the Beynon, *Working for Ford*, 2nd edn (1973; Harmondsworth: Penguin, 1984), p. 11.
86. MRC: MSS 292/571/3 'Work Study 1934–52' – 'Letter' (4 June 1948).
87. MRC: MSS 292/571/3 'Work Study 1934–52' – 'National Survey of Time Study Practice: First Interim Report' (1950).
88. MRC: MSS 292/571/3 – *Motion and Time Study*, p. 4.
89. MRC: MSS 292/571.11/3 'Industrial Research' – TUC Work Study Conference 1954; MRC: MSS 292/60.21/2b – 'Industrial Newsletter for Women 1955–58' - newsletter June 1956.
90. Department of Scientific and Industrial Research (hereafter DSIR), *Automation in Perspective* (London: HMSO, 1956), p. 80.
91. It is notable that Ford was one of the few companies to refuse to introduce payment by piece-work, a factor identified by several historians as a significant factor in industrial unrest throughout the 1960s – see S. Tolliday, 'Ford and Fordism in Post-War Britain: Enterprise Management and the Control of Labour 1937–1987', in Tolliday and Zeitlan (eds), *The Power to Manage?,* pp. 71–101, on p. 86.
92. Tolliday, 'Ford and Fordism in Post-War Britain', p. 86.
93. Cavendish, *Women on the Line*, p. 96.
94. 'The Other People's Job', *Clarks Courier*, p. 7.
95. 'The Other People's Job', *Clarks Courier*, p. 7.
96. Several examples of this type of action are recorded in the sociological studies of Caven-

dish, *Women on the Line*, and Beynon, *Working for Ford.*
97. *Big Flame Dagenham Bulletin* (July 1974).
98. Tolliday and Zeitlan (eds), *The Power to Manage?*, p. 1.
99. R. C. Browne, 'Automation and Stress', *Journal of Psychosomatic Research*, 10 (1966), p. 73.
100. A. Toffler, *Future Shock* (London: Bodley Head, 1970).
101. Modern Records Centre (MRC): MSS 126/TG/RES/X/712 A1/1 – 'Industrial Welfare 1929–57' – James Gillespie, *Dynamic Motion Study* (London, 1945).

6 Palmer, 'Cultural Change, Stress and Civil Servants' Occupational Health, *c.* 1967–85'

1. National Archives (hereafter NA), HX5/1, Thomson, 'Civil Service Sick Leave 1967', 28 January 1970.
2. E. Riska, 'From Type A Man to the Hardy Man: Masculinity and Health', *Sociology of Health and Illness,* 24 (2002), pp. 347–58.
3. A. Harrington, *The Cure Within: A History of Mind-Body Medicine* (New York: W. W. Norton and Company, 2008); C. E. Rosenberg, 'Pathologies of Progress: The Idea of Civilisation as Risk', *Bulletin of the History of Medicine*, 72 (1998), pp. 714–30; and K. Pollock, 'On the Nature of Social Stress: Production of a Modern Mythology', *Social Society of Medicine*, 26 (1998), pp. 381–92.
4. Rosenberg, 'Pathologies of Progress', p. 730.
5. Pollock, 'On the Nature of Social Stress', p. 387.
6. M. Jackson, *The Age of Stress: Science and the Search for Stability* (Oxford: Oxford University Press, 2013).
7. L. Hearnshaw, *A Short History of British Psychology* (London: Methuen & Co Ltd, 1964), p. 259.
8. J. M. M. Hill and E. L. Trist, 'A Consideration of Industrial Accidents as a Means of Withdrawal from the Work Situation', *Human Relations*, 6 (1953), pp. 357–80; and Hill and Trist, *Industrial Accidents, Sickness and Other Absences, Tavistock Pamphlet No. 4* (London: Tavistock Publications, 1962), pp. 121–52.
9. J. Chadwick-Jones, C. Brown and N. Nicholson, *Social Psychology of Absenteeism* (New York: Praeger Publishers, 1982), p. 2.
10. J. L. Halliday, *Psychosocial Medicine: A Study of the Sick Society* (London: William Heineman Medical Books Ltd, 1949), p. 185.
11. J. L. Halliday, 'The Rising Incidence of Psychosomatic Illness', *British Journal of Medicine* (2 July 1938), pp. 11–14; Halliday, 'Psychosomatic Medicine and the Declining Birth Rate', *The Lancet* (12 May 1945), pp. 601–3; and R. Hayward, 'Enduring Emotions: James L. Halliday and the Invention of the Psychosocial', *Isis* (2009), pp. 827–38.
12. Hayward, 'Enduring Emotions', p. 5.
13. D. Armstrong, 'The Rise of Surveillance Medicine', *Sociology of Health and Illness*, 17 (1995), pp. 393–404.
14. J. Calvert Spence, *Investigation into the Health and Nutrition of the Children of Newcastle upon Tyne Between the Ages of One and Five* (Newcastle upon Tyne: Co-operative Printing Society, 1934); and J. Boyd Orr, *Food, Health and Income* (London: Macmillan, 1936). See also J. Pemberton, 'Social Medicine Comes on the Scene in the United Kingdom, 1936–1960', *Journal of Public Health Medicine*, 20 (1998), pp. 149–53.

15. C. L. Cooper and P. Dewe, *Stress: A Brief History* (Oxford: Blackwell Publishing, 2004), p. 63.
16. V. Berridge, 'Jerry Morris', *International Journal of Epidemiology*, 30 (2001), pp. 1141–5
17. J. Morris and R. Titmuss, 'Epidemiology of Peptic Ulcer Vital Statistics', *The Lancet* (30 December 1944), pp. 841–5.
18. J. Morris, 'Capacity and Incapacity for Work: Some Recent History', *Proceedings of the Royal Society of Medicine*, 58 (1965), pp. 821–5; and National Archives (hereafter NA), FD12/522, Social Medicine Research Unit: Progress Report 1968–9.
19. Morris, 'Capacity and Incapacity for Work', p. 821.
20. N. G. Schenet, 'An Analysis of Absenteeism in One War Plant', *Journal of Applied Psychology*, 19 (1945), pp. 27–39; and W. A. Kerr, G. J. Koppelmeier and J. J. Sullivan, 'Absenteeism, Turnover and Morale in a Metals Fabrication Factory', *Occupational Psychology*, 25 (1951), pp. 50–5.
21. A. Myrdal and V. Klein, *Women's Two Roles: Home and Work* (London: Routledge and Kegan Paul Ltd, 1956).
22. Myrdal and Klein, *Women's Two Roles*.
23. R. Hayward, 'Desperate Housewives and Model Amoebae: The Invention of Suburban Neurosis in Inter-War Britain', in M. Jackson (ed.) *Health and the Modern Home* (London: Routledge, 2007), pp. 42–62.
24. A. Thibault, 'Comparative Examination of Male and Female Absenteeism and Turnover in the Labour Force', Unpublished study, Royal Commission on the Status of Women in Canada, 1967.
25. A. Haggett, 'Housewives, Neuroses and the Domestic Environment in Britain' in Jackson (ed.), *Health and the Modern Home*, pp. 84–110.
26. Treasury, *The Control of Public Expenditure* (London: HMSO, 1961).
27. J. Garrett, *Managing the Civil Service* (London: William Heinemann Ltd, 1980), p. 11.
28. K. Theakston, *The Civil Service Since 1945* (Oxford: Blackwell Publishing Ltd, 1995), p. 84.
29. Garrett, *Managing the Civil Service,* p. 9.
30. Garrett, *Managing the Civil Service,* p. 15; and The Civil Service, *Report of the Committee, 1966–68* (London: HMSO, 1968), vol. 2 (hereafter known as the Fulton Report).
31. Garrett, *Managing the Civil Service,* p. 2.
32. Garrett, *Managing the Civil Service,* pp. 41–63.
33. National Archive (hereafter NA), T307/10, Minutes of Establishment Officers Meeting, 29 December 1961.
34. N. Walker, *Morale in the Civil Service* (Edinburgh: Edinburgh University Press, 1961), pp. 15–26.
35. NA, T307/10, T. H. Caulcott to Establishment Officer, 2 August 1965.
36. NA, T307/10, Caulcott to Herbecq, 21 January 1966.
37. H. Parris, *Staff Relations in the Civil Service: Fifty Years of Whitleyism* (London: Allen and Unwin, 1973).
38. NA, T307/10, Caulcott to Establishment Officers, 2 August 1965: T307/23, Thomson to Morrison, 25 November 1969.
39. Theakston, *The Civil Service*, p. 88.
40. *Fulton Report*, para. 123.
41. NA, T307/23, Thomson, 'The Future of the Medical Service', 3 May 1968.
42. NA, T307/18, Thomson 'The CSD and Occupational Health', 14 November 1968, 3–8.

43. D. Thomson, 'Mass Immunisation in the Control of Infectious Disease', *British Medical Journal* (20 August 1966), pp. 427–33; 'Obituary Notices, Sir Daniel Thomson', *BMJ* (13 November 1976), p. 1204.
44. D. Thomson, 'Change in Epidemiology and Preventive Medicine', *Proceedings of the Royal Society of Medicine*, 58 (1965), pp. 831–7.
45. Thomson, 'Change in Epidemiology', pp. 831–7.
46. Thomson, 'Change in Epidemiology', pp. 831–7.
47. NA, T307/23, Thomson to Collier, 29 July 1968.
48. NA, HX6/26, Thomson, 'Work and Progress in 1967', 1967.
49. British Medical Association, *The Future of Occupational Health Services* (1961).
50. NA, T307 1/9, Jones to Hartman, 29 October 1971.
51. NA, T307 1/9, Thomson to Hartman, 9 November 1971; *BMJ,* 1 July 1961.
52. Thomson's final paper on the study, published in June 1972, is substantially different from his original unpublished introduction primarily because it lacks any discussion of stress: NA, HX5/1, Civil Service Sick Leave 1967, 28 January 1970.
53. Civil servants were allowed five days sick leave a year without medical evidence.
54. NA, HX5/1, Thomson, 'Sick Leave 1967', 2.5, 73–5.
55. NA, HX6/28, 'Review of Medical Research', 19.
56. H. Selye, *The Stress of Life* (New York: McGraw-Hill, 1956); F. Alexander, T. French and G. H. Pollock (eds), *Psychosomatic Specificity* (Chicago, IL and London: University of Chicago Press, 1968).
57. NA, HX5/1, Thomson, 'Sick Leave 1967', 1.8–10; and J. Morris, 'Capacity and Incapacity for Work: Some Recent History', Proceedings of the Royal Society of Medicine, 58 (1965), pp. 821–5, on p. 821.
58. NA, HX5/1, Thomson, 'Sick Leave 1967', 1.4.
59. NA, HX6/26, Thomson, 'Work and Progress', 1.14.
60. NA, HX6/26, Thomson, 'Work and Progress', 1.14.
61. R. Kahn et al., *Organisational Stress: Studies in Role Conflict and Ambiguity* (New York: John Wiley and Sons Inc., 1964).
62. NA, HX5/1, Thomson, 'Sick Leave 1967', 1.14.
63. NA, HX6/26, Thomson, 'Work and Progress', 23.
64. NA, HX5/1, Thomson, 'Sick Leave 1967', 1.11.
65. NA, HX5/1, Thomson, 'Sick Leave 1967', 1.15.
66. NA, HX6/26, Thomson, 'Work and Progress', 23.
67. Walker, *Morale in the Civil Service,* p. 253.
68. NA, HX6/26, Thomson, 'Work and Progress', 22.
69. NA, HX5/1, Thomson, 'Sick Leave 1967', 1:26.
70. NA, HX5/3, Thomson, 'Sickness absence in the Civil Service', 576.
71. Civil Service Department, *Civil Service Statistics 1970* (London: HMSO, 1970).
72. Civil Service Department, *Civil Service Statistics 1970.*
73. Walker, *Morale in the Civil Service*, p. 29.
74. NA, HX5/1, Thomson, 'Sick Leave 1967', 2.2.5.
75. NA, HX5/1, Thomson, 'Sick Leave 1967', 2.2.5.
76. NA, HX5/1, Thomson, 'Sick Leave 1967', 2.2.5., 1.31; 2.5.82. See also Chapter 3 'Gender, Stress and Alcohol Abuse' by A. Haggett, in this volume.
77. NA, HX5/1, Thomson, 'Sick Leave 1967', 2.2.5.
78. NA, HX5/1, Thomson, 'Sick Leave 1967', 1.16.
79. NA, HX6/26, Thomson, 'Work and Progress', 24.

80. NA, HX5/3, 'Sickness Absence 1969', 1.16.
81. NA, HX5/1, Thomson, 'Sick Leave 1967', 1:27.
82. B. Gardell, 'Technology, Alienation and Mental Health in the Modern Industrial Environment' in L. Levi (ed.), *Society, Stress and Disease* (London: Oxford University Press, 1971).
83. R. Karasek and T. Theorell, *Healthy Work: Stress, Productivity and the Reconstruction of Working Life* (New York: Basic Books, 1990).
84. J. Johnson and E. Hall, 'Job Strain, Work Place, Social Support and Cardiovascular Disease: A Cross-Sectional Study of a Random Sample of the Swedish Working Population', *American Journal of Public Health*, 78 (1988), pp. 1336–42; and J. Johnson, E. Hall and T. Theorell, 'Combined Effects of Job Strain and Social Isolation on Cardiovascular Disease Morbidity and Mortality in a Random Sample of Swedish Male Working Population', *Scandinavian Journal of Work Environmental Health*, 15 (1989), pp. 271–9.
85. M. Marmot, 2004 Balzan Prize for Epidemiology, 2012, Fondazione Internationale Balzan, Milano, p. 14 – http://www.balzan.org/upload/EstrattoMARMOT.pdf [accessed 14 November 2012].
86. M. Marmot and E. Brunner, 'Cohort Profile: The Whitehall II Study', *International Journal of Epidemiology*, 34 (2005), pp. 251–6, on p. 252.
87. M. Marmot, Interview with H. Kreisler, *Conversations with History*, 18 March 2002, http://globetrotter.berkeley.edu/people2/Marmot/marmot-con3.html [accessed 20 May 2012].
88. Marmot and Brunner, 'Cohort Profile', p. 252.
89. D. Porter, 'From Social Structure to Social Behaviour in Britain After the Second World War', *Contemporary British History*, 16:3 (2010), pp. 158–80
90. R. G. Wilkinson, *Unhealthy Societies: The Afflictions of Inequality* (London: Routledge Wilkinson 1996), p. 93.
91. Porter, 'From Social Structure to Social Behaviour', p. 75.
92. D. Black, J. Morris, C. Smith and P. Townsend, *Inequalities in Health: Report of a Research Working Group* (London: Department of Social Security, 1980).
93. V. Berridge (ed.), *Witness Seminar:* The *Black Report and the Health Divide*, 19 April 1999, http://history.lshtm.ac.uk/files/2013/07/The-Black-Report-and-the-Health-Divide-VB.pdf [accessed 14 November 2012].
94. A. Harrington, *The Cure Within: A History of Mind-Body Medicine* (New York: W. W. Norton and Company, 2008), p. 183.
95. M. Marmot, Interview with J. Al-Khalili, *Life Scientific*, BBC Radio 4, 1 November 2011.
96. R. M. Sapolsky, 'The Influence of Social Hierarchy on Primate Health', *Science*, 308 (2005), pp. 645–52; and R. M. Sapolsky, 'Endrocrinology Alfresco: Psychoendocrine Studies of Wild Baboons, *Recent Progress in Hormone Research*, 48 (1993), pp. 437–68.
97. M. Marmot, 2004 Balzan Prize for Epidemiology, 2012, Fondazione Internationale Balzan, Milano, p. 14 – http://www.balzan.org/upload/EstrattoMARMOT.pdf [accessed 14 November 2012].
98. Marmot, Interview with H. Kreisler.
99. R. Lazarus and S. Folkman, *Stress, Appraisal and Coping* (New York: Springer, 1984).
100. Marmot and Brunner, 'Cohort Profile', p. 253.
101. M. Marmot, 'Remediable or Preventable Social Factors in the Aetiology and Prognosis of Medical Disorders', in P. White (ed.), *Biopsychosocial Medicine: An Integrated Approach to Understanding Illness* (Oxford: Oxford University Press, 2005), pp. 40–1.

102. Marmot, 'Remediable or Preventable Social Factors', pp. 40–1.
103. J. Ferrie (ed.), *Work Stress and Health: The Whitehall II Study* (London: Public and Commercial Services Union, 2004), p. 6.
104. Ferrie (ed.), *Work Stress and Health*, p. 6.
105. D. Wainwright and M. Calnan, *Work Stress: The Making of a Modern Epidemic* (Buckingham: Open University Press, 2002), pp. 53–9.
106. F. North et al., 'Psychosocial Work Environment and Sickness Absence Among British CivilServants: The Whitehall II Study', *American Journal of Public Health*, 86 (1996), pp. 332–40, on p. 338.
107. J. Siegrist, 'Adverse Health Effects of High Effort-low Reward Conditions at Work', *Journal of Occupational Health Psychology*, 1 (1996), pp. 27–43.
108. Wainwright and Calnan, *Work Stress*, p. 56.
109. H. Kuper et al., 'When Reciprocity Fails: Effort-Reward Imbalance in Relation to Coronary Heart Disease and Health Functioning Within the Whitehall II Study', *Occupational and Environmental Medicine*, 59 (2002), pp. 777–84.
110. A. Feeney, et al., 'Socioeconomic and Sex Differentials in Reason for Sickness Absence from the Whitehall II Study', *Occupation and Environmental Medicine*, 55 (1998), pp. 91–8, on p. 97.
111. Feeney, et al., 'Socioeconomic and Sex Differentials', p. 97.
112. Feeney, et al., 'Socioeconomic and Sex Differentials', p. 97.
113. National Archive (hereafter NA), HX5/1, Thomson, 'Sick Leave 1967', 1.14.
114. Ferrie (ed.), *Work Stress and Health,* p. 20.
115. Ferrie (ed.), *Work Stress and Health,* p. 20
116. T. Chandola et al., 'The Effect of Control at Home on CHD Events in the Whitehall II Study: Gender Differences in Psychosocial Domestic Pathways to Social Inequalities in CHD', *Social Science and Medicine*, 58 (2004), pp. 1501–9.
117. Office for National Statistics, *Sickness Absence in the Labour Market* (15 May 2012), http://www.ons.gov.uk/ons/dcp171776_265016.pdf [accessed 14 November 2012].
118. D. Wainwright and M. Calnan, *Work Stress: The Making of a Modern Epidemic* (Buckingham: Open University Press, 2002), pp. 57–8.
119. Stress Impact Consortium, *Integrated Report of Stress Impact: On the Impact of Changing Social Structures and Quality of Life: Individual and Social Perspectives,* (August, 2006), http://www.surrey.ac.uk/psychology/projects/stress-impact/files/Stress%20 Impact%20Integrated%20Report.pdf [accessed 16 November 2012].

7 Jackson, 'Men and Women under Stress: Neuropsychiatric Models of Resilience during and after the Second World War'

1. R. R. Grinker and J. P. Spiegel, *Men Under Stress* (Philadelphia, PA: Blakiston, 1945), pp. vii–viii.
2. J. Hinton, *Women, Social Leadership, and the Second World War: Continuities of Class* (Oxford: Oxford University Press, 2002); and J. Hinton, *Nine Wartime Lives: Mass-Observation and the Making of the Modern Self* (Oxford: Oxford University Press, 2010).
3. Grinker and Spiegel, *Men Under Stress*, pp. 186–9.
4. See, for example, S. W. Davis et al., *A Study of Combat Stress, Korea 1952: Preliminary Report* (Chevy Chase, MD: Operations Research Office, Johns Hopkins University,

1953); S. W. Davis, 'Stress in Combat', *Scientific American*, 194 (1956), pp. 31–5; S. Richardson Hill et al., 'Studies in Adrenocortical and Psychological Response to Stress in Man', *Archives of Internal Medicine*, 97 (1956), pp. 269–98; D. H. Funkenstein, S. H. King and M. E. Drolette, *Mastery of Stress* (Cambridge, MA: Harvard University Press, 1957); V. H. Tompkins, 'Stress in Aviation', in Society for Psychosomatic Research, *The Nature of Stress Disorder* (London: Hutchinson, 1958), pp. 73–80; M. Friedman and R. H. Rosenman, 'Association of Specific Overt Behaviour Pattern with Blood and Cardiovascular Findings', *Journal of the American Medical Association*, 169 (1959), pp. 1286–96; F. S. Preston, 'Measurement of Pilot Fatigue', *Occupational Medicine*, 17 (1967), pp. 52–6; P. G. Bourne, *The Psychology and Physiology of Stress with Reference to Special Studies of the Viet Nam War* (New York: Academic Press, 1969); and G. Miller, R. T. Rubin, B. R. Clark, W. R. Crawford and R. J. Arthur, 'The Stress of Aircraft Carrier Landings', *Psychosomatic Medicine*, 32 (1970), pp. 581–8.

5. R. S. Lazarus, J. C. Spiesman, A. M. Mordkoff and L. A. Davison, *A Laboratory Study of Psychological Stress Produced by a Motion Picture Film* (American Psychological Association, 1962), p. 5. For a discussion of American military studies of stress, which also focused exclusively either on men or laboratory animals, see Theodore M. Brown, '"Stress" in US Wartime Psychiatry: World War II and its Immediate Aftermath', in D. Cantor and E. Ramsden (eds), *Stress, Shock and Adaptation in the Twentieth Century* (Rochester: University of Rochester Press, 2014), pp. 122–41; and T. Long, 'The Machinery and the Morale: Physiological and Psychological Approaches to Military Stress Research in the Early Cold War Era', in Cantor and Ramsden (eds), *Stress, Shock and Adaptation in the Twentieth Century*, pp. 142–85. Neither author explores the gendered nature of contemporary military stress research.
6. See Chapter 6, 'Cultural Change', by Debbie Palmer and chapter 10, 'Labouring Stress', by Joseph Melling, in this volume.
7. I. Atkin, 'Mental Disorders and External Stress', *The Lancet* (17 March 1962), pp. 581–2. In part, Atkin was mocking contemporary advice that wives should not 'contradict their husbands' in case they caused anger and stress.
8. For further discussion, see M. Jackson, *The Age of Stress: Science and the Search for Stability* (Oxford: Oxford University Press, 2013), pp. 21–55.
9. R. Hayward, 'Desperate Housewives and Model Amoebi: The Invention of Suburban Neurosis in Inter-War Britain', in M. Jackson (ed.), *Health and the Modern Home* (New York: Routledge, 2007), pp. 42–62.
10. A. Haggett, *Desperate Housewives, Neuroses and the Domestic Environment, 1945–70* (London: Pickering & Chatto, 2012).
11. J. Bourke, 'Effeminacy, Ethnicity and the End of Trauma: The Sufferings of "Shell-Shocked" Men in Great Britain and Ireland, 1914–39', *Journal of Contemporary History*, 35 (2000), pp. 57–69; J. Bourke, 'Disciplining the Emotions: Fear, Psychiatry and the Second World War', in R. Cooter, M. Harrison and S. Sturdy (eds), *War, Medicine and Modernity* (Stroud: Sutton, 1998), pp. 225–38; J. Bourke, *Fear: A Cultural History* (London: Virago, 2005); E. Showalter, *The Female Malady: Women, Madness and English Culture, 1830–1980* (London: Virago, 1987); Haggett, *Desperate Housewives*; A. Harrington, *The Cure Within: A History of Mind-Body Medicine* (New York: W. W. Norton, 2008); Hayward, 'Desperate Housewives'; A. Tone, *The Age of Anxiety: A History of America's Turbulent Affair with Tranquilizers* (New York: Basic Books, 2009); and D. Herzberg, *Happy Pills in America: From Miltown to Prozac* (Baltimore, MD: Johns Hopkins University Press, 2009). It is noticeable, however, that a recent focused

study of the history of anxiety makes little mention of gender: A. V. Horwitz, *Anxiety: A Short History* (Baltimore, MD: Johns Hopkins University Press, 2013).

12. C. L. Cooper and P. Dewe, *Stress: A Brief History* (Oxford: Blackwell, 2004); R. Kugelmann, *Stress: The Nature and History of Engineered Grief* (Westport, CT: Praeger, 1992). S. Doublet, *The Stress Myth* (Sydney: Ipsilon Publishing, 2000); A. Patmore, *The Truth About Stress* (London: Atlantic Books, 2006); I. Miller, 'The Mind and Stomach at War: Stress and Abdominal Illness in Britain, *c.*1939–1945', *Medical History*, 54 (2010), pp. 95–110; and I. Miller, *A Modern History of the Stomach: Gastric Illness, Medicine and British Society, 1800–1950* (London: Pickering & Chatto, 2011).
13. D. Freeman and J. Freeman, *The Stressed Sex: Uncovering the Truth about Men, Women, and Mental Health* (Oxford: Oxford University Press, 2013); and D. Becker, *One Nation Under Stress: The Trouble with Stress as an Idea* (New York: Oxford University Press, 2013). This recent interest is in part evident in the conference from which this volume emerged.
14. A. Young, *The Harmony of Illusions: Inventing Post-Traumatic Stress Disorder* (New Jersey, NJ: Princeton University Press, 1995); B. Shephard, *A War of Nerves: Soldiers and Psychiatrists 1914–94* (London: Pimlico, 2002); E. Jones, 'Historical Approaches to Post-Combat Disorders', *Philosophical Transactions of the Royal Society*, 361 (2006), pp. 533–42; E. Jones and S. Wessely, 'Psychiatric Battle Casualties: An Intra- and Inter-War Comparison', *British Journal of Psychiatry*, 178 (2001), pp. 242–7; and E. Jones and S. Wessely, *Shell Shock to PTSD: Military Psychiatry from 1900 to the Gulf War* (Hove and New York: Psychology Press, 2005).
15. C. Acton, 'Writing and Waiting: The First World War Correspondence Between Vera Brittain and Roland Leighton', *Gender and History*, 11 (1999), pp. 54–83.
16. There is a vast literature on shell shock and masculinity, but the most interesting and original recent exploration of these issues in the context of flying stress is the work of Michael Collins, whose doctoral thesis, entitled, 'Forging an Empire of the Air: Race and Gender in Early British Aeronautics, 1908–1933' (California State University, Sacramento), includes a discussion of traumatic neuroses in British aviators during and after the First World War.
17. 'Obituary: J. L. Birley', *British Medical Journal* (17 March 1934), p. 510.
18. J. L. Birley, 'Goulstonian Lectures on the Principles of Medical Science as Applied to Military Aviation', *The Lancet* (29 May 1920), pp. 1147–51.
19. For a study of the impact of low oxygen on performance and its measurement, see M. Flack, 'The Bag Method for the Investigation of Air Disabilities of Aviators', Air Medical Investigation Committee, in *The Medical Problems of Flying* (London: HMSO, 1920), pp. 14–17.
20. Birley, 'Goulstonian Lectures', p. 1150.
21. See the references in Birley, 'Goulstonian Lectures', p. 1151.
22. R. Cooter, 'Malingering in Modernity: Psychological Scripts and Adversarial Encounters During the First World War', in R. Cooter, M. Harrison and S. Sturdy (eds), *War, Medicine and Modernity* (Stroud: Sutton, 1998), pp. 125–48.
23. Birley, 'Goulstonian Lectures', p. 1150.
24. *Report of the War Office Committee of Enquiry into "Shell-Shock"* (London: Cmd. 1734, 1922). For further discussion, see M. Jackson, *The Age of Stress: Science and the Search for Stability* (Oxford: Oxford University Press, 2013), pp. 47–53.
25. J. Bourke, *Dismembering the Male: Men's Bodies, Britain and the Great War* (London: Reaktion, 1996); 'Effeminacy, Ethnicity and the End of Trauma: The Sufferings of

"Shell-Shocked" Men in Great Britain and Ireland, 1914–39', *Journal of Contemporary History*, 35 (2000), pp. 57–69; M. Roper, 'Maternal Relations: Moral Manliness and Emotional Survival in Letters Home During the First World War', in S. Dudink, K. Hagemann and J. Tosh (eds), *Masculinities in Politics and War: Gendering Modern History* (Manchester: Manchester University Press, 2004), pp. 295–315; M. Roper, 'Between Manliness and Masculinity: The "War Generation" and the Psychology of Fear in Britain, 1914–1950', *Journal of British Studies*, 44 (2005), pp. 343–62; J. Meyer, *Men of War: Masculinity and the First World War* (Basingstoke: Palgrave Macmillan, 2009); J. Meyer, 'Separating the Men from the Boys: Masculinity and Maturity in Understandings of Shell Shock in Britain', *Twentieth Century British History*, 20 (2009), pp. 1–22; E. Jones and S. Wessely, 'Psychiatric Battle Casualties: An Intra- and Inter-War Comparison', *British Journal of Psychiatry*, 178 (2001), pp. 242–7; and E. Jones and S. Wessely, *Shell Shock to PTSD: Military Psychiatry from 1900 to the Gulf War* (Hove and New York: Psychology Press, 2005).

26. M. Roper, *The Secret Battle: Emotional Survival in the Great War* (Manchester: Manchester University Press, 2010); and F. Reid, *Broken Men: Shell Shock, Treatment and Recovery in Britain, 1914–1930* (London: Continuum, 2011).
27. I. Miller, *A Modern History of the Stomach: Gastric Illness, Medicine and British Society, 1800–1950* (London: Pickering & Chatto, 2011); and Jackson, *The Age of Stress*.
28. J. L. Halliday, 'The Rising Incidence of Psychosomatic Illness', *British Medical Journal* (2 July 1938), pp. 11–14; and G. Draper, *Disease and the Man* (London: Kegan Paul, Trench, Trubner and Co., 1930). For more on Halliday and psychosocial medicine, see R. Hayward, 'Enduring Emotions: James Halliday and the Invention of the Psychosocial', *Isis*, 100 (2009), pp. 827–38; and A. Hull, 'Glasgow's "Sick Society"? James Halliday, Psychosocial Medicine and Medical Holism in Britain, *c.*1920–48', *History of the Human Sciences*, 25 (2012), pp. 73–90.
29. F. Twigg, 'Perforation of Duodenal Ulcer when Flying', *British Medical Journal* (25 October 1930), p. 687; and F. C. Bartlett, *Psychology and the Soldier* (London: Cambridge University Press, 1927). For further discussion, see A. D. English, *The Cream of the Crop: Canadian Aircrew 1939–1945* (Montreal: McGill-Queen's University Press, 1996), pp. 61–80.
30. M. Francis, *The Flyer: British Culture and the Royal Air Force, 1939–1945* (Oxford: Oxford University Press, 2008), pp. 121–2. See also the account of Mary Wesley's affairs with various servicemen in P. Marnham, *Wild Mary: A Life of Mary Wesley* (London: Vintage, 2007).
31. G. V. Stephenson and K. Cameron, 'Anxiety States in the Navy', *British Medical Journal* (13 November 1943), pp. 603–7, on p. 606. According to Stephenson and Cameron (p. 606), the aim of sedation was to rest 'the over-stimulated organism' and to restore 'normal functioning'.
32. S. Brandon, 'LMF in Bomber Command 1939–45: Diagnosis or Denouncement', in H. Freeman and G. E. Berrios (eds), *150 Years of British Psychiatry, Volume II: The Aftermath* (London: Athlone Press, 1996), pp. 119–29; and E. Jones, '"LMF": The Use of Psychiatric Stigma in the Royal Air Force During the Second World War', *Journal of Military History*, 70 (2006), pp. 439–58.
33. C. P. Symonds, 'The Human Response to Flying Stress: Lecture I', *British Medical Journal* (4 December 1943), pp. 703–6.
34. C. P. Symonds, 'The Human Response to Flying Stress: Lecture II', *British Medical Journal* (11 December 1943), pp. 740–4.

35. For the classic account of how to recognize and manage fear amongst soldiers, based on experiences during the First World War, see Lord Moran, *The Anatomy of Courage* (London: Constable, 1945).
36. For a discussion of 'wind up' in these terms, see W. H. R. Rivers, *Instinct and the Unconscious* (London: Cambridge University Press, 1924), discussed in Symonds, 'The Human Response to Flying Stress: Lecture II', p. 741. On Kardiner, see B. Shephard, *A War of Nerves: Soldiers and Psychiatrists 1914–94* (London: Pimlico, 2002), pp. 154–7.
37. Stephenson and Cameron, 'Anxiety States in the Navy'.
38. Lord Moran, 'Wear and Tear', *The Lancet* (17 June 1950), pp. 1099–101.
39. Moran quoted Symonds directly in *The Anatomy of Courage*, pp. 78–80.
40. D. D. Reid, 'Sickness and Stress in Operational Flying', *British Journal of Social Medicine*, 2 (1948), pp. 123–31.
41. W. R. D. Fairbairn, 'The War Neuroses: Their Nature and Significance', *British Medical Journal* (13 February 1943), pp. 183–6.
42. Fairbairn, 'The War Neuroses', pp. 183–6. See also the discussion in: English, *The Cream of the Crop*, pp. 71–2; and J. Bourke, 'Disciplining the Emotions: Fear, Psychiatry and the Second World War', in R. Cooter, M. Harrison and S. Sturdy (eds), *War, Medicine and Modernity* (Stroud: Sutton, 1998), pp. 230–1.
43. For Fairbairn's explicit application of Freudian ideas, see Fairbairn, 'The War Neuroses', p. 185. A similar framework is evident in other contemporary studies: see the review of R. D. Gillespie's *Psychological Effects of War on Citizen and Soldier*, in the *British Medical Journal* (30 January 1943), p. 133.
44. Symonds, 'The Human Response to Flying Stress: Lecture I'; Symonds, 'The Human Response to Flying Stress: Lecture II'.
45. For further discussion, see Jackson, *The Age of Stress*.
46. Reid, 'Sickness and Stress in Operational Flying', p. 130.
47. V. H. Tompkins, 'Stress in Aviation', in Society for Psychosomatic Research, *The Nature of Stress Disorder* (London: Hutchinson, 1958), pp. 73–80.
48. F. S. Preston, 'Measurement of Pilot Fatigue', *Occupational Medicine*, 17 (1967), pp. 52–6; and G. Miller, R. T. Rubin, B. R. Clark, W. R. Crawford and R. J. Arthur, 'The Stress of Aircraft Carrier Landings', *Psychosomatic Medicine*, 32 (1970), pp. 581–8. The earlier studies on which many of these assessments were based are described in Hudson Hoagland, 'Adventures in Biological Engineering', *Science*, 100 (1944), pp. 63–7. For further discussion of organismic approaches to stress and the use of steroid excretion rates to identify vulnerable personnel, see Jackson, *The Age of Stress*, pp. 56–98, 116–30.
49. R. R. Grinker (ed.), *Toward a Unified Theory of Human Behavior* (New York: Basic Books, 1956).
50. R. S. Lazarus, J. Deese and S. F. Osler, 'The Effects of Psychological Stress Upon Performance', *Psychological Bulletin*, 49 (1952), pp. 293–317; R. S. Lazarus, *Adjustment and Personality* (New York: McGraw-Hill, 1961), pp. 285–7; and R. S. Lazarus, *Psychological Stress and the Coping Process* (New York: McGraw-Hill, 1966).
51. D. H. Funkenstein, S. H. King and M. E. Drolette, *Mastery of Stress* (Cambridge, MA: Harvard University Press, 1957).
52. Funkenstein, King and Drolette, *Mastery of Stress*, pp. 282–4.
53. J. M. Tanner, *Stress and Psychiatric Disorder* (Oxford: Blackwell Scientific, 1960). The conference included contributions from leading North American scholars such as Hans Selye, Harold G. Wolff and Hudson Hoagland.

54. J. Cohen, 'Women in Peace and War', in T. H. Pear (ed.), *Psychological Factors of Peace and War* (London: Hutchinson, 1950), pp. 91–110.
55. Lord David Cecil, 'The R. A. F. : A Layman's Glimpse', in W. S. Rothenstein and Lord David Cecil, *Men of the R. A. F.* (London: Oxford University Press, 1942), p. 83.
56. W. R. D. Fairbairn, 'The War Neuroses: Their Nature and Significance', *British Medical Journal* (13 February 1943), pp. 183–6; see discussion in J. Bourke, 'Disciplining the Emotions: Fear, Psychiatry and the Second World War', in R. Cooter, M. Harrison and S. Sturdy (eds), *War, Medicine and Modernity* (Stroud: Sutton, 1998), pp. 230–1.
57. G. V. Stephenson and K. Cameron, 'Anxiety States in the Navy', *British Medical Journal* (13 November 1943), pp. 603–7, on p. 604
58. Stephenson and Cameron, 'Anxiety States in the Navy', p. 604; and R. R. Grinker and J. P. Spiegel, *Men Under Stress* (Philadelphia, PA: Blakiston, 1945), pp. 186–9. See also E. Slater, 'Psychological Aspects of Family Life', in Sir J. Marchant (ed.), *Rebuilding Family Life in the Post-War World: An Enquiry with Recommendations* (London: Odhams Press, 1945), pp. 92–106, on pp. 99–100.
59. A. D. English, *The Cream of the Crop: Canadian Aircrew 1939–1945* (Montreal: McGill-Queen's University Press, 1996); and M. K. Wells, *Courage and Air Warfare: The Allied Aircrew Experience in the Second World War* (London: Frank Cass, 1995).
60. M. Francis, *The Flyer: British Culture and the Royal Air Force, 1939–1945* (Oxford: Oxford University Press, 2008), pp. 63–84, 142–5.
61. C. Acton, 'Writing and Waiting: The First World War Correspondence Between Vera Brittain and Roland Leighton', *Gender and History*, 11 (1999), pp. 54–83. See also Francis, *The Flyer*, pp. 98–103.
62. B. E. Escott, *Women in Air Force Blue: The Story of Women in the Royal Air Force from 1918 to the Present Day* (Northamptonshire: Patrick Stephens, 1989); P. Beck, *Keeping Watch: A WAAF in Bomber Command* (Manchester: Crécy, 1989); and B. E. Escott, *Our Wartime Days: The WAAF in World War II* (Bodmin: Alan Sutton, 1995).
63. G. Whittell, *Spitfire Women of World War II* (London: Harper Perennial, 2008), pp. 22, 31–51.
64. A reference to service-women's courage is in Air Marshal Sir Andrew KcKee's foreword to: 'Archie' Hall, *We, Also, Were There: A Collection of Recollections of Wartime Women in Bomber Command* (Devon: Merlin Books, 1985), p. 9.
65. Hall, *We, Also, Were There.*
66. T. Stone, 'Creating a (Gendered?) Military Identity: The Women's Auxiliary Air Force in Great Britain in the Second World War', *Women's History Review*, 8 (1999), pp. 605–24.
67. S. I. Ballard and H. G. Miller, 'Neuropsychiatry at a Royal Air Force Centre', *British Medical Journal* (8 July 1944), pp. 40–3
68. Ballard and Miller, 'Neuropsychiatry at a Royal Air Force Centre', p. 41.
69. Ballard and Miller, 'Neuropsychiatry at a Royal Air Force Centre', p. 42.
70. Ballard and Miller, 'Neuropsychiatry at a Royal Air Force Centre', p. 42.
71. I. Atkin, 'Air-Raid Strain in Mental-Hospital Admission', *The Lancet* (19 July 1941), pp. 72–4.
72. Atkin, 'Air-Raid Strain in Mental-Hospital Admission', pp. 72–4; Anon., 'Neuroses in War-Time', *British Medical Journal* (21 January 1939), pp. 126–8; F. Brown, 'Civilian Psychiatric Air-Raid Casualties', *The Lancet* (31 May 1941), pp. 686–91; A. Harris, 'Psychiatric Reactions of Civilians in War-Time', *The Lancet* (9 August 1941), pp. 152–5; and H. Wilson, 'Mental Reactions to Air-Raids', *The Lancet* (7 March 1942), pp. 284–7.

73. Brown, 'Civilian Psychiatric Air-Raid Casualties', p. 691.
74. I. McD. G. Stewart, 'Coronary Disease and Modern Stress', *The Lancet* (23 December 1950), pp. 867–70.
75. S. I. Ballard and H. G. Miller, 'Psychiatric Casualties in a Women's Service', *British Medical Journal* (3 March 1945), pp. 293–5. See also Chapters 3 'Gender, Stress and Alcohol Abuse' and 8 'Stomach for the Peace', in this volume, by Ali Haggett and Edgar Jones, respectively.
76. Ballard and Miller, 'Psychiatric Casualties', p. 294.
77. Bourke, 'Disciplining the Emotions', pp. 233–4.
78. W. C. Menninger, 'Psychiatric Experience in the War, 1941–1946', *American Journal of Psychiatry*, 103 (1947), pp. 577–86.
79. These discussions continued an inter-war trend of explaining vulnerability partly in these terms. See, for example, M. B. Hall and F. Hopkins, 'Parental Loss and Child Guidance', *Archives of Diseases in Childhood*, 11 (1936), pp. 187–94; and R. D. Gillespie, *Psychological Effects of War on Citizen and Soldier* (London: Chapman Hall, 1942).
80. T. F. Main, 'Clinical Problems of Repatriates', *British Journal of Psychiatry*, 93 (1947), pp. 354–63.
81. J. Cohen, 'Women in Peace and War', in T. H. Pear (ed.), *Psychological Factors of Peace and War* (London, Hutchinson, 1950), pp. 91–110.
82. For inter-war and wartime discussions, see F. Hopkins, 'Attempted Suicide: An Investigation', *British Journal of Psychiatry*, 83 (1937), pp. 71–94; R. J. Bartlett, 'The Civilian Population Under Bombardment', *Nature* (7 June 1941), pp. 700–1; and H. Crichton-Miller, 'Somatic Factors Conditioning Air-Raid Reactions', *The Lancet* (12 July 1941), pp. 31–4. For an example of an advertisement for 'Menopax' linking a woman's vulnerability to the stress of air raids to menopause, see Image Number 30518628 at www.advertisingarchives.ac.uk [accessed 18 June 2014].
83. See Chapters 6, 'Cultural Change', and 3, 'Gender, Stress and Alcohol Abuse', in this volume, by D. Palmer and A. Haggett, respectively.
84. E. Wilson, *Women and the Welfare State* (London: Tavistock Publications, 1977); E. Wilson, *Only Halfway to Paradise: Women in Postwar Britain 1945–1968* (London: Tavistock Publications, 1980); P. Summerfield, *Women Workers in the Second World War: Production and Patriarchy in Conflict* (Beckenham: Croom Helm, 1984); J. Lewis, *Women in Britain since 1945: Women, Family, Work and the State in the Post-War Years* (Oxford: Blackwell, 1988); A. Holdsworth, *Out of the Doll's House: The Story of Women in the Twentieth Century* (London: BBC Books, 1988); L. A. Tilly and J. W. Scott, *Women, Work, and Family* (New York and London: Routledge, 1989); and G. Holloway, *Women and Work in Britain since 1840* (London: Routledge, 2005).
85. Wilson, *Only Halfway to Paradise*, p. 195.
86. 'Total War and the Individual', *The Lancet* (21 June 1941), pp. 791–2. For a discussion of wartime evaluations of morale during air raids, see E. Jones, R. Woolven, B. Durodié and S. Wessely, 'Civilian Morale During the Second World War': Responses to Air Raids Re-Examined', *Social History of Medicine*, 17 (2004), pp. 463–79.
87. C. Acton, 'Writing and Waiting: The First World War Correspondence Between Vera Brittain and Roland Leighton', *Gender and History*, 11 (1999), pp. 54–83; and T. Stone, 'Creating a (Gendered?) Military Identity: The Women's Auxiliary Air Force in Great Britain in the Second World War', *Women's History Review*, 8 (1999), pp. 605–24.
88. Post-war studies of stressful life events or of stress-related somatic conditions, such as gastric ulcers, rarely paid attention to either the biological or cultural underpinnings of

stress reactions, partly because many of these studies were emphasizing the occupational and psychosocial determinants of stress. See, for example: R. Doll and F. A. Jones, *Occupational Factors in the Aetiology of Gastric and Duodenal Ulcers* (London: HMSO, 1951); B. S. Dohrenwend and B. P. Dohrenwend, *Stressful Life Events: Their Nature and Effects* (New York: John Wiley and Sons, 1974).

89. Dr T. Traherne (ed.), *Healthy Minds and Bodies* (London: Waverley Book Company, 1956), p. 12.
90. F. Kerner, *Stress and Your Heart* (New York: Hawthorn Books, 1961), p. 76.
91. M. Friedman and R. H. Rosenman, 'Association of Specific Overt Behaviour Pattern with Blood and Cardiovascular Findings', *Journal of the American Medical Association*, 169 (1959), pp. 1286–96; M. Friedman and R. H. Rosenman, *Type A Behavior and Your Heart* (New York, Alfred Knopf, 1974); and M. Friedman and R. H. Rosenman, 'The Key Cause – Type A Behaviour Pattern', in A. Monat and R. S. Lazarus (eds), *Stress and Coping: An Anthology* (New York: Columbia University Press, 1977), pp. 203–16.
92. See, for example, P. M. Fine and B. O. Hartman, *Psychiatric Strengths and Weaknesses of Typical Air Force Pilots* (Texas, TX: USAF School of Aerospace Medicine, 1968), pp. 19–20.
93. K. L. McFadden, 'Comparing Pilot-Error Accident Rates of Male and Female Airline Pilots', *Omega: The International Journal of Management Science*, 24 (1996), pp. 443–50; and J. Marriott, 'Discipline is Keynote in Training the Men who can Afford No Mistakes', *The Times* (4 September 1972), p. 6. For contemporary debates about pilot fatigue, working conditions and safety, often stimulated by specific disasters, see: '"4,553 Landings" by Viscount in Crash: Inquiry Question on Stress Factor', *The Times* (13 November 1957), p. 7; 'Pilots Test System to Avoid Fatigue', *The Times* (14 May 1962), p. 6; 'Doctors Studying Pilots' Fatigue', *The Times* (13 July 1965), p. 8; 'Airline Pilots Sleep on Duty, MP Says', *The Times* (28 June 1971), p. 1; 'Ministry Inquiry Over BOAC Crew Asleep at Controls of Jet Flying at 30,000 ft', *The Times* (13 December 1972), p. 1; C. Balfour and I. George Smith, 'How Real are the Pilot's Problems?', *New Scientist* (22 March 1973), pp. 672–3; E. M. Donaldson, 'More Pilots Complain of Fatigue', *Daily Telegraph* (30 March 1973); Civil Aviation Authority, *Report of the Committee on Flight Time Limitations* (London: HMSO, 1973); and 'Call to Reduce Pilots' Hours of Work Expected', *The Times* (9 April 1973), p. 1. I am grateful to Debbie Palmer for providing me with references related to stress in commercial pilots.
94. F. S. Preston, 'Physiological Problems in Air Cabin Crew', *Proceedings of the Royal Society of Medicine*, 67 (1974), pp. 23–7.

8 Jones, 'Stomach for the Peace: Psychosomatic Disorders in UK Veterans and Civilians, 1945–55'

1. F. Assinder, 'Memoirs Collected for the Fiftieth Anniversary of the National Health Service' (1998), Royal College of General Practitioners Archive, B NHS A2-1.
2. J. Fry, 'Five Years of General Practice', *British Medical Journal*, 2 (1957), pp. 1453–7; and J. Pemberton, 'Illness in General Practice', *British Medical Journal*, 1 (1949), pp. 306–8.
3. M. J. S. Langman, *The Epidemiology of Chronic Digestive Disease* (London: Edward Arnold, 1979), p. 15; and H. Bailey and R. J. McNeill Love, *A Short Practice of Surgery* (London: H. K. Lewis, 1949), p. 248.

4. R. Doll, F. Avery Jones and M. M. Buckatzsch, *Medical Research Council Special Report Series No. 276, Occupational Factors in the Aetiology of Gastric and Duodenal Ulcers with an Estimate of their Incidence in the General Population* (London: HMSO, 1951), pp. 1–96.
5. M. Jackson, *The Age of Stress: Science and the Search for Stability* (Oxford: Oxford University Press, 2013); and H. Selye, *The Stress of Life* (New York: McGraw-Hill, 1956).
6. B. Finlay, K. Gillison, D. Hart, R. W. T. Mason, N. C. Mond, L. Page and D. O'Neill, 'Stress and Distress in General Practice', *Practitioner*, 172 (1954), pp. 183–96, on p. 183.
7. P. Addison, *Now the War is Over: A Social History of Britain 1945–51* (London: Jonathan Cape, 1985); D. Kynaston, *Austerity Britain 1945–51* (London: Bloomsbury, 2007); and D. Kynaston, *Family Britain 1951–57* (London: Bloomsbury, 2009).
8. P. Hennessy, *Never Again: Britain 1945–51* (London: Jonathan Cape, 1992); P. Hennessey, *Having it so Good: Britain in the Fifties* (London: Penguin, 2007); C. Webster, *The National Health Service: A Political History* (Oxford: Oxford University Press, 1998); and A. Digby, *Evolution of British General Practice 1850–1948* (Oxford: Oxford University Press, 1999).
9. A. Allport, *Demobbed: Coming Home after World War Two* (New Haven, CT: Yale University Press, 2009).
10. M. Harrison, *Medicine and Victory: British Military Medicine in the Second World War* (Oxford: Oxford University Press, 2004); E. Jones and S. Wessely, 'War Syndromes: The Impact of Culture on Medically Unexplained Symptoms', *Medical History*, 49 (2005), pp. 55–78; and B. Shephard, *War of Nerves, Soldiers and Psychiatrists 1914–1994* (London: Jonathan Cape, 2000).
11. For further discussion of precisely these experiences and coping strategies, see Chapter 1 'From War to Peace', in this volume, by Pamela Richardson.
12. A. Young, *The Harmony of Illusions: Inventing Post-Traumatic Stress Disorder* (Princeton, NJ: Princeton University Press, 1995); R. Leys, *Trauma: A Genealogy* (Chicago, IL: Chicago University Press, 2000); R. Hayward, 'Enduring Emotions: James Halliday and the Invention of the Psychosocial', *Isis*, 100 (2009), pp. 827–38; R. Hayward, 'Sadness in Camberwell: Imagining Stress and Constructing History in Post-War Britain', in D. Cantor and E. Ramsden (eds), *Stress, Shock and Adaptation in the Twentieth Century* (Rochester, NY: Rochester University Press, 2014), pp. 320–42.
13. G. N. Grob, 'The Rise of the Peptic Ulcer, 1900–1950', *Perspectives in Biology and Medicine*, 46 (2003), pp. 550–66.
14. I. Miller, *A Modern History of the Stomach, Medicine and British Society* (London: Pickering & Chatto, 2011).
15. Editorial, 'Dyspepsia in the Army', *British Medical Journal*, 2 (1940), pp. 836–7.
16. R. T. Payne and C. Newman, 'Interim Report on Dyspepsia in the Army', *British Medical Journal*, 2 (1940), pp. 819–21; and I. Miller, 'The Mind and Stomach at War: Stress and Abdominal Illness in Britain *c.*1939–1945', *Medical History*, 54 (2010), pp. 95–110, on pp. 99–100.
17. H. L. Tidy, 'Discussion on Dyspepsia in the Armed Forces', *Proceedings of the Royal Society of Medicine*, 34 (1941), pp. 411–17, on p. 415; and H. L. Tidy, 'Peptic Ulcer and Dyspepsia in the Army', *British Medical Journal*, 2 (1943), pp. 473–7, on p. 474.
18. C. Newman, A. Morton Gill, H. Tidy and R. S. Allison, 'Dyspepsia', in V. Z. Cope (ed.), *Medicine and Pathology* (London: HMSO, 1952), pp. 96–108.
19. H. L. Tidy, 'Peptic Ulcer and Dyspepsia in the Army', *British Medical Journal*, 2 (1943), pp. 473–7, on p. 473.

20. D. T. Davies and A. T. Macbeth Wilson, 'Observations on the Life-History of Chronic Peptic Ulcer', *The Lancet*, 2 (1937), pp. 1353–60, on p. 1353.
21. D. T. Davies and A. T. Macbeth Wilson, 'Personal and Clinical History in Haematemesis and Perforation', *The Lancet*, 2 (1939), pp. 723–7, on pp. 726, 727.
22. E. Jones, '"The Gut War": Functional Somatic Disorders in the UK During the Second World War', *History of the Human Sciences*, 25 (2012), pp. 30–48.
23. J. N. Morris and R. M. Titmuss, 'Epidemiology of Peptic Ulcer, Vital Statistics', *The Lancet*, 2 (1944), pp. 841–5.
24. Morris and Titmuss, 'Epidemiology of Peptic Ulcer', p. 845.
25. Morris and Titmuss, 'Epidemiology of Peptic Ulcer', pp. 841, 845.
26. I. Miller, *A Modern History of the Stomach, Medicine and British Society* (London: Pickering & Chatto, 2011), p. 199.
27. A. Hurst, 'Indigestion and National Health', *The Practitioner*, 152 (1944), pp. 193–6, on p. 193.
28. C. A. Hinds Howell, 'A Comparison of Dyspepsia in the Army for 1940 and 1941', *British Medical Journal*, 1 (1941), pp. 692–3.
29. G. Draper, 'The Emotional Component of the Ulcer Susceptible Constitution', *Annals of Internal Medicine*, 16 (1942), pp. 633–58.
30. Draper, 'The Emotional Component', p. 657.
31. M. Jackson, *The Age of Stress: Science and the Search for Stability* (Oxford: Oxford University Press, 2013), p. 89.
32. Jackson, *The Age of Stress*, p. 125; and H. Selye, 'The General Adaptation Syndrome and the Diseases of Adaptation', *Journal of Clinical Endocrinology*, 6 (1946), pp. 117–230.
33. H. Selye, 'Perforated Peptic Ulcer During Air-Raid', *The Lancet*, 1 (1943), p. 252; and D. N. Stewart and D. M. de R. Winser, 'Incidence of Perforated Peptic Ulcer: Effect of Heavy Air Raids', *The Lancet*, 1 (1942), pp. 259–61.
34. M. K. Wells, *Courage and Air Warfare, The Allied Aircrew Experience in the Second World War* (London: Frank Cass, 1995), p. 164.
35. E. Jones and N. Greenberg, 'Royal Naval Psychiatry: Organisation, Methods and Outcomes 1900–1945', *Mariner's Mirror*, 92 (2006), pp. 190–203, on p. 199.
36. R. C. Brown, M. J. Langman and P. M. Lambert, 'Hospital Admissions for Peptic Ulcer During 1958–72', *British Medical Journal*, 1 (1976), pp. 35–7; and J. Higham, J.-Y. Kang and A. Majeed, 'Recent Trends in Admissions and Mortality Due to Peptic Ulcer in England: Increasing Frequency of Haemorrhage Among Older Subjects', *The Gut*, 50 (2002), pp. 460–4.
37. Royal College of General Practitioners Archive, B-FRY A4-2, Practice statistics for Dr J. Fry, 1952–6.
38. J. Fry, 'Five Years of General Practice', *British Medical Journal*, 2 (1957), pp. 1453–7, on p. 1456.
39. Royal College of General Practitioners Archive, B-FRY A4-2, Practice statistics for Dr J. Fry, 1951.
40. H. Bailey and R. J. McNeill Love, *A Short Practice of Surgery* (London: H. K. Lewis, 1949), p. 248.
41. W. P. D. Logan and A. A. Cushion, *General Register Office Studies on Medical and Population Subjects No. 14, Morbidity Statistics from General Practice, Volume 1 (General)* (London: HMSO, 1958), p. 79.
42. D. Kynaston, *Austerity Britain 1945–51* (London: Bloomsbury, 2007), p. 561.
43. See also Chapter 3 'Gender, Stress and Alcohol Abuse', in this volume, by Ali Haggett.

44. The National Archives (hereafter TNA), RG16/123, 167c, R. M. S. McConaghey, 'Collective Investigation, A Historical Review', n.d.
45. TNA RG26/123, 167c, Letter to Dr R. E. Ford, Ministry of Health, 5 May 1955.
46. TNA RG26/123, 167c, Letter to Dr R. J. F. H. Pinsent, 8 June 1954.
47. Royal College of General Practitioners Archive, ACE G23-1, Memorandum, 'The Collection of Morbidity Statistics from General Practice' (n.d.), 1.
48. Research Committee of the College of General Practitioners, 'Report, The Continuing Observation and Recording of Morbidity', *Journal of the College of General Practitioners*, 1 (1958), pp. 107–28, on pp. 112–13.
49. TNA, RG26/124, Memorandum, 2 April 1957.
50. W. P. D. Logan, *General Register Office Studies on Medical and Population Studies, Vol. II, Occupation* (London: HMSO, 1960); and Research Committee of the Council of the College of *General Practitioners, General Register Office Studies on Medical and Population Studies, Vol. III, Disease in General Practice* (London: HMSO, 1962).
51. Logan and Cushion, *Morbidity Statistics from General Practice*, p. 98.
52. Logan and Cushion, *Morbidity Statistics from General Practice*, p. 94.
53. D. O'Neill, 'Dyspepsia', in *The Nature of Stress Disorder, Conference of the Society for Psychosomatic Research* (London: Hutchinson, 1959), pp. 52–60, on p. 53.
54. O'Neill, 'Dyspepsia', p. 53.
55. O'Neill, 'Dyspepsia', p. 55.
56. O'Neill, 'Dyspepsia', p. 56.
57. A. Hurst, 'Indigestion and National Health', *The Practitioner*, 152 (1944), pp. 193–6, on p. 196.
58. Hurst, 'Indigestion and National Health', p. 195.
59. J. Braine, *Room at the Top* (London: Eyre & Spottiswoode, 1957), p. 196.
60. P. Hennessy, *Never Again: Britain 1945–51* (London: Penguin Books, 2006), pp. 459–67.
61. Hurst, 'Indigestion and National Health', p. 196.
62. R. M. Titmuss, *Problems of Social Policy* (London: HMSO, 1950), pp. 55–7.
63. Titmuss, *Social Policy*, p. 201.
64. W. Beveridge, *Social Insurance and Allied Services, Cmnd. 6404* (London: HMSO, 1942), paragraph 8.
65. R. Mackay, *Half the Battle: Civilian Morale in Britain during the Second World War* (Manchester: Manchester University Press, 2002), pp. 221, 231.
66. S. Taylor, *A Natural History of Everyday Life* (London: The Memoir Club, 1988), pp. 277–8.
67. C. Webster, *The National Health Service: A Political History* (Oxford: Oxford University Press, 1998), pp. 6–7.
68. J. Prince, 'A Consumer's View of the National Health Service', in J. Farndale (ed.), *Trends in the National Health Service* (Oxford: Pergamon Press, 1964), pp. 28–41, on p. 29.
69. R. M. Titmuss, *Essays on 'The Welfare State'* (London: George Allen and Unwin, 1958), p. 196.
70. D. Kynaston, *Family Britain 1951–57* (London: Bloomsbury, 2009), pp. 625–6; and Webster, *The National Health Service*, pp. 33–5.
71. S. Taylor, *Good General Practice: A Report of a Survey* (London: Oxford University Press, 1954), p. 223–4.
72. I. Loudon, J. Horder and C. Webster, *General Practice and the National Health Service*

1948–97 (Oxford: Oxford University Press, 1998), pp. 69–70.
73. J. S. Collings, 'General Practice in England Today: A Reconnaissance', *The Lancet*, 1 (1950), pp. 555–85.
74. Taylor, *Good General Practice*, p. 416.
75. R. M. Titmuss, 'The Hospital and its Patients', in J. Farndale (ed.), *Trends in the National Health Service* (Oxford: Pergamon Press, 1964), pp. 273–82, on p. 279.
76. Quoted from Kynaston, *Family Britain*, pp. 626–7.
77. Titmuss, *Essays on 'The Welfare State'*, pp. 201–2.
78. Webster, *The National Health Service,* pp. 38–9.
79. Webster, *The National Health Service*, p. 39.
80. A. Hurst, 'Discussion on Dyspepsia in the Armed Forces', *Proceedings of the Royal Society of Medicine*, 34 (1941), pp. 411–26, on p. 423.
81. J. L. Halliday, 'Concept of a Psychosomatic Affection', *The Lancet*, 2 (1943), pp. 692–6, on p. 692.
82. J. L. Halliday, 'The Incidence of Psychosomatic Affection in Britain', *Psychosomatic Medicine*, 7 (1945), pp. 135–46.
83. Halliday, 'Concept of a Psychosomatic Affection', p. 693; and M. Jackson, *The Age of Stress: Science and the Search for Stability* (Oxford: Oxford University Press, 2013), pp. 91–3.
84. J. L. Halliday, 'Epidemiology and the Psychosomatic Affections', *The Lancet*, 2 (1946), pp. 185–91.
85. R. Hayward, 'Enduring Emotions: James Halliday and the Invention of the Psychosocial', *Isis*, 100 (2009), pp. 827–38, on pp. 827–8.
86. R. M. Titmuss, *Essays on 'The Welfare State'* (London: George Allen and Unwin, 1958), pp. 186–7.
87. J. Rickman, 'The Development of Psychological Medicine', *British Medical Journal*, 1 (1950), pp. 30–7, on p. 37.
88. M. Thomson, *Psychological Subjects: Identity, Culture and Health in Twentieth Century Britain* (Oxford: Oxford University Press, 2006).
89. Anon., 'The Society for Psychosomatic Research', in *The Nature of Stress Disorder, Conference of the Society for Psychosomatic Research* (London: Hutchinson, 1959), p. v.
90. D. K. Henderson, R. D. Gillespie and I. R. C. Batchelor, *A Textbook of Psychiatry* (London: Oxford University Press, 1958), p. 88.
91. Henderson, Gillespie and Batchelor, *A Textbook of Psychiatry*, p. 89.
92. Henderson, Gillespie and Batchelor, *A Textbook of Psychiatry*, p. 88.
93. R. Doll, F. Avery Jones and M. M. Buckatzsch, *Medical Research Council Special Report Series No. 276, Occupational Factors in the Aetiology of Gastric and Duodenal Ulcers with an Estimate of their Incidence in the General Population* (London: HMSO, 1951), pp. 79–80.
94. Doll, Avery Jones and Buckatzsch, *Occupational Factors*, pp. 79–80.
95. Henderson and Gillespie, *Textbook of Psychiatry*, p. 89
96. Jackson, *The Age of Stress*, p. 208.
97. R. M. Titmuss, *Problems of Social Policy* (London: HMSO, 1950), pp. 340.
98. The National Archives (hereafter TNA), FD1/6580, A. Lewis, 'Report on the Incidence of Neurosis, 1942'.
99. C. P. Blacker, *Neurosis and Mental Health Services* (London: Oxford University Press, 1946), p. 174.
100. E. Jones, I. Palmer and S. Wessely, 'War Pensions (1900–1945): Changing Models of

Psychological Understanding', *British Journal of Psychiatry*, 180 (2002), pp. 374–9.
101. J. Bourke, *Fear: A Cultural History* (London: Virago, 2005), pp. 191–2.
102. R. H. Ahrenfeldt, *Psychiatry in the British Army in the Second World War* (London: Routledge, 1958), p. 227.
103. B. Shephard, *War of Nerves, Soldiers and Psychiatrists 1914–1994* (London: Jonathan Cape, 2000), p. 317.
104. TNA, WO32/11125, Brigadier H. A. Sandiford, Minutes of Meeting, 27 September 1944, p. 1.
105. A. Curle, 'Transitional Communities and Social Re-Connection, Part I', *Human Relations*, 1 (1947), pp. 42–68, on p. 64.
106. E. Jones and S. Wessely, 'Prisoners-of-War: From Resilience to Psychological Vulnerability, Reality or Perception', *Twentieth Century British History*, 21 (2010), pp. 163–83.
107. D. Kynaston, *Austerity Britain 1945–51* (London: Bloomsbury, 2007), p. 190–1.
108. Quoted in S. Garfield, *Our Hidden Lives: The Everyday Diaries of Forgotten Britain 1945–1948* (London: Ebury, 2004), pp. 398, 374.
109. I. Hacking, *Rewriting the Soul: Multiple Personality and the Science of Memory* (Princeton, NJ: Princeton University Press, 1995), p. 40.
110. D. Sperber, 'Anthropology and Psychology: Towards an Epidemiology of Representations', *Man*, 20 (1985), pp. 73–89.

9 Smith, 'Food Allergy, Mental Illness and Stress since 1945'

1. R. Mackarness, *Not All in the Mind: How Unsuspected Food Allergy Can Affect Your Body AND Your Mind* (London: Pan Books, 1976).
2. Mackarness, *Not All in the Mind*, p. 18.
3. Mackarness, *Not All in the Mind*, p. 21.
4. Mackarness, *Not All in the* Mind, p. 89.
5. Mackarness, *Not All in the Mind*, p. 24.
6. Mackarness, *Not All in the Mind*, p. 24
7. For more on Feingold, see M. Smith, *An Alternative History of Hyperactivity: Food Additives and the Feingold Diet* (New Brunswick, NJ: Rutgers University Press, 2011).
8. C. Keirns, 'Better than Nature: The Changing Treatment of Asthma and Hay Fever in the United States, 1910–1945', *Studies in History and Philosophy of Science*, 34 (2003), pp. 511–31, on p. 521; and M. Jackson, '"Allergy con Amore": Psychosomatic Medicine and the "Asthmogenic Home" in the Mid-Twentieth Century', in M. Jackson (ed.) *Health and the Modern Home* (New York: Routledge, 2007), pp. 153–74.
9. Jackson, '"Allergy con Amore"', p. 154.
10. M. Smith, 'A Pre-Peanut History of Food Allergy', *Food, Culture, and Society*, 16 (2013), pp. 129–30.
11. H. Collins and T. Pinch, *Dr Golem: How to Think about Medicine* (Chicago, IL: University of Chicago Press, 2005), p. 3. Italics in original.
12. S. Sturdy, 'Looking for Trouble: Medical Science and Clinical Practice in the Historiography of Modern Medicine', *Social History of Medicine*, 24 (2011), pp. 739–59.
13. John Freeman quoted in M. Jackson, *Allergy: The History of a Modern Malady* (London: Reaktion, 2006), pp. 90–1.
14. A. H. Rowe and A. Rowe, Jr., *Food Allergy: Its Manifestations and Control and the Elimination Diets, a Compendium with Important Consideration of Inhalant (Especially Pollen), Drug, and Infectant Allergy*, 2nd edn (Springfield, IL: Charles C. Thomas,

1972), p. 339; and T. W. Clarke, 'Neuro-Allergy in Childhood', *New York State Journal of Medicine*, 42 (1948), pp. 393–7, on p. 393.
15. Clarke, 'Neuro-Allergy', pp. 393–7; and H. M. Davison, 'Cerebral Allergy', *Southern Medical Journal*, 42 (1949), pp. 712–15.
16. H. A. Abramson, 'The Present Status of Allergy', *The Nervous Child*, 7 (1948), pp. 86–101.
17. B. R. Hoobler, 'Some Early Symptoms Suggesting Protein Sensitization in Infancy', *American Journal of Diseases of Children*, 12 (1916), pp. 129–35; W. R. Shannon, 'Neuropathic Manifestations in Infants and Children as a Result of Anaphylactic Reaction to Foods Contained in their Dietary', *American Journal of Disease of Children*, 24 (1922), pp. 89–94; and G. Piness and H. Miller, 'Allergic Manifestations in Infancy and Childhood', *Archives of Pediatrics*, 42 (1925), pp. 557–62.
18. T. W. Clarke, 'The Relation of Allergy to Character Problems in Children', *Annals of Allergy*, 8 (1950), pp. 177–8.
19. Clarke, 'The Relation of Allergy', p. 178.
20. Clarke, 'The Relation of Allergy', p. 178.
21. Clarke, 'The Relation of Allergy', p. 185.
22. Clarke, 'The Relation of Allergy', p. 186.
23. Clarke, 'The Relation of Allergy', p. 183.
24. Clarke, 'The Relation of Allergy', p. 183.
25. W. Kaufman, 'Some Psychosomatic Aspects of Food Allergy', *Psychosomatic Medicine*, 16 (1954), pp. 10–40, on pp. 21, 28, 37.
26. Clarke, 'The Relation of Allergy', p. 186.
27. L. N. Gay, 'Review of *Elimination Diets and the Patient's Allergies: A Handbook of Allergy* by Arthur H. Rowe', *Quarterly Review of Biology*, 20 (1945), p. 183.
28. M. Jackson, '"Allergy con Amore": Psychosomatic Medicine and the "Asthmogenic Home" in the Mid-Twentieth Century', in M. Jackson (ed.) *Health and the Modern Home* (New York: Routledge, 2007), pp. 153–74. For one of the most influential early studies, see T. M. French and F. Alexander, *Psychogenic Factors in Bronchial Asthma* (Washington, DC: Psychosomatic Medicine Monographs, 1941).
29. Jackson, '"Allergy con Amore"', p. 157.
30. Jackson, *Allergy*, p. 89.
31. Abramson, 'Present Status of Allergy', p. 99.
32. According to one advocate of psychosomatic allergy: 'The correctness of certain psychosomatic formulations is repeatedly confirmed by clinical experience', thus emphasizing that inductive reasoning did play a role – L. J. Saul, 'The Relations to the Mother as Seen in Cases of Allergy', *The Nervous Child*, 5 (1946), pp. 332–8, on p. 332.
33. Saul, 'The Relations to the Mother', p. 334.
34. Saul, 'The Relations to the Mother', p. 334. It is interesting that maternal rejection, or fear of maternal rejection, played a pivotal role in each of these cases, since it was often parental smothering that was blamed for psychosomatic allergy – M. Sperling, 'The Role of the Mother in Psychosomatic Disorders in Children', *Psychosomatic Medicine*, 11 (1948), pp. 377–85.
35. F. Deutsch and R. Nadell, 'Psychological Aspects of Dermatology with Special Consideration of Allergic Phenomena', *The Nervous Child*, 5 (1946), pp. 339–64, on p. 339.
36. Deutsch and Nadell, 'Psychological Aspects of Dermatology', p. 355.
37. Deutsch and Nadell, 'Psychological Aspects of Dermatology', p. 355.
38. Deutsch and Nadell, 'Psychological Aspects of Dermatology', p. 344.

39. Deutsch and Nadell, 'Psychological Aspects of Dermatology', p. 463.
40. M. W. Gerard, 'Bronchial Asthma in Children', *The Nervous Child*, 5 (1946), pp. 327–31, on pp. 328, 330; and Saul, 'Relations to the Mother', p. 334.
41. M. Smith, 'Psychiatry Limited: Hyperactivity and the Evolution of American Psychiatry, 1957–1980', *Social History of Medicine*, 21 (2008), pp. 541–59.
42. W. C. Spain, 'Review of *Food Allergy*', *Quarterly Review of Biology*, 28 (1953), pp. 97–8.
43. Spain, 'Review of *Food Allergy*', p. 97.
44. A. H. Rowe, *Elimination Diets and the Patient's Allergies: A Handbook of Allergy*, 2nd edn (London: Henry Kimpton, 1944), p. 33.
45. A cooperative relationship between food allergists and patients – or the patient's parents – has a long history, pre-dating the emergence of the term allergy in 1906, and enduring to this day: A. Jamieson, 'A Discussion on Diet in the Etiology and Treatment of Diseases of the Skin', *British Medical Journal* (30 November 1895), pp. 1351–6, on p. 1353; B. Ratner, 'Diagnosis and Management of the Allergic Child', *Journal of the American Medical Association*, 96 (1931), pp. 570–5, on p. 575; W. C. Alvarez and H. C. Hinshaw, 'Foods that Commonly Disagree with People', *Journal of the American Medical Association*, 104 (1935), pp. 2053–8, on pp. 2053, 2055, 2058; and G. Pollard, 'Practical Application and Hazards of Dietary Management in Food Intolerance', in J. Brostoff and S. J. Challacombe (eds.) *Food Allergy and Intolerance*, 2nd edn (London: Saunders, 2002), p. 908.
46. T. G. Randolph, 'Human Ecology and Susceptibility to the Chemical Environment', *Annals of Allergy*, 19 (1961), pp. 518–40.
47. T. G. Randolph Papers: 1935–91, H MS c183, Harvard Medical Library in the Francis A. Countway Library of Medicine, Center for the History of Medicine, Box 7, Folder 8.
48. T. G. Randolph, 'Allergy as a Causative Factor of Fatigue, Irritability, and Behavior Problems of Children', *Journal of Pediatrics* (1947), pp. 560–72, on p. 562. See also W. Kaufman, 'Some Psychosomatic Aspects of Food Allergy', *Psychosomatic Medicine*, 16 (1954), pp. 30–1. Randolph's ideas about food allergy and fatigue were developed further by Frederic Speer in his 'Allergic Tension Fatigue Syndrome': F. Speer, 'Allergic Tension-Fatigue in Children', *Annals of Allergy*, 12 (1954), pp. 168–71.
49. Randolph, 'Allergy as a Causative Factor', p. 563.
50. C. D. May, 'Food Allergy: A Commentary', *Pediatric Clinics of North America*, 22 (1975), pp. 217–20.
51. Randolph, 'Allergy as a Causative Factor', pp. 569–70.
52. Kaufman, 'Psychosomatic Aspects', p. 31. Kaufman also found notoriety as a proponent of mega-doses of Vitamin B-3 as a treatment for arthritis.
53. Kaufman, 'Psychosomatic Aspects', p. 31.
54. A similar relationship can be identified in M. Murphy, *Sick Building Syndrome and the Problem of Uncertainty: Environmental Politics, Technoscience, and Women Workers* (Durham: Duke University Press, 2006).
55. L. W. Batten, 'Stress in Life and Medical Practice', *Journal of the College of General Practitioners*, 7 (1964), pp. 320–7; R. Viner, 'Putting Stress in Life: Hans Selye and the Making of Stress Theory', *Social Studies of Science*, 29 (1999), pp. 391–410; and M. Jackson, *The Age of Stress: Science and the Search for Stability* (Oxford: Oxford University Press, 2013).
56. N. T. McDermott and S. Cobb, 'A Psychiatric Survey of Fifty Cases of Bronchial Asthma', *Psychosomatic Medicine*, 1 (1939), pp. 203–44, on p. 205.

57. B. F. Feingold, *Introduction to Clinical Allergy* (Springfield, IL: Charles C. Thomas, 1973), p. 190.
58. Feingold, *Introduction*, p. 190.
59. S. T. Selesnick, D. B. Freedman and B. Augenbraun, 'Psychological Management of Childhood Asthma', *California Medicine*, 100 (1964), pp. 406–11, on p. 406.
60. R. H. Crede, C. T. Carman, R. D. Whaley and I. C. Schumacher, 'Dissimilar Allergic Disease in Identical Twins', *California Medicine*, 78 (1953), pp. 25–8, on p. 28.
61. Crede, Carman, Whaley and Schumacher, 'Dissimilar Allergic Disease', p. 27.
62. E. F. Freeman, et al., 'Personality Variables and Allergic Skin Reactivity', *Psychosomatic Medicine*, 29 (1967), pp. 312–22, on p. 320.
63. Freeman, et al., 'Personality Variables', p. 321.
64. B. B. Berle, et al., 'A Clinical Guide to Prognosis in Stress Diseases', *Journal of the American Medical Association*, 149 (1952), pp. 1624–8.
65. Berle, et al., 'A Clinical Guide to Prognosis'. p. 1624.
66. T. H. Holmes, T. Treuting and H. G. Wolff, 'Life Situations, Emotions, and Nasal Disease: Evidence on Summative Effects Exhibited in Patients with "Hay Fever"', *Psychosomatic Medicine*, 13 (1951), pp. 71–82, on p. 71.
67. Holmes, Treuting and Wolff, 'Life Situations, Emotions, and Nasal Disease', p. 76.
68. Holmes, Treuting and Wolff, 'Life Situations, Emotions, and Nasal Disease', p. 76.
69. Holmes, Treuting and Wolff, 'Life Situations, Emotions, and Nasal Disease', p. 76.
70. Holmes, Treuting and Wolff, 'Life Situations, Emotions, and Nasal Disease', p. 77.
71. Holmes, Treuting and Wolff, 'Life Situations, Emotions, and Nasal Disease', p. 77.
72. Holmes, Treuting and Wolff, 'Life Situations, Emotions, and Nasal Disease', p. 81.
73. Berle et al., 'Prognosis in Stress Disease', p. 1624.
74. Jackson, *Age of Stress*, p. 191.
75. R. Mackarness, *Not All in the Mind: How Unsuspected Food Allergy Can Affect Your Body AND Your Mind* (London: Pan Books, 1976), p. 42. Not all food allergists subscribed to Selye's theories. Arthur Coca, for instance, found his ideas to be 'imaginative', but also believed that he misused the term 'adaptation' and that he focused too much on the effects of adaptation, rather than the causes. Randolph Papers: 1935–91, H MS c183, Harvard Medical Library in the Francis A. Countway Library of Medicine, Center for the History of Medicine, Box 7, Folder 11.
76. T. G. Randolph, 'Human Ecology and Susceptibility to the Chemical Environment', *Annals of Allergy*, 19 (1961), pp. 518–50, on pp. 520–1.
77. T. G. Randolph, 'Clinical Ecology as it Affects the Psychiatric Patient', *International Journal of Social Psychiatry*, 12 (1966), pp. 245–54, on p. 248; and Randolph Papers, Box 7, Folder 8.
78. Randolph, 'Human Ecology', p. 523.
79. Randolph, 'Clinical Ecology', p. 248. Italics in original.
80. Randolph Papers, Box 2, Folder 3.
81. Randolph Papers, Box 2, Folder 6.
82. Randolph, 'Human Ecology', p. 530 and pp. 245–54.
83. Randolph Papers, Box 2, Folder 13.
84. Randolph Papers, Box 7, Folder 8. Randolph did offer to present his research to psychiatrists, though most of his overtures went unrewarded.
85. K. Ishizaka, T. Ishizaka, M. M. Hornbrook, 'Physico-Chemical Properties of Human Reaginic Antibody. IV. Presence of a Unique Immunoglobulin as a Carrier of Reaginic Activity', *Journal of Immunology*, 97 (1966), pp. 75–85; and G. Mitman, *Breathing*

Space: How Allergies Shape Our Lives and Landscapes (New Haven, CT: Yale University Press, 2007), p. 194.

86. M. Smith, 'A Pre-Peanut History of Food Allergy', *Food, Culture, and Society*, 16 (2013), pp. 125–43.
87. P. Radetsky, *Allergic to the Twentieth Century* (Boston, MA: Little, Brown and Company, 1997), pp. 113–35.
88. J. S. Lebovidge, H. Strauch, L. A. Kalish and L. C. Schneider, 'Assessment of Psychological Distress Among Children and Adolescents with Food Allergy', *Journal of Allergy and Clinical Immunology*, 124 (2009), pp. 1282–8; A. J. Cummings, R. C. Knibb, M. Erlewynn-Lajeunesse, R. M. King, G. Roberts and J. S. Lucas, 'Management of Nut Allergy Influences Quality of Life and Anxiety in Children and their Mothers', *Pediatric Allergy and Immunology*, 21 (2010), pp. 586–94; and K. M. Roy and M. C. Roberts, 'Peanut Allergy in Children: Relationships to Health-Related Quality of Life, Anxiety, and Parental Stress', *Clinical Pediatrics*, 50 (2011), pp. 1045–51.
89. B. F. Feingold, *Introduction to Clinical Allergy* (Springfield, IL: Charles C. Thomas, 1973), pp. 189–95.
90. Some new research in this area can be found here: C. Liezmann, B. Klapp and E. M. J. Peters, 'Stress, Atopy and Allergy', *Dermatoendocrinology*, 3 (2011), pp. 37–40.
91. R. Mackarness, *Not All in the Mind: How Unsuspected Food Allergy Can Affect Yours Body AND Your Mind* (London: Pan Books, 1976), p. 103.

10 Melling, 'Labouring Stress: Scientific Research, Trade Unions and Perceptions of Workplace Stress in Mid-Twentieth-Century Britain'

1. University College Union, *Tackling Stress in Higher Education* (London: UCU Publications, 2012), p. 8.
2. M. Jackson, *The Age of Stress: Science and the Search for Stability* (Oxford: Oxford University Press, 2013), pp. 69–75.
3. See, for example, C. L. Cooper and P. J. Dewe, *Stress: A Brief History* (London: Blackwell, 2004).
4. A. Young, *The Harmony of Illusions: Inventing Post-Traumatic Stress Disorder* (Princeton, NJ: Princeton University Press, 1995); and D. Cantor and E. Ramsden, 'Introduction', in D. Cantor and E. Ramsden (eds), *Stress, Shock, and Adaptation in the Twentieth Century* (Rochester, NY: University of Rochester Press, 2014), pp. 9–35.
5. Jackson, *Age of Stress*, pp. 14–18, 40–3.
6. J. Kitanaka, 'Work, Stress, and Depression: The Emerging Psychiatric Science of Work in Contemporary Japan', in Cantor and Ramsden (eds), *Stress, Shock, and Adaptation*, pp. 342–65.
7. A. Booth and J. Melling, 'Workplace Cultures and Business Performance: British Labour Relations and Industrial Output in Comparative Perspective', in J. Melling and A. Booth (eds), *Managing the Modern Workplace: Productivity, Politics and Workplace Culture in Postwar Britain* (Aldershot: Ashgate, 2008), pp. 1–26.
8. Modern Record Centre, Warwick University, Trades Union Congress Papers (hereafter TUC), MSS 292, D/847.38/2, Minutes of Social Insurance Committee (SIC), 'Mental Stress at Work', 10 October 1973. By 1972 mental illness accounted for 36.5 million working days lost 'through industrial injuries and diseases', a figure that had increased significantly in the fifteen years to 1968 – TUC MSS 292 D/847.38/2, Memorandum

of Peter Jacques of Social Insurance Department to Len Murray, 7 March 1974.

9. C. Sellers and J. Melling, 'Towards a Trans-national Industrial Hazard History: Charting the Circulation of Workplace Dangers, Debates and Expertise', *British Journal of the History of Science*, 45 (2012), pp. 401–24.
10. J. Melling, 'Making Sense of Workplace Fear: The Role of Physicians, Psychiatrists, and Labor in Reframing Occupational Strain in Industrial Britain, *c.*1850–1970' in Cantor and Ramsden (eds), *Stress, Shock, and Adaptation*, pp. 292–341.
11. National Archives (hereafter NA), Medical Research Council (hereafter MRC), FD 9/4158, A. Macauslan to Dr R. C. Norton of MRC, 11 October 1974; FD 9/4392, 'Commissions from the Department of Employment: Occupational Stress and Well-Being', 'DE/MRC Specific Commission No. 227: Occupational Stress and Well-Being' (Draft, *c.* March 1977); and Gilbert Jessup to A.V. Dalton, 16 March 1977, regarding SAPU.
12. FD 9/4367, 'Literature Survey of Mental Stress in Industry', 'Minutes of an Informal Meeting at MRC to Discuss the Survey of the Literature on Mental Stress in Industry', 27 January 1976 (minutes dated 18 February 1976); John Alwen to K. F. H. (Hywel) Murrell, 20 February 1976, following meeting of Alwen and Jessup, 27 January 1976; and Alwen to Jessup, 27 February 1976.
13. FD 9/4158, Notes on Visit to Cambridge 16 December 1974, dated 18 December 1974.
14. FD 9/4160, 'Me[n]tal Stresses in Industry: Potential Commissions for the Department of Employment', 'Background Note' (dated 9 September 1980).
15. FD 9/4367, 'Literature Survey', 'Minutes' 27 January 1976; and FD 9/4158, F. B. Loder of MRC to Dr Harry Kay, 26 February 1975. Kay was, at this period, Vice-Chancellor of the University of Exeter.
16. TUC, 292 D/847.38.7, David Basnett to Victor Feather, 5 September 1973; TUC, Larry Whitty to Trevor Mawer, 22 September 1975; TUC, 292 D/847.38/2, Harry Unwin of Transport and General Workers' Union to Jacques, 13 January 1976; and Alan Fisher of National Union of Public Employees to Jacques, 29 January 1976.
17. TUC, 292 D/847.38/2, Minute 'Mental Stress at Work', Minutes of SIC, 10 October 1973.
18. TUC, 292 D/847.38/2, Minutes of Social Insurance Committee, 8 May 1974; and Meeting at Employment Medical Advisory Service (EMAS), with Confederation of British Industry and TUC to discuss 'Mental Stress', 22 August 1974. Jacques and Rea pressed for research into production lines at British Leyland.
19. Minutes of Social Insurance Committee, Minutes of Meeting on Mental Stress in Industry at MRC, 18 April 1975.
20. Minutes of Social Insurance Committee, D. E. Broadbent to Mawer, 20 August 1975, emphasizing that he was 'purely interested in having a look at the sort of job which worries people'.
21. Minutes of Social Insurance Committee, Mawer to Jacques, re. Memorandum: 'Mental Stress in Industry', 21 April 1975. W. B. Spry of the HSE and Jessup advised the DE's Scientists' Committee on 'psychological stress' and mental illness, including assembly lines 'commonly identified' as 'areas of high stress'. J. A. Tannahill, EMAS, to Jacques, 7 October 1974; Spry to T Moores [sic], 30 September 1975, regarding the 'Goldberg Questionnaire'; Extract of Minutes of Social Insurance Committee of TUC, 9 March 1976; and Clive Jenkins of Association of Scientific, Technical and Managerial Staffs (ASTMS) to Peter Jacques of TUC's SIC, 8 January 1976, enclosing report from

ASTMS Research Department which noted that there were no satisfactory agreed indicators of 'stress'.

22. FD 9/4367, 'Literature Survey of Mental Stress in Industry', 'Minutes of an Informal Meeting at MRC to Discuss the Survey of the Literature on Mental Stress in Industry', 27 January 1976 (minutes dated 18 February 1976). See also J. Alwen to G. Jessup, 27 February 1976, noting their interest in 'The Physiological and Behavioural Correlates of Psychological Well-Being at Work'.
23. FD 9/4158, A. Macauslan (Secretary to DE Chief Scientists' Committee) to Dr R. C. Norton of MRC, 11 October 1974; FD 9/4392, 'Commissions from the Department of Employment: Occupational Stress and Well-being', 'De/MRC Specific Commission No. 227: Occupational Stress and Well-being' (Draft, *c.* March 1977); and Jessup to A. V. Dalton, 16 March 1977, regarding funding for research at the MRC's Social and Applied Research Unit (SAPU). The DE statement in the 'Research Statement' defining stress measured by 'psychophysiological symptoms' can be clearly distinguished from the MRC 'summary of research to be undertaken'.
24. FD 9/4158, Notes on Visit to Cambridge, 16 December 1974, notes dated 18 December 1974, unsigned but probably composed by Dr Faulkner of MRC.
25. FD 1/7303, MRC Committee on Industrial Psychology, Minutes of CIP Meeting, 8 February 1935; MRC, 'Proposals for Further Work in Industrial Psychology', 17 April 1935; and F. C. Bartlett to D. Munro, 17 February 1936.
26. LAB 19/10, Ministry of Labour and National Service, 'Joint Experiment in the Application of Psychological Method to Vocational Guidance by the Industrial Health Research Board and the Ministry of Labour', copy of letter of James Drever to Munro (no date but *c.* June 1935); B. R. Hunter to J. D. Blake, 4 July 1935; Emmerson to Matson, 19 July 1935; Gordon Lee to Wolfe, Ministry of Labour, 11 December 1934; and Eric Farmer [to Munro?] 29 May 1935. L. Gordon Lee to Tribe at office of Commissioner for Special Areas, 12 February 1935, noted that 'Dunfermline experiment' had been carried out at 'the Institute', possibly the NIIP, as well as conflict of Myers and Munro over Juvenile Advisory Councils. To smooth over Myers, who agreed to re-join the IHRB, the Ministry of Labour suggested research in Kent – Gordon Lee to Emmerson, 18 February 1935, 'Industrial Psychology. Memorandum by the Secretary on Scheme of Research ... for the Industrial Health Research Board' (unsigned but written by Munro, December 1934), 1–3; Memorandum of Lee for Humbert Wolfe, Ministry of Labour, 11 December 1934; Lee to B.R. Hunter, 14 December 1934; and B.R. Hunter to Gordon Lee, 15 December 1934. By 1937 the IHRB was chaired by the Glasgow physiologist, Professor E. P. Cathcart. The Psychology Committee included Burt as Chairman, Bartlett, Myers, Sherrington, P. E. Vernon, S. Wyatt and Munro.
27. LAB 19/10, Ministry of Labour and National Service, 'Joint Experiment in the Application of Psychological Method to Vocational Guidance by the Industrial Health Research Board and the Ministry of Labour', 'Industrial Psychology. Memorandum by the Secretary on Scheme of Research ... for the Industrial Health Research Board' (unsigned but written by Munro, December 1934), 5. The IHRB Committee on Industrial Psychology, Minutes, 8 February 1935, FD 1/7303, noted that Rosenfield was 'no longer anxious' to carry out this research. See also FD 3/77, S. Wyatt and J. N. Langdon, 'Preface', in *MRC, IHRB, Report 77: Fatigue and Boredom in Repetitive Work.*
28. FD 3/77, Wyatt and Langdon, *Fatigue and Boredom in Repetitive Work,* p. 28. The study (p. 49) noted that fear of unemployment was the greatest single factor influencing workers, yet the statistics suggested 'Fatigue caused by work' as well as room

temperature was a more important specific cause of dissatisfaction (p. 56).

29. FD 3/82, S. Wyatt and J. N. Langdon, 'Preface', in *MRC, IHRB, Report 82: The Machine and the Worker: A Study of Machine-Feeding Processes,* pp. 11, 13, 16, 18, 39–40, 44.
30. Wyatt and Langdon, *The Machine and the Worker,* pp. 20, 34–5.
31. FD 1/4006, 'Selection of Industrial Workers in War Time', Bartlett, 'Psychological Laboratory Cambridge, Progress Report, 1940–41', 7 August 1941; and Munro to Farmer, 5 October 1939.
32. FD 1/4006, 'Selection of Industrial Workers in War Time', E. F[armer], 'Note on a Visit to the Brush Engineering Works, Loughborough', 27 May 1942. Farmer annotated his report with the comment that the firm was 'now applying our test'. See also Chapter 6, 'Cultural Change', by Debbie Palmer, and Chapter 7, 'Men and Women Under Stress', by Mark Jackson in this volume.
33. NA, Ministry of Labour and National Service, LAB 19/10, 'Joint Experiment in the Application of Psychological Method to Vocational Guidance by the Industrial Health Research Board and the Ministry of Labour', J. G. S[pens?] to Emmerson, 28 May 1937; FD 1/4006, 'Selection of Industrial Workers in War Time' [File inscribed 'Psychological Work – Cambridge: General']; F. Bartlett, 'Progress Report, 1940–41', in which he noted that Farmer and Botopf's army testing had been assisted by Rodger, Anstey and Davies and that 'experience gained from this work has gradually converted the Army from scepticism on the matter of psychological selection tests'; and Farmer to Landsborough Thomson at MRC, 2 March 1942.
34. FD 1/4006, E. F[armer], 'Selection of Industrial Workers in War Time', [File inscribed, 'Psychological Work – Cambridge: General'], 3–4, 8–9; E. F[armer], 'Note on a Visit to the Brush Engineering Works, Loughborough', 27 May 1942; and Farmer, 'Progress Report', 7 July 1942.
35. FD 1/4006, Eric Farmer to Munro, 5 October 1939 and Farmer to Landsborough Thomson at MRC, 2 March 1942, bemoaning the failure to apply the test developed by him and Alice Heim for Ministry of Labour. Employers such as Brush Electrical Engineering (BEE) were keen to utilize the test – F. Simmonds of BEE to IHRB, 15 April 1942.
36. FD 1/4006, 'Selection of Industrial Workers in War Time'. Farmer's army experiments were assisted by Rodger, Anstey and Davies, all army personnel, though Rodger was previously employed by the NIIP. See: Bartlett to Mellanby, 27 April 1941; Mellanby to Bartlett, 13 May 1941; Eric Farmer to Munro 5 October 1939; and Farmer to Landsborough Thomson at MRC, 2 March 1942.
37. FD 1/7303, MRC Committee on Industrial Psychology, Bartlett to Munro, 23 February 1937.
38. FD 1/7307, Minutes of Occupational Psychology Committee of MRC, 18 January 1949, with Bartlett as Chair, where Bartlett said of the Tavistock research, 'if at the end of another year, a similar report were submitted, he himself would certainly not recommend that the Medical Research Council should continue to be responsible for the work'.
39. LAB 14 /315, 'Industrial Health Advisory Committee, Minutes', Meeting 5 April 1943; Charles Hill of BMA to D. C. Barnes of Ministry of Labour, 23 February 1944; C. Hill, 'The Future of Medical Services in Industry'; Hill to Barnes, 19 September 1944; IHAC Minutes, 7 November 1944; and Hill to Barnes, 4 December 1944.
40. FD 1/4027, 'Satisfaction and Discontent Among Production Workers, 1946–50', by

R. Marriott (31 May 1948); J. Wyatt and R. Marriot, 'Vauxhall Motors Ltd. Results of Interviewing a Sample of Men on Production Work', pp. 12–24, 36, 52–5, 65–7; and note by 'R. M[arriott]', 20 December 1946. The research was conducted from November 1946 to June 1947. Initial reports were read by Joan Faulkner of the MRC, who also figured in 1970s research discussions – Marriott to Faulkner, 23 December 1946. Marriott noted the concern was not with 'individual reaction' to working conditions since this would involve a careful (probably 'psychiatric') analysis of personal, domestic and non-work environment as well as working life. See Memorandum, 10 February 1950, to the Secretary of MReC on the decision not to publish results in a formal report.

41. FD 1/4027, Wyatt and Marriott, 'Vauxhall Motors Ltd. Results of Interviewing', pp. 42, 69–71.
42. FD 1/4027, Wyatt and Marriott, 'Vauxhall Motors Ltd. Results of Interviewing', pp. 56–8.
43. FD 1/4027, 'Satisfaction and Discontent Among Production Workers, 1946–50', 'Interim Report' (no date); and Marriott to Joan Faulkner, 6 October 1947. Wyatt and Marriott cooperated with Morris Motor Company rather than reluctant Austin. Marriott to Faulkner, 15 October 1947, 29 November 1947; and J. Melling, 'Fordism and the Foreman: Labour Relations and Supervisory Trade Unionism in the American and British Automobile Industries, 1939–1970', in J. Melling and A. Booth (eds), *Managing the Modern Workplace: Productivity, Politics and Workplace Culture in Postwar Britain* (Aldershot: Ashgate, 2008), pp. 27–48.
44. FD 9/4367, 'Literature Survey of Mental Stress in Industry', Hywel Murrell, 'Work STRESS and Mental STRAIN', 27 January 1976, pp. 35–9.
45. J. Melling, 'Making Sense of Workplace Fear: The Role of Physicians, Psychiatrists, and Labor in Reframing Occupational Strain in Industrial Britain, *c.* 1850–1970', in D. Cantor and E. Ramsden (eds), *Stress, Shock, and Adaptation in the Twentieth Century* (Rochester, NY: University of Rochester Press, 2014).
46. D. E. Broadbent, *Decision and Stress* (London: Academic Press, 1971).
47. Modern Records Centre, TUC 292 D/847.38.7, Larry Whitty to Trevor Mawer, 22 September 1975.
48. National Archives, MRC, FD 9/4160, 'Me[n]tal Stresses in Industry: Potential Commissions for the Department of Employment', 'Background Note' (dated 9 September 1980).
49. FD 9/4367, 'Literature Survey of Mental Stress in Industry', 'Minutes of an Informal Meeting at MRC to Discuss the Survey of the Literature on Mental Stress in Industry', 27 January 1976 (minutes dated 18 February 1976).
50. FD 9/4367, 'Literature Survey of Mental Stress in Industry', Hywel Murrell, 'WORK STRESS and Mental STRAIN', pp. 3–4, 5–6, 10–11, 15, 20–1. Murrell emphasized the limited utility of applying the physiological idea of homeostasis to psychology ('psychology does not have its Selye'), where no settled state can be said to exist, arguing in favour of descriptions of 'work pressures' and 'strain'. Lazarus's concern with 'coping' moved attention to personality traits and response to different life experiences. Murrell commended Kornhauser's Detroit study of workers' mental well-being rather than mental illness.
51. Murrell, 'Literature Survey of Mental Stress in Industry', pp. 15, 20–1, 27–31. Fraser's wartime study had discovered that 8.5 per cent of males and 12.7 per cent of females showed 'definite neurosis', and an additional one fifth of males and slightly more females displayed 'minor neuroses'. See FD 9/4159, MRC, 'Mental Stress in Industry:

Potential Commissions from Department of Employment', Report of a Meeting of 14 December 1976, Murrell presentation, 'Survey of the Literature on Mental Stress in Industry', pp. 3–4.

52. FD 9/4159, 'Mental Stress in Industry: Potential Commissions from Department of Employment', Report of a Meeting of 14 December 1976, Draft Minutes of the Meeting and Discussion, pp. 2–5 – proposed projects included 'the foreman' and 'the woman'. Sylvia Shimmin argued for laboratory as well as fieldwork study of physiological and psychological changes among workers, while Dennis Gath (a hospital psychiatrist who collaborated with Broadbent of the Experimental Psychology Department at Oxford) suggested an analysis that combined a survey of psychiatric medical records with screening of workers. Tom Cox, from Nottingham, outlined 'Psychological Models of Occupational Stress' as a research proposal.
53. FD 9/4392, 'Commissions from the Department of Employment: Occupational Stress and Well-being', File Note 'Telephone Conversation with Mr. Sell (DE) – 5 January 1977'.
54. FD 9/4392, 'Commissions from the Department of Employment: Occupational Stress and Well-being', 'Note of a Meeting Held on 23 February 1977 ... [re] DE Commissioning Work on Occupational Stress at the MRC Social and Applied Psychology Unit'; and FD 9/4159, MRC, 'Mental Stress in Industry: Potential Commissions from Department of Employment', John Alwen to Ivor Batchelor, 14 March 1977.
55. FD 9/4159, 'Mental Stress in Industry: Potential Commissions from Department of Employment', Report of a Meeting of 14 December 1976: Dennis Gath, 'A Psychiatrist's Approach to Mental Stress in Industry', pp. 2–3; and Sylvia Shimmin, 'Difficulties Attaching to the Formulation and Implementation of Research on Mental Stress in Industry'.
56. For discussion of their transactional model of occupational stress, see T. Cox and C. Mackay, 'A Psychological Model for Occupational Stress', p. 8, in FD 9/4159, 'Mental Stress in Industry: Potential Commissions from Department of Employment', Report of a Meeting of 14 December 1976.
57. FD 9/4159, 'Mental Stress in Industry: Potential Commissions from Department of Employment', Report of a Meeting of 14 December 1976: Donald Broadbent, 'Proposed Study of Assembly-Line Workers'.
58. TUC 292 D/847.38.7, D. E. Broadbent to Mawer, 20 August 1975.
59. TUC 292 D/847.38.7, W. B. Spry (SEMA Mental Health) of HSE to T Moores (sic), 30 September 1975. Goldberg wrote *The Detection of Psychiatric Illness by Questionnaire*.
60. TUC 292 D/847.38.7, Alan Fisher of National Union of Public Employees (NUPE) to Jacques, 29 January 1976; Extract of Minutes of SIIWC of 9 March 1976; and Len Murray, General Secretary of TUC, to J. M. Service of Confederation of Shipbuilding and Engineering Unions, 3 May 1976, requesting cooperation.
61. TUC 292 D/847.38.7, Harry Unwin of Transport and General Workers' Union (TGWU) to Jacques, 13 January 1976. TGWU suggested Ford plants at Dagenham and Halewood as well as the Joseph Lucas plant and the British Steel Corporation plant at Ebbw Vale.
62. FD 9/4159, 'Mental Stress in Industry: Potential Commissions from Department of Employment', John Alwen to Ivor Batchelor, 14 March 1977; FD 9/4392, 'Commissions from the Department of Employment: Occupational Stress and Well-being', Note by D.R. James, 'Telephone Conversation with Mr Sell (DE) – 18 August 1978'. F. J. Bayliss of Department of Employment (DE) to R. C. Norton of MRC, 27 September 1978.
63. FD 9/4159, 'Mental Stress in Industry: Potential Commissions from Department of

Employment', Report of a Meeting of 14 December 1976, Joan Faulkner to Alwen, 4 March 1977.

64. FD 9/4160, 'Me[n]tal Stresses in Industry: Potential Commissions for the Department of Employment', Report on commissioned research for Neurosciences Board (dated February 1981). Neurosciences Board Meeting Minutes, 17 February 1981, noted that reports indicate research was 'interesting', though 'the quality was rather variable'.
65. J. Melling and A. Booth, 'Waiting for Thatcher? Trade Unionism, Labour Politics and Shop Floor Bargaining in Post-war Britain', in J. Melling and A. Booth (eds), *Managing the Modern Workplace: Productivity, Politics and Workplace Culture in Postwar Britain* (Aldershot: Ashgate, 2008), pp. 125–63.
66. http://www.hse.gov.uk/stress, 'Making the Stress Management Standards Work: How to Apply the Standard in your Workplace'; and http://www.tuc.org.uk/stress [both accessed 20 February 2010]. Impacts of stress include high absenteeism, increased labour turnover, poor morale, difficult labour relations and increased risk of accidents and illness.
67. J. Melling, 'Making Sense of Workplace Fear: The Role of Physicians, Psychiatrists, and Labor in Reframing Occupational Strain in Industrial Britain, *c.*1850–1970', in D. Cantor and E. Ramsden (eds), *Stress, Shock, and Adaptation in the Twentieth Century* (Rochester, NY: University of Rochester Press, 2014), pp. 189–221.
68. C. Sellers and J. Melling, 'Towards a Trans-national Industrial Hazard History: Charting the Circulation of Workplace Dangers, Debates and Expertise', *British Journal of the History of Science*, 45 (2012), pp. 401–24.

11 Creating 'The Social': Stress, Domesticity and Attempted Suicide

1. J. Butler, *Bodies that Matter: On the Discursive Limits of Sex* (London: Routledge, 1993); and T. Dixon, *From Passions to Emotions: the Creation of a Secular Psychological Category* (Cambridge: Cambridge University Press, 2003).
2. I. Hacking, *Rewriting the Soul* (Princeton, NJ: Princeton University Press, 1995), p. 236.
3. J. Moncrieff, *Myth of the Chemical Cure* (Basingstoke: Palgrave Macmillan, 2007), p. 6.
4. Moncrieff, *Myth of the Chemical Cure*, p. xi.
5. D. S. Goldstein and I. J. Kopin, 'Evolution of Concepts of Stress', *Stress: The International Journal on the Biology of Stress*, 10 (2007), pp. 109–20, on p. 110.
6. R. S. Lazarus and S. Folkman, *Stress, Appraisal and Coping* (New York: Springer, 1984), p.1.
7. W. B. Cannon, *Bodily Changes in Pain, Hunger, Fear and Rage* (New York: D. Appleton & Co., 1929); and W. B. Cannon, 'Organization for Physiological Homeostasis', *Physiological Reviews*, 9 (1929), pp. 299–431.
8. For example, T. H. Holmes and R. H. Rahe, 'The Social Readjustment Rating Scale', *Journal of Psychosomatic Research*, 11 (1967), pp. 213–18.
9. Holmes and Masuda quoted in C. L. Cooper and P. Dewe, *Stress: A Brief History* (Oxford: Blackwell, 2004), p. 42.
10. M. Jackson, *The Age of Stress: Science and the Search for Stability* (Oxford: Oxford University Press, 2013).
11. A. Young, *The Harmony of Illusions: Inventing Post-Traumatic Stress Disorder* (Princeton, NJ: Princeton University Press, 1995).
12. D. Armstrong, *Political Anatomy of the Body: Medical Knowledge in Britain in the Twentieth Century* (Cambridge: Cambridge University Press, 1983), p. 8.

13. Armstrong, *Political Anatomy*, p. 10
14. J. Donzelot, *The Policing of Families*, trans. R. Hurley (Baltimore, MD: Johns Hopkins University Press, 1979).
15. Armstrong, *Political Anatomy*, p. 100.
16. C. Webster 'Review: David Armstrong, *Political Anatomy of the Body*', *Medical History*, 28 (1984), pp. 335–6, on p. 335
17. T. Pearce, 'From "Circumstances" to "Environment": Herbert Spencer and the Origins of the Idea of Organism-Environment Interaction', *Studies in History and Philosophy of Biological and Biomedical Sciences*, 41 (2010), pp. 241–52.
18. M. Poovey, *Making a Social Body: British Cultural Formation, 1830–1864* (Chicago, IL: University of Chicago Press, 1995).
19. M. Jones, *Social Psychiatry in Practice: The Idea of the Therapeutic Community* (Harmondsworth: Penguin, 1968).
20. T. Harrison and D. Clarke, 'The Northfield Experiments', *The British Journal of Psychiatry*, 160 (1992), pp. 698–708.
21. A. Curle and E. L. Trist, 'Transitional Communities and Social Reconnection (part 1)', *Human Relations*, 1:2 (1947), pp. 42–68.
22. G. Rose and D. J. P. Barker, 'What is Epidemiology?', *British Medical Journal*, 2 (1978), pp. 803–4, on p. 803.
23. M. Shepherd, 'Prologue: A Critical Appraisal of Contemporary Psychiatry', in M. Shepherd (ed.), *The Psychosocial Matrix of Psychiatry: Collected Papers* (London: Tavistock, 1983), p. 20.
24. M. Parascandola, 'Epidemiology in Transition: Tobacco and Lung Cancer in the 1950s', in G. Jorland, A. Opinel and G. Weisz (eds), *Body Counts: Medical Quantification in Historical and Sociological Perspective* (Ithaca, NY: McGill-Queen's University Press, 2005), p. 226.
25. Jorland et al. (eds), *Body Courts*, p. 227.
26. A. D. Gardner, 'Debauchery of Honest Words', *British Medical Journal*, 1 (1952), p. 715.
27. A. Clare, 'Obituary: Professor Michael Shepherd', *The Independent*, 30 August 1995.
28. M. Shepherd, 'Epidemiology and Clinical Psychiatry', *British Journal of Psychiatry*, 133 (1978), pp.289–98, on p. 289.
29. R. de Alarcón, 'The Spread of Heroin Abuse in a Community', *Bulletin on Narcotics (United Nations)*, 21:3 (1969), pp.17–22, on p. 21.
30. Letter from G. M. Carstairs to H. Himsworth (MRC Secretary) dated 1 July 1959, The National Archives (TNA): PRO FD 7/1043.
31. G. Rosen, 'Social Stress and Mental Disease from the Eighteenth Century to the Present: Some Origins of Social Psychiatry', *Milbank Memorial Fund Quarterly*, 37:1 (1959), pp. 5–32, on p. 28.
32. R. Hayward, 'Sadness in Camberwell: Imagining Stress and Constructing History in Postwar Britain', in D. Cantor and E. Ramsden (eds), *Stress, Shock, and Adaptation in the Twentieth Century* (Rochester: University of Rochester Press), p. 320–42.
33. M. Jackson, *The Age of Stress: Science and the Search for Stability* (Oxford: Oxford University Press, 2013), p. 171.
34. A. Lewis, 'Social Aspects of Psychiatry: Part I', *Edinburgh Medical Journal*, 58:5 (1951), pp. 214–47, on p. 215.
35. Armstrong, *Political Anatomy*, p. 102.
36. Armstrong, *Political Anatomy*, p. 114.

37. Hayward, 'Sadness in Camberwell', p. 320.
38. O. Anderson, 'Prevention of Suicide and Parasuicide: What can we Learn from History?', *Journal of the Royal Society of Medicine*, 82 (1989), pp. 640–2, on p. 642.
39. C. Millard, 'Reinventing Intention: "Self-Harm" and the "Cry for Help" in Postwar Britain', *Current Opinion in Psychiatry*, 25 (2012), pp. 503–7.
40. E. Stengel and N. Cook, *Attempted Suicide: Its Social Significance and Effects* (London: Chapman and Hall, 1958), p. 22. Original emphasis.
41. Stengel and Cook, *Attempted Suicide*, p. 116; and M. Woodside, 'Attempted Suicides Arriving at a General Hospital', *British Medical Journal*, 2 (1958), pp. 411–14, on p. 411.
42. N. Kessel, 'Self-Poisoning (2)', *British Medical Journal*, 2 (1965), pp. 1336–40, on p. 1336.
43. N. Kessel and W. McCulloch. 'Repeated Acts of Self-Poisoning and Self-Injury', *Proceedings of the Royal Society of Medicine*, 59:2 (1966), pp. 89–92, on p. 91.
44. I. S. Kreeger, 'Initial Assessment of Suicidal Risk', *Proceedings of the Royal Society of Medicine*, 59:2 (1966), pp. 92–6, on p. 92.
45. Kreeger, 'Initial Assessment', p. 93.
46. W. McCulloch and A. E. Philip, *Suicidal Behaviour* (Oxford: Pergamon, 1972), p. 31. Original emphasis.
47. N. Kessel, 'Self-Poisoning (1)', *British Medical Journal*, 2 (1965), pp. 1265–70, on p. 1269.
48. J. Ruesch and G. Bateson, *Communication: The Social Matrix of Psychiatry* (New York: W. W. Norton, 1951), p. 3.
49. Ruesch and Bateson, *Communication*, pp. 50, 78.
50. Ruesch and Bateson, *Communication*, p. 79.
51. R. Jack, *Women and Attempted Suicide* (London: Lawrence Erlbaum, 1992), p. 21.
52. N. Kessel, 'Self-Poisoning (1)', *British Medical Journal*, 2 (1965), pp. 1265–70, on p. 1270.
53. V. Long, '"Often There is a Good Deal to be Done, but Socially Rather than Medically": The Psychiatric Social Worker as Social Therapist, 1945–70', *Medical History*, 55 (2011), pp. 223–39, on p. 225.
54. J. Stewart, '"I Thought you Would Want to Come and See his Home": Child Guidance and Psychiatric Social Work in Inter-War Britain', in M. Jackson (ed.), *Health and the Modern Home* (New York: Routldege, 2007), pp. 111–12.
55. N. K. Hunnybun, 'Psychiatric Social Work', in C. Morris (ed.), *Social Case-Work in Great Britain* (London: Faber and Faber, 1950), p. 105.
56. Hunnybun, 'Psychiatric Social Work', p. 103.
57. Long, '"Good Deal to be Done"', p. 226.
58. E. L. Younghusband, *Social Work in Britain: A Supplementary Report on the Employment and Training of Social Workers* (Dunfermline: Carnegie United Kingdom Trust, 1951), p. 81.
59. E. L. Younghusband, *Social Work in Britain, 1950–1975: A Follow-up Study* (London: Allen and Unwin, 1978), p. 165.
60. R. M. Titmuss, 'Community Care: Fact or Fiction?', in R. M. Titmuss (ed.), *Commitment to Welfare* (1961; London: George Allen and Unwin, 1968), p. 105.
61. J. Bowlby 'Maternal Care and Mental Health' (Geneva: World Health Organization, 1951).
62. A. Storr, 'Bowlby (Edward) John Mostyn (1907–1990)', in *Oxford Dictionary of Na-*

tional Biography (Oxford: Oxford University Press, 2004).
63. A. Lewis, 'Social Aspects of Psychiatry: Part I', *Edinburgh Medical Journal*, 58:5 (1951), pp. 214–17, on p. 215.
64. Younghusband, *Social Work in Britain, 1950–1975*, p. 165.
65. J. P. Nursten 'Editor's Foreword' to A. Munro and J. W. McCulloch, *Psychiatry for Social Workers*, 2nd edn (Oxford: Pergamon Press, 1975), p. xiii.
66. G. W. Brown et al., 'Influence of Family Life on the Course of Schizophrenic Illness', *British Journal of Preventive & Social Medicine*, 16:2 (1962), pp. 55–68.
67. F. Post, 'Mental Breakdown in Old Age', *British Medical Journal*, 1 (1951), pp. 436–40.
68. F. Post and J. Wardle, 'Family Neurosis and Family Psychosis', *British Journal of Psychiatry*, 108 (1962), pp.147–58, on p. 147.
69. N. Rose, *Governing the Soul: The Shaping of the Private Self* (London: Free Association Press, 1999), p. 171.
70. Rose, *Governing the Soul*, p. 175.
71. M. Thomson, *Psychological Subjects: Identity, Culture, and Health in Twentieth-Century Britain* (Oxford: Oxford University Press, 2006), p. 269.
72. G. Eghigian, A. Killen and C. Leuenberger, 'The Self as Project: Politics and the Human Sciences in the Twentieth Century', *Osiris*, 22 (2007), pp. 1–25, on p. 22.
73. Rose, *Governing the Soul*, pp. 155–81, 205–13.
74. Rose, *Governing the Soul*, p. 178.
75. Stewart, '"See his Home"', p. 117.
76. Stewart, '"See his Home"', p. 118.
77. Stewart, '"See his Home"', p. 118.
78. J. Faulkner 'Note on Visit to the Unit for Research on the Epidemiology of Psychiatric Illness Edinburgh', 9 November 1962, dated 29 January 1963 pp. 1–2, The National Archives (TNA): PRO FD 12/408.
79. E. Irvine, 'Psychiatric Social Work', in Younghusband, *Social Work in Britain, 1950–1975*, p. 180.
80. N. Kessel and E. M. Lee, 'Attempted Suicide in Edinburgh' *Scottish Medical Journal*, 7 (1962), pp. 130–5, on p. 130.
81. Kessel and Lee, 'Attempted Suicide in Edinburgh', p. 130n.
82. N. Kessel, W. McCulloch and E. Simpson, 'Psychiatric Service in a Centre for the Treatment of Poisoning', *British Medical Journal*, 2 (1963), pp. 985–8, on p. 987.
83. Kessel, McCulloch and Simpson, 'Psychiatric Service', p. 985.
84. Kessel, McCulloch and Simpson, 'Psychiatric Service', p. 985.
85. N. Kessel, 'Attempted Suicide', *The Lancet*, 281 (1963), p. 448.
86. Kessel, 'Self-Poisoning (1)', p. 1267.
87. J. Lewis, 'Public Institution and Private Relationship: Marriage and Marriage Guidance, 1920–1968', *Twentieth Century British History*, 1 (1990), pp. 233–63.
88. E. Heimler, *Mental Illness and Social Work* (Harmondsworth: Penguin, 1967), p. 55.
89. Irvine, 'Psychiatric Social Work', p. 194.
90. Kessel and Lee, 'Attempted Suicide in Edinburgh', p. 134.
91. N.Timms, *Psychiatric Social Work in Great Britain (1939-1962)* (London: Routledge & Kegan Paul), p. 117.
92. Kessel, 'Self-Poisoning (2)', *British Medical Journal*, 2 (1965), pp. 1336–40, on p. 1337.
93. W. McCulloch and A. E. Philip, *Suicidal Behaviour* (Oxford: Pergamon, 1972), p. 20.
94. J. H. Wallis, *Marriage Guidance: A New Introduction* (London: Routledge & Kegan Paul, 1968), p. 105.

95. Kessel, 'Self-Poisoning (2)', pp. 1336–7.
96. Kessel and Lee, 'Attempted Suicide in Edinburgh', p. 134.
97. Kessel, 'Self-Poisoning (1)', p. 1267.
98. Kessel, 'Self-Poisoning (1)', p. 1267.
99. E. Slater and M. Woodside, *Patterns of Marriage: A Study of Marriage Relationships in the Urban Working Classes* (London: Cassell, 1951), p. 15.
100. A classic statement is E. Showalter, *The Female Malady: Women, Madness and English Culture 1830–1980* (London: Virago, 1987).
101. A. Haggett, 'Housewives, Neuroses and the Domestic Environment in Britain, 1945–1970', in Jackson (ed.), *Health and the Modern Home* (New York: Routledge, 2007), p. 84.
102. Kessel, 'Self-Poisoning (1)' p. 1267.
103. Stewart, '"See his Home"', p. 117.
104. Timms, *Psychiatric Social Work*, p. 126.
105. Timms, *Psychiatric Social Work*, pp. 112–13.
106. Timms, *Psychiatric Social Work*, p. 113.
107. I. Hacking, *Rewriting the Soul* (Princeton, NJ: Princeton University Press, 1995), p. 236.
108. T. Szasz, *Myth of Mental Illness* (New York: Dell, 1962), pp. 265–6.
109. Szasz, *Myth of Mental Illness*, p. 266.
110. E. Fuchs and G. Flügge, 'Chronic Social Stress: Effects on Limbic Brain Structures', *Physiology & Behavior*, 79 (2003), pp. 417–27.

INDEX

For Product Safety Concerns and Information please contact our EU
representative GPSR@taylorandfrancis.com
Taylor & Francis Verlag GmbH, Kaufingerstraße 24, 80331 München, Germany

www.ingramcontent.com/pod-product-compliance
Ingram Content Group UK Ltd.
Pitfield, Milton Keynes, MK11 3LW, UK
UKHW020012200926
475702UK00014B/1842
* 9 7 8 1 1 3 8 6 3 0 1 3 0 *